Interaction for Practice in Community Nursing

Edited by
ANN LONG

Foreword by Philip Burnard

MACMILLAN

First published 1999 by
MACMILLAN PRESS LTD
Houndmills, Basingstoke, Hampshire RG21 6XS
and London
Companies and representatives throughout the world

ISBN 0–333–72779–7

A catalogue record for this book is available
from the British Library.

This book is printed on paper suitable for recycling and
made from fully managed and sustained forest sources.

10 9 8 7 6 5 4 3 2 1
08 07 06 05 04 03 02 01 00 99

Copy-edited and typeset by Povey–Edmondson
Tavistock and Rochdale, England

Printed in Malaysia

I would like to dedicate this book to the profession of community nursing of which I am truly honoured to be a part.

CONTENTS

LIST OF FIGURES

LIST OF BOXES

Communication and interaction have, appropriately, become the cornerstone of effective health care. This exciting text brings together a wide range of approaches to thinking about interaction in practice. The book also offers practical guidance – the 'how' of communication.

Too often, perhaps, writers on these topics have taken a fairly straightforward 'skills' approach to discussing how to communicate with others. As Ann Long indicates in her introduction, there is, of course, much more to it than this. We communicate at different levels, both verbally and non-verbally, but also *beyond* these two dimensions. A meeting between two people, in health-care contexts, as in others, can never be reduced to the bare bones of words and gestures. This is the *human* level of communication and it is a feature that is admirably addressed within this volume.

It is on this, human, level that the book speaks to the reader. What is both admirable and valuable about the work is its ability to allow each of the writers to adopt his or her own 'voice'. We are not offered a particular 'party line' on communication but a personal and insightful essay from each of the contributors.

I enjoyed reading this book and I know it will be both useful and of great practical and intellectual value to other readers. It manages to convey those most important features of the nursing communication: humanity and the frailty of the human condition.

PHILIP BURNARD
Vice Dean
School of Nursing Studies
University of Wales College of Medicine
Cardiff

Successive governments have indicated their commitment to enhancing the health of the nation and, in recent years, the focus of care delivery has shifted with escalating speed into the community. In so doing, it has become evident that community nurses and health visitors provide the focus for the promotion of health gain, and for the maintenance of positive health status for individuals, groups and local communities. Community nurses and health visitors are destined, therefore, to become leaders in the design, delivery and evaluation of effective health care interventions, informed by academic discovery, and advanced practice skills and competencies.

The changes that confront the contemporary community nursing practitioner are characterised by the diverse nature of the context within which community care is transacted, with an increasing emphasis on inter-sectoral co-operation, interprofessional collaboration, community action and development, and reduced reliance on the acute sector and residential care provision for longer stay client groups.

The impact of change, pushed by a growing demand for flexible, high-quality services provided within local communities, will inevitably shape the NHS of the future. Resources have already been shifted to the community (although at a pace that is all too often criticised as being grossly inadequate to meet client need). Commissioners and providers are now required to demonstrate that the care they purchase and deliver is effective and responsive to the needs of local practice populations. To complement this, community nurses will be required to ensure that their activities make a significant impact on health gain for their practice population and, as such, must become seriously involved in structuring the political agenda that ultimately governs their practice environment.

In order for the community workforce to respond to these challenges, it will be necessary to ensure that community workers are equipped with the necessary skills and knowledge base to be able to function effectively in the 'new world of community health practice'. Nurses will be required to develop and change, drawing upon the very best of their past experience, and becoming increasingly reliant upon the production of research evidence to inform their future practice.

This series is aimed at practising community nurses and health visitors, their students, managers, professional colleagues and commissioners. It has been designed to provide a broad-ranging synthesis and analysis of the major areas of community activity, and to challenge models of traditional practice. The texts have been designed specifically to appeal to a range of professional and academic disciplines. Each volume will integrate contemporary research, recent literature and practice examples relating to the effective delivery of health and social care in the community. Community nurses and health visitors are encouraged towards critical exploration and, if necessary, to change their own contribution to health care delivery – at the same time as extending the scope and boundaries of their own practice.

Authors and contributors have been carefully selected. Whether they are nurses or social scientists (or both), their commitment to the further development and enrichment of health science (and nursing as an academic discipline in particular) is unquestionable. The authors all demonstrate knowledge, experience and excellence in curriculum design, and share a commitment to excellence in service delivery. The result is a distillation of a range of contemporary themes, practice examples and recommendations that aim to extend the working environment for practising community nurses and health visitors and, in so doing, improve the health status of their local consumer populations.

Interaction for Practice in Community Health Nursing, edited by Ann Long, has been written by a range of carefully selected authors. Between them, they provide a breadth of creative vision informed by a range of research and practice perspectives applied to advanced interaction. The book challenges community practitioners to replace conventional methods of interaction and engagement with clients with a new paradigm characterised by partnership with clients and their carers. The authors provide an excellent synthesis of interaction related to health promotion, therapeutic encounters and counselling. In addition the authors focus attention on the need to dismantle existing barriers to effective communication, and examine the ethical, societal and cultural determinants of human relationships. The text is based on a vision for advanced interaction to assist community health care practitioners to demonstrate effective partnerships in health care delivery. The text is imbued with examples gleaned from practice. Readers will be challenged to adopt a proactive approach to care delivery and act as change facilitators in their area of specialist practice.

DAVID SINES
University of Ulster
Belfast

ACKNOWLEDGEMENTS

I would like to thank my friends and colleagues who contributed to this book, including David Sines, the Series Editor, for his continuous support and guidance. I would also like to thank my family and partner, all of whom are in the caring professions. They have all given me courage and help in their own unique way.

ANN LONG

Owen Barr, RGN, RNMH, JBCNS, Course 805, CNMH, Adv. Dip. Nursing, BSc (Hons) Nursing is a Lecturer in Nursing in the School of Health Sciences, University of Ulster, Coleraine, Northern Ireland.

Rosario Baxter, RSCN, RGN, BSc nursing, RNT, Cert HCIAE, MEd (Ed Management), MPhil is a Lecturer in Community Children's Nursing and Ethics in the School of Health Sciences, University of Ulster, Jordanstown, Newtownabbey, Northern Ireland.

David Dickson, BA (Joint Hons) Psychology/Philosophy, Dip. Education, Ma (Ed), PhD, Associate Member BPsS, Associate Fellow BPsS, Chartered Psychologist BPsS is a Senior Lecturer in Communication in the School of Behavioural and Communication Sciences, University of Ulster, Jordanstown, Newtownabbey, Northern Ireland.

Paul Fleming, ATVL, BEd, LGSM, ALCM, PGDHE, MIHE, MSc is a Lecturer in Health Promotion and Course Director for the BSc/MSc Health Promotion in the School of Health Sciences, University of Ulster, Newtownabbey, Northern Ireland.

Sara Groogan, BSc (Hons) Communication, Advertising and Marketing is a Research and Information Officer at the Northern Health and Social Services Board, County Hall, Galgorm Road, Ballymena, Northern Ireland.

Diane Hazlett, BSc, MSc, CHSM, MRCSLT is a Lecturer in Speech and Language Therapy in the School of Behavioural and Communication Sciences, University of Ulster, Jordanstown, Newtownabbey, Northern Ireland.

Pauline Irving, BSc, (Hons) Psychology, Dip. Careers Guidance, MSc Occup. Psychology BPsS, Chartered Psychologist, MSc Public Relations, DPhil is a Lecturer in Counselling in the School of Behavioural and Communication Sciences, University of Ulster, Jordanstown, Newtownabbey, Northern Ireland.

Raman Kapur, BSc (Hons), MSc, MPhil, PhD, is an Individual and Group Psychotherapist, Consultant Clinical Psychologist and Assistant Director (Clinical) with Threshold (Richmond Fellowship, Northern Ireland). He is also an Honorary Lecturer with Queen's University, Belfast, and the University of Ulster.

Ann Long, BSc Psychology, MSc Counselling, Post Graduate Certificate in Research Methods, Certification in Psychodynamic Therapy, RGN, RMN, HV, Dip. Nursing, RNT, RHVT is a psychotherapist, writer, Senior Lecturer in the School of Health Sciences, University of Ulster. She is also Course Director for the BSc (Hons) in Community Health Care Nursing, University of Ulster, Jordanstown, Newtownabbey, Northern Ireland.

Eamonn Slevin, PG Dip. Nursing, BSc (Hons) Nursing, Dip. Nursing, Adv. Dip. Education, RGN, RNMH, RNT is a Lecturer in Nursing in the School of Health Sciences, University of Ulster, Jordanstown, Newtownabbey, Northern Ireland.

Oliver Slevin, BA, MA, PhD, Nurse Tutor's Dip., RMN, RGN, RNT is Chief Executive of the National Board for Nursing, Midwifery and Health Visiting (Northern Ireland) and Visiting Professor of Nursing at the University of Ulster and Centre House, Belfast.

Dennis Tourish, BSc (Hons) Human Communication, MSc Health and Social Services Management, DPhil is a Lecturer in Communication in the School of Behavioural and Communication Sciences, University of Ulster, Jordanstown, Newtownabbey, Northern Ireland.

Introduction

Ann Long

The amazing and enigmatic world of communication is a world we cannot touch and yet it touches every aspect of our being. It is a world that surrounds us like a transparent veil and yet it helps us to reach out and be touched by, as well as to touch, the hearts, minds, feelings and souls of others. Through the channel of communication we make the decision either to 'be receptive' and enter communion with others, thus becoming emotionally intimate, or to withdraw and distance ourselves from other human beings.

This book has not been written with the intention of examining communication networking through the impersonal world of the computer, internet or any other high-technology invention. Computers allow people to correspond to others all over the planet–with their fingers. Yet sometimes those very same people may not have the skills, let alone the will, to communicate with the person sitting at the next computer terminal. It is even more disconcerting to realise that those very same people may be members of our 'family'.

The purpose of the book is to examine and explore from philosophical as well as empirical evidence all those deep and meaningful theoretical issues involved in the development, maintenance and closure of human relationships. The book is also about community nursing so each chapter resonates with the need to integrate the art and skill of sensitive, compassionate communication with the art and science of therapeutic nursing practice. The chapters emphasise the importance of nurses *being human*, hence bringing inherent core, human care qualities with them to the therapeutic relationship, thus enlightening their nursing practice. It attempts to unravel the concepts that are embraced within

1

specific human care qualities that nurses, as human beings, bring with them to the healing relationship.

Theoretical evidence related to self-acceptance, unconditional positive regard for self and others and other higher-level modes of feeling, thinking and relating are skilfully embroidered within the tapestry of the text. The book also speaks to the value and dignity of life and of each of us having a life that although like billions of others is also unique.

From a metaphysical perspective, being like so many others means that nurses may be looking at the moon or a star and realise that this same sky can be seen in other countries at the same time by other human beings, thus connecting all of us together as one family, in one universe (Kome and Crean, 1986; Long, 1997). Being like other human beings also means that each of us can communicate through the channels of our senses: by looking and being looked at; by hearing and being heard; and by touching and being touched.

From an existential perspective touching means that we can touch and be touched intuitively and spiritually. We have the ability to make connections with other human beings, to touch their lives, to leave our compassionate silhouette imprinted on the minds and hearts of others, to form relationships through entering into dialogue and communion with them and to 'let go' of them, in silence, with grace and dignity. Through life experiences and by demonstrating empathy and compassion with other human beings, we can make intuitive connections with their pain and suffering regardless of where they live on this planet. For example, when atrocities occur in other countries, as well as our own, people's suffering may have an impact on the self of the person who chooses to make a connection with his or her brothers and sisters at that moment of history (Walsh, 1984; Long 1997).

Conversely, being unique implies that each one of us has an individual way of communicating that we care and of making a statement that we belong to the human species in the knowledge and understanding that we have a special place on this planet. As nurses we are in an advantaged position.

As the chapters unfold the aim is to open the reader's mind to acknowledging the honour and privilege it is for us, as nurses, to be greeted and accepted into the personal, familial and social world of other human beings in need of health and social care. As community health nurses we are also invited into all the intricacies of other people's eccentricities, culture, community, ethnicity and homes.

Realising that and being on the receiving side of such trust and acceptance may sometimes be overwhelming. Consequently, being invited across the doorstep of another human being's internal and external world is something that we should never respond to in a frivolous or light-hearted manner.

Chapter 1 by Sara Groogan aims to set the scene by providing a critical appraisal of the value of sensitive and effective communication for enhancing the quality of the health and social care provided within the current NHS. Sara begins by giving a historical overview of the emergence of community care and speaks to the advancement of multidisciplinary teamwork and of working together alongside clients in the community. She proposes ways of improving communication systems with clients and others, by utilising and analysing the nature and process of communication and adroitly linking the theoretical concepts involved in communicating with the provision of effective nursing care. In this chapter the carer's requirements for honest and accurate complementary communication with professionals have not been forgotten. The chapter concludes by postulating that real empowerment of service users and their carers can only be realised by involving them in the assessment of needs at individual, family and community levels and at all stages of service delivery including forward planning. Sara contends that in order to do this successfully, more meaningful and genuine communication must be utilised regarding clients' true health and social needs as well as their aspirations.

Analysed and eloquently debated by Eamonn Slevin in Chapter 2 is the axiom which suggests the fundamental need for the use of 'presence' in community health care nursing. Eamonn draws from the theoretical work of existential philosophers such as Buber (1977), Marcel (1967) and Sartre (1958) and advances perspectives that are analogous with the philosophical standpoint of the centrality of human relationships in nursing. He concludes the chapter by proposing that the concept of 'presence' is always best accomplished in the real world such as that experienced in the practice of community health care nursing and more exclusively within the nurse–client relationship. However, Eamonn has deep aspirations that the written words in this book will encourage community health care nurses to recognise and embrace the value of relating with self and others in their own unique ideology of caring for people. Eamonn's chapter is best encapsulated by a citation he uses to support one of his propositions: 'For above the world of objects the presence of Thou is suspended like the spirit upon the waters

3

. . . this vapour is not inactive, it puts itself forth as beneficent rain' (Marcel, 1967, p.47).

Oliver Slevin's Chapter 3 on 'The Nurse-Patient Relationship: Caring in a Health Context' leads readers in a competent and compassionate manner from Chapter 2 into the world of 'care'. He enters into a dialogue with readers and speaks of a philosophy of 'care', proposing that it begins with nurses making a decision to enter into a responsible and intentional engagement with others by fully attending to, confronting and coming into relation with them. He extrapolates from the works of Sartre (1958) stating that 'caring' is an 'authentic way of being-in-the-world'. Throughout the chapter Oliver advances a theoretical framework for care which is drawn from research and encompasses a triad of caring. On one axis of the configuration he sees caring as skilled intervention, on another axis as compassion, while on the third axis he perceives caring as negotiation of health choices. Oliver concludes by asserting that the theoretical framework of care he is promoting is particulary relevant to community health care nursing which, in a future primary-led service, will be at the forefront of health care provision.

Chapter 4 by David Dickson examines and explores barriers to communication. David makes a scientific investigation into the role and function of communication in health care delivery. His research clearly details some of the respects in which communicating convincingly seems to fail the recipient of the service. Using empirical evidence David highlights, for example, semantic, emotional and relational areas of concern which give clues to the actual barriers that get in the way of effective communication which should be appropriately open, honest, comfortable and respectful. David's analysis of research findings shows that the path of communication between carer and patient is decidedly barrier-strewn. He concludes the chapter by stating that attempts to improve levels of communication with patients are unlikely to be particularly successful unless each of these barriers is acknowledged and steps taken to remove them. David soundly contends that quality health care delivery demands no less.

Owen Barr's Chapter 5 propels readers into the nature of counselling. He postulates that communication can be viewed on a continuum which ranges from interpersonal skills at the one end and follows distinct yet overlapping stages through to the use of helping skills (Heron, 1986), counselling skills and finally to the provision of counselling *per se*. Owen examines definitions of

4

counselling and recounts and challenges three specific schools of counselling thought, namely, the psychoanalytic, behavioural and person-centred approaches to counselling. Owen continues the chapter by examining the theoretical basis underpinning the combined approaches to counselling. Throughout the chapter Owen has related his theoretical arguments to the practice of community health care nursing. Owen concludes by inviting nurses to reflect on the types and range of interpersonal and counselling knowledge and skills they use when working with clients and their carers. The principles highlighted in the *Scope of Professional Practice* (UKCC, 1992) are utilised by Owen to emphasise that nurses are required to ensure that nursing interventions are always directed in a coordinated manner to meet identified needs and serve the best interests of clients. The guidance also highlights the need to honestly acknowledge any limits of personal knowledge and skill and take steps to remedy deficits. Owen reminds readers that these principles apply equally to counselling as they do to any other nursing activity and he petitions readers to clarify the wider professional and local procedural guidelines and make ethical and moral decisions prior to embarking on either using counselling skills or committing themselves to a counselling relationship.

This chapter dovetails with Raman Kapur's Chapter 8 on unconscious communication processes that are forever alive and active thus continuously sending 'unconscious' messages within human relationships. Raman examines the work of Freud (1935, 1936), Klein (1932) and other analysts and speaks specifically to the nature and meaning of processes such as transference, countertransference and projection within the nurse–patient relationship. Raman concludes with an illustration of how unconscious communication processes may reveal and ignite themselves in practice and tentatively highlights important skills nurses may use to explore and 'contain' them within the therapeutic relationship.

Chapter 6 by Rosario Baxter explores the proposition that there exists a profound and complex dimension to communication which is concerned primarily with the principle of truth-telling or the 'wholesomeness' of community health care nurses' communion with patients. Rosario asserts that it is impossible to separate the technical aspects of information exchange from the ethical responsibilities with which they are bound. From an analysis of the literature, Rosario proposes the need to develop a philosophy of ethical communication that places individual patient's needs, ambitions and dreams above all other considerations, including perceived professional role boundaries. The philosophy of ethical communication, Rosario suggests, could begin with the development of an interprofessional alliance among medical and nursing staff whose primary aim would be to commit themselves to designing and practising a philosophy of care which embraces the moral and ethical aspects of communication in health care as its mission statement. A 'friendship' among professionals such as the one envisaged by Rosario should remain mindful of recognising the valuable contribution of clients and carers. The scope and depth of worthwhile human interaction, Rosario believes, is a more appropriate channel for delivering care than any that other current models can offer.

Dennis Tourish, in Chapter 7, 'Communicating Beyond Individual Bias', examines research which highlights the uniqueness of human beings. He contests convincingly that instead of perceiving people as unique individuals we tend to view them as representative of a broader social category possessed of certain qualities which we dislike and which we assume are shared by most or all members of that particular social group. Dennis examines research on the nature of prejudice and stereotypical generalisations and purports that the categorisation of people into in-groups and out-groups enables us to perceive order in the world rather than random chaos and in many respects is, therefore, necessary. Redressing the challenge of communicating beyond individual bias, Dennis contends, requires effective communication and great care on the part of trainers, sensitivity to feelings and strong diplomatic skills combined with a willingness to acknowledge their own biases. Dennis continues by asserting that perceiving and accepting differences between and among groups can be recognised as a general cultural enrichment of society rather than a threat. He advocates the need for training in this area primarily to promote healing in communities through working together to achieve common health and social goals.

Paul Fleming's Chapter 9 gives a critical overview of the communication skills and qualities that are essential for community nurses to fulfil their role as health promoters. Paul provides readers with an innovative and creative model of health promotion which incorporates facilitating individuals, families and communities to identify their own health and social needs and, through utilising Paul's model of health promotion, to take steps to make health changes in their lives. This imaginative health promotion model forwarded by Paul could, when utilised, benefit individuals, families and communities as well as the present and future population. Proficiently composed within the chapter is an in-depth examination of the key communication skills and qualities that are essential for community health care nurses to fulfil their role as health promoters.

Chapter 10 by Pauline Irving and Diane Hazlett takes a close look at the community nurse's role in dealing with challenging clients. Included in this chapter are evaluations of research which support the authors' contention about the painful yet enlightening need for community health care nurses to examine the part they play in creating and maintaining challenging situations and experiences. Pauline and Diane submit a theoretical and pragmatic model of challenging communication and examine in detail the concepts and phenomena that may be implicated in challenging situations regarding the client, the nurse and the communication process itself. The chapter continues by illustrating examples of challenging communication and the authors draw from empirical research to detail ways of working with two specific groups: clients with communication difficulties and clients who are aggressive or angry. The communication principles proposed, the authors contend, should have a positive effect on all caring interventions. However, they assure readers that the skills of the helper are most severely tested in challenging situations.

The book closes with a chapter by the editor Ann Long. Ann attempts to synthesise some of the key points that have been illustrated in the previous chapters. This was not an easy task as the book glides and changes from one chapter to the next. While this change instilled an air of excitement the magnitude of the task of trying to extrapolate key communication areas was somewhat daunting. This is one of the reasons why readers are encouraged to read all of the chapters. However, specific chapters have been identified which relate to the concepts being emphasised in this chapter. The main aim of Chapter 11 was to demonstrate that communication rests most comfortably at the heart of nursing care and that without integral communication skills and qualities essential for health-giving relationships all other care becomes obsolete. Ann concludes the chapter by examining and exploring some of the subtle and complex dynamics that are involved in the totality of health-enriching, health-nurturing communication. Some of the difficulties involved in understanding complex concepts such as being receptive and interpreting and responding to communication messages are worked through in a sensitive and adroit manner.

In conclusion, this book has been written with the intention of inviting readers into the caring ethos of communication in community health care nursing. It also requests that readers explore their own private, personal and professional worlds and accept and embrace that we, as nurses, have much to offer to clients in terms of core human care qualities, knowledge and skills. More important, and equally meaningful, is the fact that clients continue to enrich and nurture our lives also.

References

Buber, M. (1977) *I and Thou*. New York: Scribner.

Freud, S. (1935) *An Autobiographical Study*. London: Hogarth Press.

Freud, S. (1936) *The Problem of Anxiety*. New York: W.W. Norton.

Heron, J. (1986) *Six Category Intervention Analysis*. 2nd edn. Human Potential Research Project, University of Surrey.

Klein, M. (1932) *The Psychoanalysis of Children*. London: Hogarth Press.

Kome, P. and Crean, P. (1986) *Peace: A Dream Unfolding*. San Francisco, Calif.: Sierra Club Books.

Long, A. (1997) Nursing: a spiritual perspective. *International Journal of Nursing Ethics*, 4(6), pp. 496–510.

Marcel, G. (1967) *The Philosophy of Existentialism*. Secaucus, NJ: Citadel Press.

Sartre, J. P. (1958) *Being and Nothingness*. London: Methuen.

United Kingdom Central Council for Nursing, Midwifery and Health Visiting (UKCC) (1992) *The Scope of Professional Practice*. London: UKCC.

Walsh, R. (1984) *Staying Alive: The Psychology of Human Survival*. Boston, Mass: Shambala.

CHAPTER ONE

Setting The Scene

Sara Groogan

THE EMERGENCE OF COMMUNITY CARE

The NHS and Community Care Act 1990 and its associated White Papers have emphasised the importance of caring for people in the community, which will be accompanied by reduced dependency on secondary health care provision. Subsequently a new philosophy of care has emerged, based on the principle that care should be shared with individuals and that whenever possible, care should be provided as close to the person's home as possible (Sines, 1995).

The Department of Health has defined community care as providing the right level of intervention and support to enable people to achieve maximum independence and control over their lives (DoH, 1989). The DoH, in *New World, New Opportunities* (1993), has stated that the best way to meet the health needs of the local population is to focus health care services within the very heart of naturally occurring communities. In doing so opportunities for the further advancement of multidisciplinary teamwork and improved communication systems with clients would be provided.

Community care is about helping clients and carers in or near their homes rather than in hospitals and away from the community in which they live. Community care is about supporting individual and family responsibility and about clients' rights and choices. Care in the community can empower the disadvantaged and the marginalised, thus resulting in the provision of more flexible and responsible services that are planned, designed, evaluated and controlled in partnership with users (Øvretveit, 1993).

However, the reality of care in the community has not always matched this ideal. As Øvretveit (1993) has pointed out, the history of community care is one of competition for finance between acute hospital care and primary health care. It is, according to Øvretveit, a history of division between health and social care and one of few fragile alliances. An accusation which is often levied at community care is that whilst it can be highly successful in meeting the need of a client with only a single need, it very often fails those clients with multiple and complex needs. Quite often this can be attributed to poor communication among professionals and between the professional and the client.

Dickson (1995) drew attention to the dramatic effects of providing care in the community on community nursing. He deems them to be profound due to the different patterns of contact with clients and families in the community, coupled with the often long-term involvement necessitated by chronic conditions and the care of the dying. According to Dickson, all of these put an added premium upon effective communication given the growing body of empirical evidence that suggests not only that patients demand more and better standards of communication from health carers but that they actually benefit from it.

THE COMMUNICATION PROCESS

Early models of communication such as those forwarded by Shannon and Weaver (1949) present communication as a simple linear process. In its most general sense communication may be defined as a process involving the transmission of information from sender to receiver (Forgas, 1985). From this definition it follows that any communication involves:

- A *sender* or source who *encodes*
- the *message* to be *transmitted*
- through a particular *channel*
- to a *receiver* who *decodes* the message.

In this model communication is viewed as something one person *does* to another. The sender encodes ideas and feelings into a message and then injects them by means of a channel into a receiver.

Any interference in the process is termed as *noise* (Adler *et al.*, 1989). This perspective does provide some useful information. The characteristics of the sender, the message, the channel and the receiver all have important influences on the communication process. For example, each channel, such as using the telephone or face-to-face contact with a client, does have its differences. The characteristics of the sender and receiver, such as status and power, also feature. This can be particularly relevant in health care if we are to try to empower clients and involve them in their care. Finally, the nature of the message itself can be very important in determining how we communicate. We will use a very different language when discussing social issues, such as the weather, with clients than when we are breaking bad news.

The linear model also shows how *noise* can interfere with a message. Adler *et al.* (1989) identify two types of noise which can block communication: physical and psychological. With physical noise it may be that we simply cannot hear what the client is saying or it may be that the chair on which we are sitting is uncomfortable. All of this can detract from the message. Psychological noise is a force within the sender or receiver which makes them less likely to communicate effectively. For example, the form of address we use towards a client, or that we request a client to use towards the professional, can disempower the client and affect communication from the outset.

However, despite the advantages of the linear model, it inaccurately suggests that communication flows in one direction: from sender to receiver. This may be the case with print and broadcast messages but interpersonal communication is a two-way exchange. Communicators usually send and receive messages simultaneously so that they are not doing only one or the other but rather both are superimposed and redefined as participants communicate (Rogers and Kincaid, 1981).

At a given moment we are capable of receiving, decoding and responding to another person's behaviour, while at the same time the other person is receiving and responding to ours. Adler *et al*, (1989) suggest that it is difficult to isolate a single discrete act of communication from the events that precede and follow it. Communication is not something that people do to one another, but rather a process in which they create a relationship by interacting *with* each other. Adler *et al*, (1989, p. 12), thus defines communication as:

11

'a continuous, transactional process involving participants who occupy different but overlapping environments and create a relationship by simultaneously sending and receiving messages, many of which are distorted by physical and psychological noise.'

Two elements of this definition which are particularly pertinent to community care are 'different but overlapping environments' and 'creating a relationship'. All interpersonal communication relies to some extent on shared social knowledge, but we can take much of this shared knowledge for granted. For example, when interacting with clients we may take for granted the use of some medical terminology or we may assume that a client has understood a process we have explained. This may not be the case as medical jargon is an element of the practitioner's environment which may be unfamiliar to the client. In order for the environments to overlap and harmonise we must ensure that the message has been understood, otherwise it becomes lost and the client may be left feeling bewildered and confused.

The idea of communication creating a relationship is also an important concept in community health care. It is vital for the community practitioner to distinguish between *treating* clients in the community and *caring* for clients in the community. The term 'care' encompasses much more than simply administering treatments. Rather it is about using a holistic approach to the individual and to their social, psychological and physical needs. In community health care, nursing care is also about promoting healthy communities and involves working to eliminate disadvantages in health and social care. It also means community nurses should nurse 'sick' communities and promote peace and reconcilation.

The UKCC (1996) states that building a trusting relationship will greatly improve care and help to reduce anxiety and stress for patients and clients, their families and carers. They stress that it is important to create an environment for effective communication so that a relationship of trust can be built with the client.

THE SKILL OF COMMUNICATION

As early as 1967 Argyle suggested that there was a useful analogy between motor skills and social skills. In each case the person is goal-directed and makes moves which are intended to further these

12

goals, observes what effect he or she is having and takes corrective action as a result of feedback.

Argyle (1983) outlines the social skills model as follows:

1. *Goal-directed action* Goals and subgoals are the basic motivation in a motor skill. For example, when our goal is to learn to drive a car, we have subgoals such as learning to steer the car, learning to stop the car, learning to start the car and so on. This is also the case in the social skills situation. Social skills operators will be motivated by a combination of professional and social motivations. For example, they may wish the client to learn from the knowledge they are imparting and as a result of the learning alter aspects of their health behaviour. Communication is thus goal-directed.

2. *Hierarchical structure of social acts* These goals are organised in a hierarchical structure. When one subgoal has been met, the sequence leading to the next subgoal begins, until the main goal is attained. Most of the goals at the lower end of the structure become habitual and automatic and we tend to concentrate more on the higher-level units. An example from practice may show the professional dealing with a client who has a phobia about going to the shop. The main goal is to help the client to overcome the phobia. Thus the first subgoal may be to help the client to reach the front door. When this has been achieved the next goal may then be to help the client to reach the end of the garden path, then visit the shops with the nurse and finally unattended. When the first series of goals have been met, they become habitual and so we concentrate more on the later goals. When the client is reaching the shops unattended we hope that reaching the front door has now become automatic.

3. *The perceptions of others' reactions* When utilising a motor skill, attention is concentrated on certain stimuli – we learn which cues to attend to and become highly sensitive to them. For example, in learning to drive a car we learn to make use of visual and aural stimuli and to focus on those connected to the practice of driving the car, such as other traffic, traffic lights, a car horn. The perceptual channels used in social interaction include hearing the literal content of the speech, hearing the paralinguistic, emotive aspects of the speech, and observing facial expressions and other visual clues. Failure of social performance can result from not looking in the right place at the right time or not being able to interpret what is seen or

13

heard. The practitioner may be unaware of the cues which the client is presenting in their paralinguistic and facial expression for example, but may also be unaware of the cues they are presenting to the client through their own social behaviour. This can result in the client receiving a mixed message or becoming confused or even afraid of the practitioner.

4. *Feedback and corrective action* Feedback can be both verbal and non-verbal. Clients may indicate that they do understand the information that the practitioner is presenting to them by simply stating this. However, a practitioner may also be able to gauge this through non-verbal behaviour such as a confused facial expression or an insecure posture. As a result of this feedback the social skills operator can take corrective action. For example, if our goal is to try to get the client to talk more and feedback has indicated that this is not the case, then we can take corrective action to attempt to resolve this. For example, we can talk less, we can ask more open-ended questions and we can reward what is said, for example by head-nodding. Argyle (1983) believes that taking the right corrective action may require some knowledge and understanding of people and social situations.

5. *Timing of responses* The timing of a response is important in even the simplest type of interaction, a conversation between two people. In such an interaction the participants must speak in turns, the length of speech may have to be adjusted and the speed of reaction may be an important factor. There may also be a tendency on the part of practitioners (or clients) to interrupt. A synchronised set of responses should develop which will facilitate effective communication.

Thus, Argyle (1967) purports that the social skill is analogous to a motor skill, that it is learned and, therefore, it can be taught. Practitioners should be aware that effective client communication is achievable and is not an inherent trait that one does or does not possess. Argyle (1983) also points out that social competence is not a general factor – a practitioner may be more effective at the skill of listening than the skill of self-disclosure and may be a more effective social skills operator in one situation than another. It is inappropriate to assume that all patients have the same nurse–client relationship needs and thus that they will all be satisfied with the same communication approaches during visits.

COMMUNICATION IN COMMUNITY HEALTH CARE PROVISION

Øvretveit (1993) purports that for clients and carers to be involved in decision-making, they need to be able to obtain and understand information at all stages of the caring process. People cannot choose or give consent if they do not know that they have the right to choose or what those choices are. They cannot make an informed choice if they do not understand the information they are given, or if they do not get the information they need to understand the advantages and disadvantages of each option. Øvretveit also goes on to suggest that in order to increase choice we have to not only develop alternatives but also change the way we communicate and relate with clients to enable them to choose and make decisions about services. Further, we need to be able to work with clients and carers to create new choices, choices which may not occur in the minds of professionals alone and which are more satisfactory ways to meet their needs within the constraints Øvretveit (1993, p. 164) states: 'Client choice, involvement and participation are not just a matter of handing out a menu and explaining it, but about cooking with clients and carers.'

The majority of complaints which reach the NHS Ombudsman are the result of poor communication (Health Service Commissioner, 1997). Martin (1997) believes that coordinating multidisciplinary health care and involving patients and their families in decisions about care and treatment can be extremely difficult and that it is not surprising that failings occur. How much patients understand is compromised by the use of jargon or by a failure to recognise that their comprehension has been blocked or distorted by stress and anxiety. Martin points to the use of ambiguous social phrases such as 'feeling comfortable' and concludes that communicating in a simple direct language is a skill that must be learned and used.

Øvretveit (1993) asks two key questions regarding community health care provision: how far is it the responsibility of the sender to ensure that the receiver not only receives but also understands what the sender intends him to; and how far is it the responsibility of the receiver to make sure he or she has understood? However, it remains the responsibility of teams and practitioners to make sure that clients and carers are provided with and understand the right information at each phase of the communication process.

15

Another common communication problem which Øvretveit (1993) draws attention to is that of too much information. The receiver can get lost in detail. Often too much information is sent or recorded because the sender does not know what the receiver needs to know or indeed what is significant.

All these problems arise because senders do not think about the receiver, how they receive the information, how they interpret it and what they need and want to know. To work as an effective practitioner means understanding the receiver (Øvretveit, 1993).

Empirical findings have largely corroborated the popular impression of the practitioner as someone who tends to do things rather than say things, being essentially concerned with the functioning of some part of the body rather than the client as a person (Dickson *et al.*, 1989). Dickson *et al.*, have identified four areas of deficiency in health care practitioners' communication. They are: getting information; providing information; time; and the nature of communication.

1. *Getting information* Practitioners have been found to neglect important areas when interviewing or they collect detail in such a way that it is likely to be inaccurate or incomplete.
2. *Providing information* The giving of information often invites criticism because the amount provided is inadequate or alternatively is delivered in an insensitive or unintelligible way.
3. *Time* Practitioners have been accused of having little time to listen to what the client wants and needs to say.
4. *Nature of communication* Communication which does take place tends to be primarily functional, addressing physical aspects of a condition. Comfort and support often tend to be neglected.

Moreover, previous research has been critical of the quality and quantity of nurse–client communication, describing it as brief and superficial, and nurses are depicted as controlling and restricting the course and topics of conversation with clients (Jarrett and Payne, 1995). However, Sieko and Greeff (1995) state that therapeutic communication remains the quintessential element in all nurse–client interactions. The UKCC (1996) state that to ensure that practitioners gain the trust of patients and clients they should recognise them as equal partners, use language that is familiar to them and make sure that they understand the information practioners are giving.

Above all, people want to be seen by practitioners as individuals with problems, not as problems *per se*. People who are respected and treated as active participants in their own care are more likely to respond positively to care (Welsh Health Planning Forum, 1993).

INVOLVING RECEIVERS OF CARE AND THEIR CARERS

Traditionally the health service has been criticised for not involving the receivers of care. The 1983 Griffiths Management Inquiry in England and Wales condemned the NHS for this failure, while as long ago as 1978 the World Health Organisation articulated the right and duty of people to participate individually and collectively in the planning, implementation and evaluation of services. A further push for users and carers has been the development of the Patient's Charter (1991) which has not only set local and national targets but has also raised user expectation of service delivery. The charter is not a mechanism for involvement, rather a response to the public's expressed concerns about the current services provided (Winkler, 1996).

The concept of patients as 'consumers' has been closely associated with the UK health reforms of the 1980s and the introduction of a quasi-marketplace in the health services (Balogh *et al.*, 1995). While there has been criticism of such commercially derived language, Long, 1997 points out that it does convey the idea of a more active participant than the word 'patient'.

Ignatieff (1984) has stated that there are few presumptions in human relations more dangerous than the idea that one knows what another human being needs better than they do themselves. There has been an increasing acceptance of the value of involving the receivers of care in planning and monitoring health services and an acknowledgement that such involvement empowers communities and provides useful information for service providers (Kelson, 1995). Demands for greater accountability of the health service and for measures which enable patients and carers to judge the quality of care according to improved health are championed not only by client groups and policy-makers but also by an alliance of researchers, social scientists, doctors and other health professionals (Frater, 1992).

Tangible benefits include: improved prospects of recovery if clients are happy with the care provided; the use of patients' opinions to maintain and improve levels and type of service;

17

community and general practice population profiling to determine those most in need of attention; and the use of public opinion to make the case for increased funding (Frater, 1992). Those seeking to involve the receivers of care often fail because they are not clear about why they *should* be involved, or why people might *want* to be involved (Winkler, 1996).

Involving the receivers of care seems to be an essential element of good professional practice at all levels of service provision (Campbell, 1997). The traditional health and welfare state culture is based mainly on one group of service providers making decisions for another group of service users with little overlap between the two (Simpson, 1997). This has traditionally been very disempowering for service users so a move has taken place from providing services based on professional judgement to a culture of real partnership between service providers and recipients of care (Croft and Beresford, 1993).

Developing partnership with people does not mean coercing clients to contribute more fully when they may not wish to take such an active role. Care is individualised in that it recognises that some clients would prefer to remain passive (Simpson, 1997).

Rigge (1994) highlights the fact that when getting users to take more responsibility in health and service planning and delivery it is important to stress that partnership is in a health service rather than an illness service. Without success in this area involvement will only lead to a downward spiral of clamouring demand being met mainly with clinical refusal, leading to dissatisfaction. Clients as partners in health care must be alert to the current political and managerial climate in NHS developments, hence understanding the professionals' constraints when focusing on their own needs. A key dilemma in the NHS is that changes are driven by central directives, while the public are consulted on their local implementation (Winkler, 1996).

CARERS

Carers have become increasingly important in supporting the concept of care in the community. Studies have shown that carers generally feel that they have no option but to provide care (Finch, 1985; Bell *et al.*, 1987). Very few have made a conscious decision to become carers or indeed fully understand what they are undertaking.

Providing care has a number of implications. It is associated with meeting the physical needs of the dependent relative and involves getting and maintaining support from other members of the family and professionals. It also involves coping with the financial implications of caring and at times the emotional stress of the potential death of the dependent relative (Comerasamy, 1997). Professionals and lay carers lack awareness of the two different worlds. There are traditions in the NHS of professional power and control and a lack of value placed by professionals on the experiential knowledge of carers experiencing the effect of care delivery. Both professionals and lay carers lack interaction with each other on an equal level and lack knowledge and an understanding of their different roles in caring (Wilson, 1995). By working with carers it is possible for health professionals to build up a picture of patients' lives, to assess their needs more effectively and to be able to evaluate their preferred options for their overall care and future management (Simpson, 1997).

A study conducted by Warner (1995) found that there was dissatisfaction from carers about support from service agencies, and 80 per cent of the carers surveyed felt that community care has made no difference. The advent of the Carers (Recognition and Services) Act 1995, which took effect in England and Wales on 1 April 1996, should prompt carers' needs to be addressed more vigorously as it allows for an individual assessment of carers' needs in their own right (Firth and Keerfoot, 1997).

ADVOCACY

Full user involvement should engage all types of receipients of care who have a vested interest in a service. However, some individuals or groups such as children, people with learning difficulties, older people or those with a mental illness may have difficulties expressing their own needs and interests. In these instances advocacy is an important activity in achieving involvement (Kelson, 1995). The UKCC (1996) states that advocacy is concerned with promoting and protecting the interests of patients or clients many of whom may be vulnerable and incapable of protecting their own interests or who may be without the support of family or friends. In addition, the UKCC suggests that this can be done by practitioners providing information and making patients and clients feel confident that they have a right to make their own decisions. They also state that practitioners must not practise in a way which assumes that they know what is best for clients, as this can only create a dependence and interfere with the clients' right to self-determination.

COMPLAINTS

Complaints can be understood as an opportunity to improve services or they can be seen as threatening, trivial or part of an illness (Welsh Health Planning Forum, 1993). Traditionally professionals have steered away from clients' grievances and have discouraged them from making complaints.

The Wilson Report (1994) formed the basis for the establishment of a new complaints procedure in the NHS, which took effect on 1 April 1996. The main thrust of the Wilson Report was that complaints should be dealt with quickly and where possible on the spot. It also advocated a policy of openness on how a formal complaint can be made. The guidelines on the new procedure are entitled *Listening, Acting, Improving* (HPSS Executive, 1996) which is the essence of what complaints represent. Practitioners should listen to clients, hear and acknowledge their grievances, and take some action to redress the situation. Ultimately this should lead to service improvement.

Martin (1997) believes that nurses can often prevent matters escalating into a formal written complaint. An explanation of what happened or even a reassuring manner can often be sufficient. Complainants often fear and suspect a cover-up, so a full coherent explanation can help to overcome this. The new complaints procedure encourages professionals to deal with complaints at their level and to offer explanations and solutions to clients. However, if the complaint is unresolved at this level the professional should not feel threatened by a formal written complaint. Cole (1996) states: 'The them and us culture will never change unless we encourage users to tell us what they expect and what we could do better' (p. 21).

Treating complaints seriously means being prepared to challenge the assumption that professionals always act in the best interests of the patient. Too much of what exists is provided on the basis of what professionals think users want. To provide responsive high quality services we must be able to react positively to patients' concerns and criticisms and where necessary change existing services (Thomas, 1996).

CONCLUSION

The importance of effective communication to the community practitioner is no longer in any doubt. Effective communication at an interpersonal level is essential so that clients are able to fully understand all information they are given and as a result are fully aware of the choices that are available to them. Sensitive and effective communication at an interpersonal level also allows the client to be valued as an individual each with their own ideas and concerns. However real empowerment of service users and their carers can only be realised by involving them in the assessment of needs at individual, family and community levels, and in the planning and improvement of services utilising meaningful communication regarding their true needs and aspirations.

References

Adler, R., Rosenfeld, L. and Towne, N. (1989) *Interplay, The Process of Interpersonal Communication*. Orlando, Fla: Holt, Rinehart & Winston.

Argyle, M. (1967) *The Psychology of Interpersonal Behaviour* (1st edn). Middlesex: Pelican Books.

Argyle, M. (1983) *The Psychology of Interpersonal Behaviour*, (4th edn.) Middlesex: Pelican Books.

Balogh, R., Simpson, A. and Bond, S. (1995) Involving clients in clinical audits of mental health services. *International Journal for Quality in Health Care*. 7(4), pp. 343–55.

Bell, R., Gibbons, S. and Pinchen, I. (1987) *Patterns and Process in Carers' Lives: Action Research with Informal Carers of Elderly People*. London: Health Education Council.

Campbell, P. (1997) Citizen Smith. *Nursing Times*, 93(41), pp. 31–2.

Carers (Recognition and Services) Act 1995. London: HMSO.

Cole, A. (1996) Satisfied customers. *Nursing Times*, 92(10), pp. 20–1.

Comerasamy, M. (1997) Invisible carers. *Nursing Times*, 93(41), pp. 54–5.

Croft, S., and Beresford, P. (1993) Getting involved – a practical manual. Cited in P. Simpson (1997) Carers as equal partners in care planning. *Journal of Psychiatric and Mental Health Nursing*, 4, pp. 345–54.

Department of Health (1983) *NHS Management Inquiry Report*. London: DHSS.

Department of Health (1989) *Caring For People: Community Care in the Next Decade and Beyond.* London: HMSO.

Department of Health (1991) *The Patient's Charter.* London: HMSO.

Department of Health (1993) *New World. New Opportunities.* London: HMSO.

Dickson, D. Hargie, O. and Morrow, N. (1989) *Communication Skills Training for Health Professionals. An Instructor's Handbook.* London: Chapman & Hall.

Dickson, D. (1995) Communication and interpersonal skills. In D. Sines (ed.) *Community Health Care Nursing.* Oxford: Blackwell Science.

Finch, H. (1985) *Health and Older People: Attitudes Towards Health in Older Age and Caring for Older People.* London: Social and Community Planning Research.

Firth, M. and Keerfoot, M. (1997) *Involving Users and Carers in Commissioning and Delivering Mental Health Services,* Ed. R. Williams, G. Emerson and Z. Muth. The NHS Health Advisory Service. London: HMSO.

Forgas, J. P. (1985) *Interpersonal Behaviour: The Psychology of Social Interaction.* Oxford: Pergamon Books.

Frater, A. (1992) Health outcomes. A challenge to the status quo. *Quality in Health Care,* 1(1), pp. 87–8.

Health Service Commissioner (1997) *First Report of Session 97–98. Annual Report for 1996/97.* London: HMSO.

HPSS Executive (1996) *Complaints. Listening, Acting, Improving. Guidance on the Implementation of the HPSS Complaints Procedure.* London: HPSS.

Ignatieff, M. (1984) *The Needs of Strangers.* Slough, Berks: Vintage.

Jarrett, N. and Payne, S. (1995) A selective review of the literature on nurse–patient communication: has the practioner's contribution been neglected. *Journal of Advanced Nursing,* 22(1) pp. 72–8.

Kelson, M. (1995) *Consumer Involvement Initiatives in Clinical Audit and Outcomes. A Review of Developments and Issues in the Indentification of Good Practice.* London: DoH.

Long, A. (1997) *Avoiding abuse amongst vulnerable groups in the community – people with a mental illness.* in C. Mason (ed.) Achieving Quality in Community Health Care Nursing, pp. 160–81. London: Macmillan.

Martin, L. (1997) Talking point. *Nursing Standard,* 11(45), p. 19.

NHS and Community Care Act 1990 London: HMSO.

Øvretveit, J. (1993) *Coordinating Community Care. Multidisciplinary Teams and Care Management.* Buckingham: Open University Press.

Rigge, M. (1994) Sharing power. *The Health Service Journal.* Health Management Guide 1, pp. 1–3.

Rogers, E and Kincaid, D. (1981) *Communication Networks.* New York: Free Press.

Shannon, C. and Weaver, W. (1949) *The Mathematical Theory of Communication.* Princeton, Illinois: University of Illinois Press.

Sieko, C. and Greeff, M. (1995) Psychiatric nurses' communication with psychiatric patients. *Curationis,* 18(4), pp. 15–19.

Simpson, R. (1997) Carers as equal partners in care planning. *Journal of Psychiatric and Mental Health Nursing,* 4, pp. 345–54.

Sines, D. (1995) *Community Health Care Nursing.* Oxford: Blackwell Science.

Thomas, B. (1996) Welcome complaints. *Nursing Times.* 92(24), p. 54.

United Kingdom Central Council for Nursing, Midwifery and Health Visiting (UKCC) (1996) *Guidelines for Professional Practice.* London: UKCC.

Warner, N. (1995) *Better Tomorrows: A Report of the National Study of Carers and the Community Care Changes.* London: Carers National Association.

Welsh Health Planning Forum (1993) *Welsh Office NHS Directorate – Protocol for Investing in Health Gain – Mental Health.* Wales: Welsh Health Planning Forum.

Wilson (1994) *Being Heard – the Report of a Review Committee on NHS Complaints Procedure.* London: HMSO.

Wilson, J. (1995) *Two Worlds: Self Help Groups and Professionals.* Birmingham: British Association of Social Workers.

Winkler, F. (1996) Involving Patients. In M. Meads (ed.), *A Primary Care Led NHS: Putting It Into Practice.* Edinburgh: Churchill Livingstone.

CHAPTER TWO

Use of Presence in Community Health Care Nursing

Eamonn Slevin

'A community is built upon a living, reciprocal relationship, but the builder is the living, active centre.'
(Martin Buber, 1970, p. 94)

INTRODUCTION

The Nurses Registration Act (Ministry of Health, 1919) instigated the beginning of a movement which precipitated nursing on a journey towards professional status. Many changes have taken place in health care since this Act. There has been a steady retraction in the number of large hospitals that for many years were seen as places of 'asylum' for people with mental health problems and those with learning disabilities. The increase in the number of older people who require health and social care and people who have chronic illnesses or disabilities, and the ever shortening period that people now stay in general hospitals have led to an increased focus on community care. There has also been a philosophical shift in health care provision from what was previously amelioration of illness to a more preventative health-promoting focus.

One of the major responses that nursing has made to the above social and health policy changes has been the development of community health care nursing. Community health care nursing has developed into eight distinct specialisms to meet current needs: children, learning disability, mental health, district, occupational health, school, public health and general practice nursing (UKCC, 1994).

Godin (1996) provides a developmental account of community psychiatric nursing since the turn of the twentieth century. Two of the main ideologies which Godin suggests have influenced the development of community psychiatric nursing have been 'physicalism' and the 'psychosocial' approach to care. Physicalism is the development of physical treatments such as major tranquillisers and the administration of these drugs by 'depot' injections for people with mental health problems. The psychosocial model emphasises the psychological and social causation of mental illness, thus supporting a health promotion focus in mental health care employing social, environmental and educational interventions.

Both models which Godin refers to are known to influence all specialists of community health care nursing. Physicalism is evident in the technological advances in general medicine and surgery which have led to much shorter stays in hospital by patients followed by their rapid discharge to community care. Indeed many individuals are now receiving treatment in the community who previously would have been admitted to hospital. The psychosocial model has been an influencing factor on the aims of the report *Caring for People* (DoH, 1989), which recognises the benefits to individuals in all client groups of remaining in their own community when they require health or social care.

However, a sceptical view, which will not be debated here, would be that government had other agendas in mind when they pushed for community care.

The emphasis of this chapter is to suggest that community health care nurses should focus, or perhaps refocus, on an additional ideology or model which is based on the philosophy of dialogicalism, as presented by thinkers such as Martin Buber (1970) and Gabriel Marcel (1949). The work of existentialist philosophers such as Sartre (1958) will also receive attention. The issues which these philosophers have deliberated on relate to the perception of 'self', the 'self' and 'others' and 'presence' with others. These premises have been debated and written on extensively (whole texts addressing them) by philosophers, and in a chapter of this size all that can be provided is an overview of some of their central ideas. This chapter links very closely with Chapter 3, both advancing a 'relationship'-focused approach to community health care nursing.

Nursing theorists who forward perspectives which are analogous with the philosophical standpoint of the centrality of human relationships in nursing will be presented. The mergence of relation-ship-focused nursing theories with the ideas of the philosophers mentioned above will be suggested as an additional human caring foundation to be used by community health care nurses in conjunction with (not to replace) the physical and psychosocial models. For example, it will be suggested that whether a community health care nurse is providing physical or clinical care 'to' a person in need of such, cognitive therapy 'to' a person with mental health problems, or behavioural therapy 'to' a child with learning disabilities, in each situation care may be viewed as being provided 'with' the other person and not 'to' him or her.

PHILOSOPHIES OF HUMAN EXISTENCE

We live in a materialistic world. Self-perception is often affirmed in terms of the cars we drive, the size of our houses and where they are located, the possessions we own, as well as our financial status and occupations. All these material things have become status symbols which individuals strive to obtain in modern society. And yet, when illness or disability befalls us, when a mother gives birth to a disabled child or when a diagnosis of a terminal illness is confirmed, these material status possessions become less significant. At these times the fundamentals of life – *relationships* – take on a prominent position.

Therapeutic (or healing) caring relationships with clients can be enhanced by community health care nurses following philosophical examples when they communicate and relate with their clients. It seems appropriate, therefore, that nurses have an understanding of philosophies which may guide and underpin how they relate with themselves and with the people they care for.

According to Dallmayr (1984), philosophical writers on human existence fall within two major conceptions: transcendental phenomenology (or 'transcendentalism') and the philosophy of dialogue (or 'dialogicalism'). An oversimplified explanation of these two perspectives now follows.

Transcendentalism

Transcendentalism is based on intersubjectivity and the view that individuals can discover their true self (the 'I') by a process of transcendental reflection. When human beings achieve this they can then understand the other as 'another I' or an alter ego. The best-known proponent of this view is Husserl (1962). Other philosophers such as Heidegger (1962) and Sartre (1958) are sometimes associated with the views of Husserl (Theunissen, 1984), but they did reject many of his ideas. For example, Heidegger did not believe that individuals can use the process of totally 'bracketing' life experiences to gain access to the intersubjective true self, as did Husserl. The perspectives of Husserl and those of Heidegger are basically analogous except for their differing views on bracketing. Sartre, although influenced by Husserl and, most profoundly, by Heidegger, was an existentialist. His existentialism is depicted in his book *Being and Nothingness* (1958). The book's central theme contests the conflict that exists between objective things and human consciousness. Sartre's view was that humans are free in their actions, they can determine their own destiny and that not to acknowledge this is a dishonesty to self or, as he saw it, 'bad faith'.

Broadly speaking, transcendentalism views human beings and identity by internal intersubjective processes. It should be pointed out, however, that the distinction between transcendentalism and dialogicalism is not clear-cut. For example, the views of Sartre (1958) could be seen as spanning both perspectives. In his view, 'being' exists as an immediate presence – others help me find my true self – but self-determination also has a place. Immediacy in relationship interactions is also central to dialogicalism. Sartre further asserted that we can be dehumanised or objectified through materials. As will be explored below, this is quite similar to dialogicalism.

Dialogicalism

Dialogicalism, the second major philosophical conception of human existence, according to Theunissen (1984), is based not so much on the intersubjective self but on the self which is interpreted through encounters with others. It is sometimes referred to as the philosophy of the 'between'. The best-known proponents of this perspective are Martin Buber (1970) and Gabriel Marcel (1949).

Buber suggested two fundamental ways of relating with another person based on expressive and receptive modes of communication – 'I–it' and 'I–thou' relationships. I–it relationships are charac-terised by domination and subservience, by relating to other people as objects rather than human beings, and by using others for self-advancement. I–thou relationships on the other hand are characterised by genuine human respect, reciprocity and equality. According to Buber people can only really know their true self by interacting with others. He contended that oscillation between I–it and I–thou ways of relating take place in life encounters. In fact he proposed that to be really able to enter an I–thou encounter, individuals need to know the reality of relating both with self and with another, in an I–it manner. Immediacy of relationship is central to this position which is displayed in that moment of encounter between two persons through the spoken word, a touch, eye contact and body posture. Reading these cues shows if people are being related to in either an I–thou or an I–it fashion.

Marcel (1949), another philosopher asserting the dialogicalism perspective, forwarded the theory of 'presence' with another person. Presence is seen by Marcel as similar to an I–thou encounter, although he adds a spiritual element to being in presence with another person, or with one's self. He further exhorted two types of human existence – 'being and having'. 'Being' is 'presence' with self and others, it is similar to the 'I–thou' relationship. 'Having', alternatively, is related to material possessions and with other affluence. It is also associated with taking rather than giving in human encounters. It is more aligned with I–it relationships.

'Being', according to Marcel, is represented by two self-participation manners – 'disposability' and 'engagement'. Disposability is the capacity to be available to self and to other people, and to enter their 'presence', thus demonstrating a willingness to engage with them. An indisposable person lacks self-awareness and exists behind a socially constructed shield which creates a barrier to true engagement with another human being (Cain, 1963).

Dialogicalism can be briefly summarised as human existence taking place through the quality of relationships between people, and it is through the channel of such relationships that we come to know our true selves. The 'self' would not exist without the 'other' for it is the relationship 'between' them which constitutes human existence.

Conclusion to philosophies of existence

Having briefly discussed dialogicalism and transcendentalism, which are difficult concepts to grasp and which have been debated by philosophers for many years, a wise decision may be to assert that 'truth' most likely exists in both perspectives. In addition, there are many overlapping themes highlighted within the views of philosophers from both schools of thought. Both perspectives have much to offer community health care nursing.

Transcendentalism has inspired innovations in education, and many religious and social reforms have been guided by these perspectives. The feminist movement and feminist research owe much to the critical thinkers of this school. Transcendentalism has much to offer the caring professions. For example, research into community living and many areas of nursing has been guided by this movement. The influence of transcendentalism is evident in the work of contemporary nurse theorists such as Benner (1984) and Parse (1995). Followers of this tradition are principally committed to intuition as a way of knowing, to introspection, and to the essence of human goodness in both humanity and nature.

In most of the discussion in the following sections of this chapter, the therapeutic effects of dialogicalism as a way of relating with other people, as forwarded by Buber and Marcel, will be discussed. However, it must be noted that the writings of transcendentalist philosophers also offer perspectives which may be used to underpin caring relationships.

THERAPEUTIC CARING IN COMMUNITY HEALTH CARE NURSING

When the mist of depression descends upon a person, or where an individual has a learning disability, or a physical disability or illness which prevents them from obtaining or maintaining material possessions (which as stated previously seem to have gained prominence in modern life), they become more dependent on relationships with others for their self-affirmation. Under these conditions 'caring relationships' take on a new meaning, and in fact can end up being therapeutic or non-therapeutic, depending on how the person is related to. Thus the primary aim of community health care nurses should be to form therapeutic caring relationships with their clients. This in itself can be justified in terms of respect for others, dignity and human rights. Theoretical support for this viewpoint has been presented by many nurse theorists who claim that 'mind' can affect 'body' (Peplau, 1952; Watson, 1979, 1988; Rogers, 1990; Parse, 1995). As Rogers (1996, p. 174) states:

'basic science has provided unequivocal evidence that mind–body relationships exist, nurses have been slow to recognize their ability to affect these relations and enhance healing.'

When community health care nurses visit people in their own homes at least one therapeutic encounter takes place. It does not matter whether the reason for a visit is to provide technical or physical care, psychological support, education, information or social guidance. In all cases nurses can relate to the other person with humanity (this term is used here to mean Buber's I–thou stance), or inhumanity (this term is used here to mean Buber's I–it stance). Relating to others with humanity involves community nurses having the values and ways of 'being with', or entering 'presence' with another which are presented in Figure 2.1. These values and ways of being with another human being, which capture and convey values inherent in the use of presence in the therapeutic relationship that exists between nurses and people, are supported by an eclectic range of literature on caring relationships (Mayeroff, 1971; Watson, 1988; Montgomery, 1993). Each of these values is now discussed in terms of how therapeutic presence is utilised when relating to people with humanity, hence contributing to therapeutic care which aids healing, growth and development.

In the following discussion the values listed in Figure 2.1 are discussed individually to facilitate explanation but in the real world they merge in terms of a holistic 'way of being' with another person.

Equality

Community health care nurses may find difficulty relinquishing the power they hold in terms of their professional position and specialist knowledge. But if they wish to show solidarity and allegiance to the people they care for, an equal relationship should exist. The fact that the nurses are in possession of professional knowledge which benefits the person they care for, and their family, need not mean inequality in status. It is not the possession of professional knowledge *per se* which may lead to inequality, but how the knowledge and skills possessed by a professional are used. A tradition exists in professions such as medicine and law of guarding knowledge in a cloak of mystique. This leads to members of such professions placing themselves in a self-created stratum which in turn creates

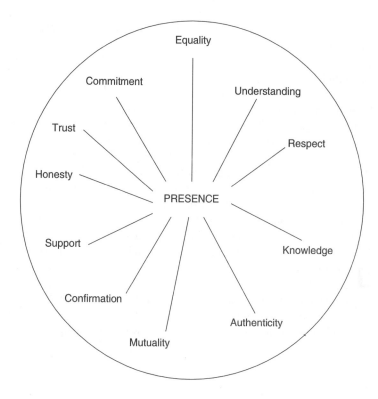

Figure 2.1   Values associated with therapeutic presence

distance between them and those they provide a service for. Cain (1963, p. 39) states:

> 'Marcel's view of thou does not require the physician, lawyer, or other professional practitioners in human affairs to abandon objective analysis . . . [when relating with people] but insists that to treat them as mere "cases" does not touch the true being.'

Community health care nurses should avoid professional guarding which creates distance from those they care for. One example of this is in the use of language. Professional jargon can disempower people who do not understand it, while a shared language between a service provider and service user empowers the user and leads to equality. By endorsing equal relationships with the people they care for, community health care nurses can enter human presence with them.

Authenticity

Authenticity or genuineness is an essential value for a community health care nurse to have when relating with others. Authenticity is one of the quintessential elements of care and presence with another person. It involves being genuine with the people you care for. As Montgomery (1993) proposes, authenticity involves genuine demonstrations of thoughts and feelings that are displayed with affection or humour by the professional. Montgomery further suggests the professional should be able to express anger and frustration in the 'here and now' and at times enter into confrontation with those they care for. However, such confrontations must remain caring as:

'the difference between a caring and a noncaring confrontation is that a caring confrontation is motivated by a sincere desire to stay in relationship, to stay involved in a way that is helpful to the patient.'
(Montgomery, 1993, p. 56)

Community health care nurses may show authenticity to those they care for by sincere expression. For example, the use of humour has been mentioned above but it should be remembered that humour should involve laughing 'with' and not 'at' people. Displays of affection can be shown by appropriate verbal exchanges, non-verbal expressions and use of touch. In all such authentic caring relationships, nurses should have knowledge of appropriate communication skills and when to use these. This knowledge would include being aware of when it is appropriate to enter a person's private space, when the use of humour is suitable, when and what type of verbal affection is fitting in an interaction, and also when such expressions of affection would not be fitting.

There is a growing body of literature that supports touch as a healing therapeutic interaction in nursing (Rogers, 1990; Heidt, 1991; France, 1993; Van Sell, 1996). Touch can be a very useful means of communicating authenticity when used sensitively. Touch can be 'instrumental', which may involve nurses touching a person to provide such care as personal hygiene, or it may be 'affective', which could involve the nurse sensitively placing a hand on the person's shoulder or gently holding his or her hand. It is in these moments that the nurse can demonstrate an authentic 'presence' with the other person. When this presence is felt between nurse and client, therapeutic caring will take place and so healing will be promoted.

Trust

Trust is fundamental to most human relationships because if it does not exist then the relationship will break down. Wilmot (1995) suggests that trust is an attribute which is associated with many types of relationship. When a person is in distress due to illness or disability, they may become dependent on the care provider. Under such circumstances trusting the person who provides the care is essential. Therefore, if you as a community health care nurse make a promise to a person you care for, it should always be kept. Breaking a promise to another person is hurtful to them and the more dependent that person is on you the more severe the hurt will be. It follows that nurses should not make promises to another person unless they know they will be able to keep it.

An example from practice illustrates how breaking a promise can sabotage a relationship. A mother of a hyperactive child with a learning disability had reached a state of not being able to cope with her child due to physical and mental exhaustion. The community health care nurse visited the family and made a promise to the mother that she would arrange for her child to spend the weekend in a respite residence to give the mother a much-needed rest. The mother was extremely grateful for this. However, the nurse had made this promise without first checking on the availability of a respite place, and after trying and failing to obtain a place for the child she had to return to the mother before the weekend and inform her that she could not keep the promise. The outcome to this was that the mother lost trust in the nurse and requested to have the community health care nurse changed.

Honesty

Honesty is closely associated with trust in that honesty in caring relationships can build trust, or alternatively dishonesty can diminish trust. As Burgoon *et al.* (1994) suggest, the credibility of a communicator is effected by honesty and trustworthiness. A dishonest communicator will not cultivate confidence in the person he or she communicates with. The health promotion aspect of community health care nursing often requires the nurse to be able to effectively encourage people to adopt a more health-oriented lifestyle. If the person receiving care does not have confidence in the honesty of the nurse then they will be less likely to follow their advice. Community health care nurses practise within multidisciplinary teams which provide caring services. At times conflict may occur in these teams if a decision has been made not to be totally honest with clients. For example, the medical member of the team may believe that it is right to withhold a diagnosis from a client.

Community nurses could find themselves in regular contact with a person who asks about their prognosis, and nurses may be placed in the difficult position of having to be dishonest by withholding information. It is difficult to see how nurses could enter presence with another person while not being honest with them. Most people are dishonest about minor things at some time in their life, but to be dishonest about something major that has the power to influence other people's perceptions of their lives presents an ethical dilemma.

Brown *et al.* (1992) discuss the issue of deliberation on truth-telling. They suggest that truth is important because of its connection with autonomy and the dignity of planning one's life. Brown *et al.* further suggest that truth is also relevant to group autonomy in that if all those in the group do not have access to the truth then they will not be co-deliberating as equals. In mutuality (to be discussed later), shared planning of care with clients will be considered, but if such sharing involves withholding information from the care recipient then it has to be questioned as to how much it really is sharing.

Brown *et al.* propose that even though individuals know that truth is a foremost consideration, there are times when they still decide to be deceptive for another reason that they strongly believe in as passionately as the righteousness of truth. Brown *et al.* suggest some of these reasons might be that: truth will in some way harm the person; they may not be ready to be told the truth; enough time is not available to tell them in the manner in which they should be told; they cannot cognitively grasp an understanding of what they may be told; and there are some clients who may not actually want to be told. However, if nurses choose to follow the road of deception for whatever reason, then they must accept responsibility for making this decision and be able to defend it as well as the consequences of it on moral grounds.

A final word on honesty is that the 'right' decision will rest with you as a community health care nurse. But it should be kept in mind that if you encounter true presence with the other person, much of what is communicated between you will take place at an intuitive or spiritual level. Verbal deception will not always hide the truth which is communicated more deeply by various other modes.

Understanding

Understanding in the context of therapeutic relationships is about understanding the other person's feelings. It is about reaching out to the other person and being with them. It is about reaching a state of presence with the other person, and with them entering your presence. Unlike empathy, which is associated with psychological counselling theories and encourages the therapist to stand back while endeavouring to enter the client's world, thus encouraging a dualistic affiliation (Montgomery, 1993), understanding in therapeutic caring relationships is about merging with the feelings of the other.

Granted, all people are unique and one person can never fully understand the absolute condition of another person, as Callaghan (1990, p. 22) states: 'the person who says 'I know exactly how you feel' is repeating a nonsense . . . He or she cannot know how you feel because he or she is not you.' But in a therapeutic caring relationship there is an affiliation which demonstrates the wish to understand. Sometimes understanding may even be shown by stating that 'no one can understand what you are going through'. The paradox embedded within this saying may be that you actually let the person know that you do understand how they feel because, in reality, only that person alone, at that moment in time and in this context, can truly experience what they feel. Just by being in their presence, a spiritual and psychological wealth circulates between them. Similarly, listening in silence to the total person – to what they say as well as what they do not say – their silence is touched by your silence and they understand that you are with them.

Knowledge

Knowledge is closely associated with understanding. Community health care nurses need to have 'knowledge' of their client. It is quite obvious that this knowledge relates to clinical knowledge of the client's condition, the family dynamics and various theories, but at a deeper and more meaningful level it involves knowledge of the person. In turn, according to the philosophy of dialogicalism discussed above, knowledge of the other person is intrinsically affiliated to self-knowledge. When we have self-knowledge and true knowledge of the other person, and they of us, what exists between each person in an encounter is therapeutic. McKenna (1997, p. 42) states:

> 'most nurses are not able to prescribe medication nor do they possess an arsenal of surgical instruments: what we have is ourselves and we can use this therapeutically to make a difference to the welfare of clients.'

According to Benner's (1984) perspective, through experience nurses develop an intuitive knowledge of the people they care for. Benner sees this intuitive understanding as the hallmark of an 'expert' practitioner. When nurses develop this degree of expertise a fusion of knowledge and doing takes place. Such a nurse will know the person he or she cares for, and this knowing in itself will be therapeutic because it will guide the care that is delivered.

Respect

Respect for personhood is needed if humanistic therapeutic relationships are to filter through encounters between community health care nurses and those they care for. Respect is shown when nurses convey the values mentioned above: trust, honesty, understanding and authenticity. Other ways of being with another person, such as compassion, mutuality and commitment, to be discussed later, are means of showing respect for people. These ways of being are integral to nursing theories of human caring (Watson, 1988; Parse, 1995).

Community health care nurses who show respect for others will instil self-worth in them. By showing that you respect someone you are showing them that they matter, that you care and that they are important in themselves as human beings. No matter how debilitating the disability or illness is, it is the individual who matters and all human beings should be respected for their personhood. The key ways of conveying respect for self and others are demonstrated by how you as a nurse communicate and relate with the person, especially at the initiation, maintaining and closing of relationships. Some ways by which respect may be shown in relationships are:

- Addressing the other person by their preferred name or title and finding out what the person's preferences are in social discourse.
- Respecting the person's right to self-determination.
- Always maintaining the person's dignity when caring tasks are being undertaken.
- Sharing time equally during interactional encounters and noting that at times of emotional need the other person may require more time to explore and express feelings.
- Being open to the other person in encounters and showing this by verbal and non-verbal acknowledgement.
- Showing acceptance of people – individual differences should be respected even when the other person's values, beliefs and feelings are not in harmony with your own.
- Giving people the time, space and recognition to show their emotions, including anger.

True respect leads to mutuality in that when you as a nurse show compromise and accommodation to another person without conditions, they will come to afford you respect for the person you are.

Mutuality

Mutuality is the term used here to cover various different ways of humans 'being with' each other in therapeutic caring relationships. It involves community health care nurses 'sharing' all (or as much as possible) of the total care planning and care provision with the care receiver. Kendall (1996) suggests that partnership between professionals and carers, clients and other professionals is strongly supported in contemporary health care policies. She forwards as examples of these policies: *The Patient's Charter* (DoH, 1990a), The Children Act (DoH, 1990b), *The Health of the Nation* (DoH, 1992) and *Changing Childbirth* (DoH, 1993). Support for partnership models of practice in many settings is also provided by Courtney *et al.* (1996). This tendency towards partnership and sharing in health care is guided by principles and ideologies such as empowerment, autonomy and self-advocacy. Referring to self-advocacy, Sines (1996, p. 477) states: 'the key to ensuring that people do speak for themselves lies in the extent to which they are empowered to express their views both individually and collectively'.

Therefore, community health care nurses should empower their clients by being prepared to abrogate professional demarcation lines and barriers which exclude those they care for from involvement in self-determination. By adhering to these values nurses can encourage true mutual sharing relationships between themselves and people who use their services.

Another element of mutuality in therapeutic caring is 'reciprocity'. In the past this idea was frowned upon in nursing. Nurses were educated to keep their distance and avoid any emotional cohesion with clients. But there has been a movement in nursing which is referred to by Stevens Barnum (1994, p. 226) as 'New Age paradigm images' which are transcending many nursing theories. For example, while there are differences between nursing interaction theories such as those of Orlando (1990) and Watson (1988) who promote a transpersonal intersubjective human caring model, and the existentialist perspectives of Paterson and Zderad (1988) they all share a belief in the principle of mutuality between nurse and client as well as the integrity of reciprocity in therapeutic caring relationships. Moreover, recent trends in nursing literature promote the need to incorporate therapeutic humanistic caring relationships into all aspects of the nursing curriculum and subsequently integrate this knowledge with all areas of practice (Kirby and Slevin, 1992; Taylor, 1993; Higgins, 1996; Dillon and Wright-Stines, 1996). Reciprocity in community health care nursing, therefore, involves a mutual sharing or 'being with' the other person. In therapeutic caring encounters nurse and client mutually experience each other's presence and are touched by it. Nurses should be 'real' with those they care for and should not hide their emotions. At times this will mean expressing anger, laughing with and even sometimes crying with those you care for. Community health care nurses who open themselves up and express their emotions and who do not hide behind a façade will encourage those they care for to self-disclose and this mutuality will lead to positive growth in both nurse and client.

Support

In therapeutic caring relationships community health care nurses provide support by being with the other person. This means a total 'presence', not only words of support. In fact there are times when just being there, or a touch, a smile, or a shared experience at a significant moment will provide support. In the words of a client expressing personal experiences of depression, cited by Jambunathan (1996, p. 29), the power of presence as support is illustrated:

'In very bad times I was desperate for someone to sit with me . . . Depressed people need someone to be there. Actions speak louder than words . . . Never underestimate the power of being there.'

As nurses we use our humanness as a therapeutic agent and when we enter a mutual presence with the other we can encourage their healing. Sometimes this can be done by words, by silence, by non-verbal communication or by touch. At other times support can be present in a supporting media such as music, drama or art, or in complementary therapies such as aromatherapy. These aesthetic media can add richness to therapeutic relationships and when appropriate may provide emotional support. As Cain (1963) pointed out, Gabriel Marcel in his life-work has followed three paths: the way of music and spontaneous improvisation; the way of meditative thought and phenomenological analysis of spirituality; and the way of drama to find meaning in metaphysical meditations. By these modes a person may find the answers to their inner despair, or possibly come to realise that there are no answers other than that fate has taken its course, which in itself can lead to contentment. As a nurse you can share and support the person in these very precious experiential moments.

Commitment

Commitment is seen as a caring action by Montgomery (1993, p. 61) when she states that 'commitment is evidenced by going beyond the call of duty'. In other words it involves nurses extending the boundaries of the care they provide when this is required. Many community health care nurses work beyond their contracted hours, or make their phone number available to clients. These extra endeavours indicate a deep commitment to care. Commitment is also about being committed to a way of relating with other human beings. It is about embracing and owning the values mentioned above such as trust, honesty, respect and so on. When one is committed to this way of responding to others a genuineness will emanate from such a person and reach out to touch those they relate with. Therapeutic caring relationships guide nurses com-mitted to humanistic values, and in so doing they subsequently change to that of an ethical caring position (Kitson, 1993). Kitson continues by suggesting that nurse theorists such as Watson (1988) and Benner (1984) highlight caring relationships as ethical virtues.

When community health care nurses are fully committed to the humanistic mode of relating with people, therapeutic encounters take on a moral rightness.

Confirmation

There is a need to confirm in the other person all of the above values, actions and ways of knowing people which, it is suggested here, guide therapeutic caring relationships. According to Montgomery (1993), there is a significant overlap between caring and confirmation. When we 'confirm' our presence with others they feel that we 'care' for them and thus confirmation of the other is integral to caring. Rather than confirmation being a value in itself, it can be viewed as an indication of you, as a community health care nurse, entering a therapeutic presence with the other person. Thus, confirmation is seen here as an outcome and it is evidenced in the other person by affirmation and growth, and likewise in confirmed affirmation and growth in the nurse. This may be something which is not tangible (existing at a spiritual level, which will be discussed later) or it may be present in the mood and emotions of clients which may be communicated by showing:

- an increased interest in personal appearance;
- more confidence in social encounters;
- a raised mood;
- contentment with one's life and condition;
- more openness in social discourse;
- a deepened faith in the goodness of humanity, and
- physical healing being hastened by the serenity of the mind.

In nurses confirmation may manifest in self-satisfaction which brings forth growth and well-being, and the knowledge that they have an enhanced ability to therapeutically relate with others.

PRESENCE

Presence is a way of being with another human being as in the 'I–thou' relationship of Buber (trans. 1970). No one could ever live their life in total presence with others at all times, as it may lead to a state of mental and physical exhaustion. There is a need to move between I–it and I–thou relating. But as stated at the beginning of this chapter, when people are vulnerable, ill or disabled it is then that they rely on relationships with others. Community health care nurses, therefore, are frequently in contact with people who will reach out to receive their presence.

All the values mentioned above, and many more which are intangible or invisible, come together and unite in human caring under the concept of 'presence'. Spirituality is one such abstraction which involves a higher level of presence between people. Here I am referring not only to religious beliefs but to the spiritual harmony which can exist between people. Neither do I exclude religious beliefs which may mean so much to a person. According to Price *et al.* (1995) spirituality can encompass a broad range of religious views, philosophies and world-views. Thus, the presence which is reached through spirituality has to do with personal mind/body unison, with unison between people, and with unison with one's universe, beliefs, or a God of our understanding. This presence can lead to healing. The concept of presence is perhaps beyond that which can be explained by words but I will attempt this in the remainder of this chapter with the use of illustrative examples.

Illustrative example one – reaching out through turmoil

Ann is a community health care nurse who knows and has visited Alison, a young mother who has recently given birth to her third child. Ann has been visiting the family since the birth and formative years of the first two children in the family. Alison and her husband's first two children are very healthy young girls now aged four and six. On the birth of their latest child, a little boy whom they named Simon, the couple were so happy and they felt their family was now complete. But very soon after the birth their elation changed to shock, disbelief and dismay as they were informed that Simon had Down's syndrome. It is now a few months since Simon's birth and Ann has been making regular visits to the home. Alison has good and bad days and on this particular day she feels in very low spirits when Ann calls to visit. After the initial discussion on Simon's general condition Ann notices Alison's low mood so she asks, 'What about yourself?' She looks into Alison's eyes and sees the despair before the flood of tears. Alison sobs uncontrollably, opening the floodgates of her emotions. 'Why did it happen to us? Why us?' she cries. Ann knows that there is no answer to this question which will reconcile Alison in her despair, so she moves forward and puts her arms around her. Ann gently hugs Alison as she says, 'I have no answer for you but I will be here when you need me.' The embrace only lasts for a moment or so but within these brief moments each feels the 'presence' of the other. Alison feels much better following the encounter, the emotional release has helped her, and as she dries the tears from her eyes she says 'I feel really silly.' Ann places her hand on top of Alison's and gently squeezes as she says, 'You are not silly at all, you should never be afraid to show your emotions.' On this particular day the presence of Ann made a difference to Alison.

Illustrative example two – meeting in the darkness

Sarah is a 65-year-old woman who has lived much of her later adult life with periodic episodes of depression. With her husband John she lived on a small farm in a beautiful rural area. They never had children and Sarah's depression could always be managed with John's help. But John died two years ago and since then the cloud of depression has fallen more frequently on Sarah, and periods of remission have been few. On occasions hospital care was suggested to her, but she declined, wishing to stay in the home she had always shared with John. At times Sarah has felt that life was not worth continuing and indeed thoughts of ending her life had crossed her mind. She felt very low on this particular Monday afternoon, even though she knew Peter, her community nurse, was calling to see her and his visit always made her feel better. Peter had been visiting Sarah on and off during the past five years and he was a strength to her during John's illness and subsequent death.

At around 4 o'clock Peter turns into the narrow winding lane which leads to Sarah's house. He likes calling on Sarah in these pleasant surroundings, and it is even more enjoyable on this warm summer afternoon. Peter thinks to himself that it has been a long day, but he looks forward to finishing his working day with a visit to Sarah. Monday evenings are a time of great enjoyment for Peter, he plays football for a local team and afterwards goes to the pub with his friends. He is looking forward to the evening. Peter knocks and enters Sarah's house and on seeing her he knows she is not well. He has a deep knowledge of Sarah, and she of him, and as they glance at each other they communicate before they speak. Peter knows the torturous sadness he sees in Sarah's creased and weathered face as well as he knows his own feelings. He sits on the chair remaining silent for a while before saying, 'You don't seem to be feeling much better Sarah?' They converse and sit in periods of silence for the next hour and a half, and slowly Sarah comes round a bit. Peter asks, 'Have you gone outside lately?' Sarah replies 'I haven't crossed the door in days.' 'Come on then,' says Peter, 'let's take a walk down the lane.' With some encouragement from Peter, Sarah agrees. Peter and Sarah walk down the lane in the warm summer evening in each other's 'presence'. Peter talks about the wild flowers on the verge of the lane and shows excitement when he sees an occasional rabbit in the fields. This brings a smile to Sarah's face as she recalls, 'If John was here now he would be looking to get his gun to shoot the rabbits, but I wouldn't let him, many an argument we had over that.' They walk on and as the birds sing and the sun begins to fall in the sky, there is a 'spiritual presence' between these two people that can only be felt; it cannot be seen, but it exists between them. They have both been touched by it. Eventually they return and Peter leaves after having a cup of tea. He promises Sarah he will be back the next day, as he knows the depth of her depression. As Peter turns his car to leave Sarah waves goodbye to him from the door and she feels a lot better. She marvels at how the young nurse can make her feel good, and she laughs to herself as she thinks of what John used to say about him – 'That's a young man with an old man's head and wisdom on his shoulders.'

Peter has forgotten the time; he looks at his watch and sees it is 7.30. Too late for the football, he thinks, but no matter, there will be plenty of other Monday evening games. Peter too feels good about the encounter and how he, at least temporarily, lifted Sarah's spirits. In fact he thinks to himself, 'I wouldn't feel as good if I had played in the game tonight and scored the winning goal.'

Illustrative example three – a touching of souls at life's end

Mary, a young student nurse, enters a home with the community health care nurse – Angela – who is her preceptor during her community placement. They have been visiting this home frequently where the father – Bill – is dying from a terminal illness. Angela knows the end is very near for Bill. The family take turns at sitting with him. Angela and the student have been calling twice daily for the past two weeks attending to Bill's physical hygiene, turning him and administering and monitoring his analgesics by the infusion pump. At first, the student felt awkward in Bill's company because he could still speak. But she was full of awe at the rapport which had developed between Angela and Bill, and found she was drawn into the interactions. Bill even joked with Angela and they all laughed together. At other times Bill would say, 'I don't have long left', and Angela would sit and hold his hand. She would say positive things to him such as, 'But you have great sons and daughters and grandchildren who will be here.' The student noticed that Angela was always truthful to Bill, even when it seemed dishonesty would have been an easier option. But as Angela had often told her, 'Yes, it would be easier to be dishonest, easier for me though, not for Bill.' The student greatly admired Angela for making such a choice. As they made Bill comfortable Angela worked with the student in silence, for she recognised that death was near for Bill. She knew the sound of the rattle in his chest, the long pauses in his breathing, and the irregular fall and rise of his chest. She recognised the almost transparent colour of his skin and his frail skeletal form that she had cared for on many occasions. When they had finished making Bill comfortable Angela sat at his bedside and held his hand in silence for a brief moment. She then stood up and before leaving she leaned over and kissed Bill on the forehead. As she lifted her head the student saw the sparkle of a tear in Angela's eye. Outside the room Angela told Bill's daughter that 'it will not be long now' and, as they hugged tears appeared again in Angela's eyes.

The student had not realised that a nurse could, or should, be so emotionally involved. Her education to date had not prepared her for this. But the student too had felt the 'presence' in this house between Angela, Bill and his daughter. This 'way of being' with another person was impregnated on her soul, and it was something she would never forget. In future years this student, like Angela, would enter presence with others because she now realised that this is the essence of nursing.

CONCLUSION

The material content of this chapter has been difficult to write about. I have attempted to put into words that which exists between people in a therapeutic caring relationship. I feel confident that I have captured many of the central components inherent in the use of presence in 'therapeutic relationships'. However, I am equally confident that there is a myriad of understandings on this topic which preclude the use of words. There is also a sense that when one attempts to expound concepts such as 'being with another', 'presence' and spirituality', as I have attempted to, that the very thing which Buber, Marcel and others stringently opposed – objectification – will raise its head. But as Long (1997, p. 173) states:

> 'The nurse–patient relationship is the most vital therapy of all. A consistent, structured, therapeutic encounter is the greatest catalyst a nurse can bring to healing.'

This being the case, it seems vital that there are continuing attempts to explicate the concept of 'therapeutic relationships' in nursing. Granted, a concept such as 'presence' will always be best experienced in the real world, as with the student in the final illustration above, but if written words can at least encourage community health care nurses to recognise the value in relating with self and others, as I suggest throughout this chapter, then my efforts will not have been in vain. Most nurses enter their profession with a strong belief in the ideology of caring for other people. And even though various factors seem to operate to harden or even break the caring ideology within many nurses, it is commendable that we, as a profession, hold on dearly to these values. This is evident in the reemergence of 'therapeutic caring relationships' presented in the nursing literature on practice, research and theory in nursing. The work of humanist nurse theorists such as Watson (1988), Parse (1995) and others is receiving ever increasing interest in nursing circles. This interest must surely provide an indication of the profession's view of the centrality of 'human presence' as a therapeutic core in nursing. It seems that the humanist nursing theories, combined with the philosophical thinking of philosophers such as Buber (1970) and Marcel (1949), can provide direction for therapeutic caring relationships in all settings in nursing. I would suggest that this is a wise direction for nursing to follow. Many eminent philosophers on human existence have written on relationships between people. I feel the words of one such philosopher best encapsulate what I have attempted to say in this chapter and I will conclude with his words. Gabriel Marcel (1967, p. 47), commenting on the work of Buber, stated:

> 'he reminds us, with an insistence which never excludes this notion, of the subtlety that above the world of objects the presence of the Thou is suspended like the spirit upon the waters. . . this vapour is not inactive, it puts itself forth as a beneficent rain. Through its agency, man can resist the oppressive force which emanates from the object'.

References

Benner, P. (1984) *From Novice to Expert: Excellence and Power in Clinical Nursing.* Menlo Park, Calif.: Addison-Wesley.

Brown, J. M., Kitson, A. L. and McKnight, T. J. (1992) *Challenges in Caring Explorations in Nursing and Ethics.* London: Chapman & Hall.

Buber, M. (1970) *I and Thou: Martin Buber A new translation, with prologue and notes,* trans W. Kaufmann. Edinburgh: T. & T. Clark.

Burgoon, M., Hunsaker, F. G. and Dawson, E. J. (1994) *Human Communication,* 3rd edn. London: Sage Publications.

Cain, S. (1963) *Gabriel Marcel.* London: Bowes & Bowes.

Callaghan, W. S. (1990) *Good grief.* London: William Collins.

Courtney, R., Ballard, E., Fauver, S., Gariota, M. and Holland, L. (1996) The partnership model: working with individuals, families, and communities toward a new vision of health care. *Public Health Nursing,* 13(3), pp. 177–86.

Dallmayr, F. R. (1984) Introduction. In M. Theunissen (ed.), *The Other Studies in the Social Ontology of Husserl, Heidegger, Sartre, and Buber.* Boston, Mass.: MIT Press, pp. ix–xxv.

Department of Health (1989) *Caring for People: Community Care in the Next Decade and Beyond.* London: HMSO.

Department of Health (1990a) *The Patient's Charter.* London: HMSO.

Department of Health (1990b) *The Care of Children.* London: HMSO.

Department of Health (1992) *The Health of the Nation.* London: HMSO.

Department of Health (1993) *Changing Childbirth.* London: HMSO.

Dillon, R. S. and Wright-Stines, P. (1996) A phenomenological study of faculty student caring interactions. *Journal of Nursing Education,* 35(3), pp. 113–18.

France, N. E. M. (1993) The child's perception of the human energy field using therapeutic touch. *Journal of Holistic Nursing,* 11(4), pp. 319–31.

Godin, P. (1996) The development of community psychiatric nursing: a professional project? *Journal of Advanced Nursing,* 23(5), pp. 925–34.

Heidegger, M. (1962) *Being and Time,* trans. J. Macquarrie and E. Robinson. New York: Harper & Row.

Heidt, P. (1991) Helping patients to rest: clinical studies in therapeutic touch. *Holistic Nursing Practice*, 5(4), pp. 57–66.

Higgins, B. H. (1996) Caring as therapeutic in nursing education. *Journal of Nursing Education*, 35(3), pp. 134–6.

Husserl, E. (1962) *Ideas: General Introduction to Pure Phenomenology*, trans. R. B. Goodman, New York: Collier.

Jambunathan, J. (1996) Depression: dealing with the darkness. *Perspectives in Psychiatric Care*, 32(1), pp. 26–9.

Kendall, S. (1996) Partnership in care. In S. Twinn, B. Roberts and S. Andrews (eds), *Community Health Care Nursing: Principles and Practice*. Oxford: Butterworth-Heinemann, pp. 419–30.

Kirby, C. and Slevin, O. (1992) A new curriculum for care. In O. Slevin and M. Buckenham (eds), *Project 2000: The Teachers Speak. Innovations in the Nursing Curriculum*. Edinburgh: Campion Press, pp. 57–88.

Kitson, A. (1993) Formalising concepts related to nursing and caring. In A. Kitson (ed.) *Nursing: Art and Science,* (pp. 25–47). London: Chapman and Hall.

Long, A. (1997) Avoiding abuse amongst vulnerable groups in the community: people with a mental illness. In C. Mason (ed.), *Achieving Quality in Community Health Care Nursing*. London: Macmillan, pp. 160–81.

McKenna, H. (1997) *Nursing Theories and Models*. London: Routledge.

Marcel, G. (1949) *Being and Having*, trans. K. Farrer and M. Friedman, Westminster: Dacre Press.

Marcel, G. (1967) I and thou. In P. A. F. Schilpp (ed.), *The Philosophy of Martin Buber*. London: Cambridge University Press, pp. 41–8

Mayeroff, M. (1971) *On Caring*. New York: Harper & Row.

Ministry of Health (1919) *Nurses Registration Act (9 & 10 Geo. 5 Ch 94)*. London: HMSO.

Montgomery, C. L. (1993) *Healing Through Communication: The Practice of Caring*. London: Sage Publications.

Orlando, I. J. (1990) *The Dynamic Nurse–Patient Relationship*. New York: National League for Nursing.

Parse, R. R. (1995) *The human becoming theory in nursing*. In R. R. Parse (ed.), *Illuminations: the Human Becoming Theory in Practice and Research*. New York: National League for Nursing Press, pp. 147–57.

Paterson, J. G. and Zderad, L. T. (1988) *Humanistic Nursing*, New York: National League for Nursing.

Peplau, H. E. (1952) *Interpersonal Relations in Nursing*, New York: G. P. Putnam's Sons.

Price, J. L., Stevens, H. O. and LaBarre, M. C. (1995) Spiritual caregiving in nursing practice. *Journal of Psychosocial Nursing*, 33(12), pp. 5–9.

Rogers, M. E. (1990) Nursing: science of unitary, irreducible, human beings: update 1990. In E. A. M. Barrett (ed.), *Visions of Rogers' Science Based Nursing*. New York: National League for Nursing, pp. 5–11.

Rogers, S. (1996) Facilitative affiliation: nurse–client interactions that enhance healing. *Issues in Mental Health Nursing*, 17(3), pp. 171–84.

Sartre, J. P. (1958) *Being and Nothingness*. London: Routledge.

Sines, D. (1996) Advocacy. In S. Twinn, B. Roberts and S. Andrews (eds), *Community Health Care Nursing: Principles and Practice*. Oxford: Butterworth-Heinemann, pp. 471–9.

Stevens Barnum, B. J. (1994) Theories focusing on the nurse–patient relationship. In B. J. Stevens Barnum (ed.), *Nursing Theory, Analysis, Application and Evaluation*. Philadelphia: J. B. Lippincott, pp. 215–27.

Taylor, M. (1993) The nurse–patient relationship. *Senior Nurse*, 13(5), pp. 14–18.

Theunissen, M. (1984) *The Other Studies in the Social Ontology of Husserl, Heidegger, Sartre, and Buber,* trans C. Macann, Boston, Mass.: MIT Press.

United Kingdom Central Council for Nursing Midwifery and Health Visiting (UKCC). (1994) *The Future of Professional Practice – The Council's Standards for Education and Practice Following Registration*. London: UKCC.

Van Sell, S. L. (1996) Reiki: an ancient touch therapy. *RN*, 59(2), pp. 57–9.

Watson, J. (1979) *The Philosophy and Science of Caring*. Boston, Mass.: Little, Brown.

Watson, J. (1988) *Nursing: Human Science and Human Care: A Theory of Nursing*. New York: National League for Nursing.

Wilmot, W. W. (1995) *Relational Communication*. New York: McGraw-Hill.

CHAPTER THREE

The Nurse-Patient Relationship: Caring in a Health Context

Oliver Slevin

'One must rid oneself of all prejudice and let the mind of the other act on one without restraint. Thus can one establish contact with him and understand him.'
(Wilhelm, 1924/1987, p. 122)

INTRODUCTION

You must look first to the title. It speaks to you of a nurse and a patient, and it connects them with a hyphen. This hyphen means that they are one; the word 'nurse-patient' is one word not two, and it is joined. The nurse-patient when so joined is one. It was two entities who were separate persons. But they have now been placed together and become different from the two apart. The title speaks to you also of the nature of this joining. The word 'relationship' is used, and this word means connection. It alludes to this coming together of the entities 'nurse' and 'patient', the existence of some connection between them. But what is the nature of this connection?

The title speaks to you again. It is extended and speaks the words, 'caring in a health context'. This you now see is the connection. It is a connection, a relationship, characterised by caring for someone. The title calls us to an acknowledgement that within the relationship there is care. As such it is a bond between the carer and the cared for. It speaks of more than a relationship that is merely a state of being. It implies a bond which may be more accurately described as being *in relation,* as something which is being lived dynamically.

This having of care is something we will explore later. It is variously described. The existential philosopher Heidegger (1962) spoke of it as *Sorge*, the translation from German of which is care as a responsible and intentional engagement with the other, be it person or object. Both he and Sartre (1958) saw it as an authentic way of being-in-the-world. For them, care implied fully attending to, confronting, coming into relation. To fail to address the other in this way, to relate to another human being as an object, a role, a configuration of symptoms, rather than a person, shows a lack of care, a lack of authentic being-in-the-world with that other. In failing to confront the person as whole we in effect withhold our own person as whole from that person. This is why the two main dictionary meanings of the word 'relate' are 'to tell' and 'to connect' (see for example Collins Concise English Dictionary, 1978). That form of relating which is telling – giving and receiving information, exchanging some other commodity – is a relating only in part. We withhold from the other, and there is no full coming into relation, no connection of person with person. Heidegger described this as 'inauthentic being', and Sartre (perhaps more dramatically) spoke of 'bad faith' in the relation.

Others, such as the theologian Matthew Fox (1990) and the nursing scholars Roach (1987, 1991) and Watson (1985, 1988, 1992), speak of care as a state of compassion. This is more than the mere intentional countenancing of the other. It intrinsically involves a condition of being for and with the other, a true experiencing with and understanding of the joys and pains of that other, a feeling of concern for their plight which is in essence a sharing of their pain, and an unconditional reaching out to help. It is these additional attributes which extend the notion of care as a commitment to authentic being with the other to the level of a commitment to action as informed and moral helping. It is perhaps true that when care exhibits its compassion it is best described by the Hebrew concept of *hesed* or 'deeds of love'. In nursing, care is a call to action for and with others. It embraces a will to help and a capability to do so through expertise and competence, which can not be separated from compassion but becomes an obligation intrinsic to it in all acts of caring. This is artfully encapsulated in Watson's (1990) notion of 'informed moral passion'.

To have care is a way of being which is realised in *an act of caring*, of going out to the person for the person, to act in their interest and not in your own or any other person's interest. Furthermore, in the context of which we speak this is a specific way of going out. It is going out in a health context. Health sets the parameters. So, it is a going out to the other not in his or her context as your son, or mother, or friend, or lover, but in the context of his or her health and well-being. Behind the word mother–baby is a relation in which a mother fondles and feeds and a baby responds, a baby cries and a mother responds. Behind the word nurse–patient is a nurse who attends to a person's health needs and a person called patient or client who responds, a patient who fevers and a nurse who cools. So, in our title, we have the four key words. These are:

Nurse–Patient + Relationship + Caring + Health

The title could be shortened. It speaks to you one word, the word 'nursing'. It does in effect define this word.

THE TWO CULTURES

For and against care

The chapter builds on the earlier chapters, particularly Chapter 2 which addresses the professional–human interface and the therapeutic use of self. The concern here is not with interpersonal communication skills, which are adequately addressed in other chapters. This chapter is concerned instead with the nature of the relation between nurse and patient or client. The term 'relation' is profoundly significant, because nursing is in essence an intensely relational human activity which involves the giving and receiving of care between one and another.

Much of the literature on nursing as caring centres on a conflict between the view that nursing must be understood as a compassionate, sharing, person-centred relation and an opposing view that nursing is a highly skilled technical and therapeutic activity which requires, if not indeed demands, a less personal relationship. The caring perspective, as explicated by various nursing writers (for example, Bevis, 1981; Roach, 1987; Watson, 1988; Kirby and Slevin, 1992; Watson, 1992; Taylor, 1994; Kirby, 1995; Kirby and Slevin, 1995a), emphasises an intensely personalised and humanistic approach which speaks of presence, authenticity, intentional helping and compassion. Indeed, for some scholars in the idiom, the concept of caring is indivisible from ethical professional practice. This view, as expressed particularly in the work of Carper (1979),

Gilligan, (1982), Noddings (1984), Gadow (1996) and Kirby and Slevin (1995b), is that care in itself is intrinsically ethical, that when we relate to others with a caring intent this is by definition ethical. In simple terms, if our intention towards others is exclusively directed to their individual or collective good or well-being, our actions are never intentionally harmful and always morally justified.

Within the alternative viewpoint, the emphasis is on a technical, role-orientated perspective in which the patient is viewed as a health or disease problem or at very best a bio-psycho-social entity who will respond to the right interventions based on the best objective empirical evidence. Apart from the recognition of a biomedical ethic based on what is known as the four principles of beneficence, non-maleficence, respect for autonomy and justice (Beauchamp and Childress, 1979; Gillon, 1994; Beauchamp, 1994) all other humanistic and subjective knowledge is rejected as irrelevant. This does not necessarily mean that the patient or client is completely dehumanised in the process. But the emphasis is on a professional role that warns against 'personal involvement'. The concern here is with the establishment of a clearly delineated role which does not impose the person of the nurse upon the patient or client, a view also expressed in the work of Peplau (1952, 1969) in her conceptualisation of 'professional closeness'. The argument here is that the nurse or therapist does not bring 'self' to the relation. Indeed, it would be argued that in situations where relationships are part if not the whole of a patient's problems, the imposition of an additional personal relationship as opposed to a professional or role-limited arrangement may be dysfunctional.

This dichotomy is often viewed as a situation of treatment versus care, science versus art, role versus person, doing to versus being with and for, task-centredness versus person/client-centredness, or variations of these more or less apparently dichotomous positions. Those who subscribe to the more humanistic, caring perspective often decry the mechanistic and limited objective–analytic–scientific approach. Similarly, those opposed to the caring perspective have mounted powerful criticisms in attempts to negate that perspective as being unscientific, lacking in sound objective evidence, excessively drawing on theological and New Age philosophies, and so on (see for example the extreme critique by Barker et al. (1995) of the work of Watson (1988) and Kirby and Slevin (1992)).

It has long been recognised, as evidenced in the seminal essay by Snow (1959) almost forty years ago, that there is a split in society and in human thinking into what has become known as 'The Two

Cultures', those who subscribe to a scientific and those who subscribe to a humanistic mode of thinking and being. The dichotomy within nursing mirrors this wider split within society. A danger here is that one or other perspective may hold dominance and deprive our practice of the other. What is of even more concern is that one or other viewpoint, through being the darling of academics and nursing pundits, might be imposed on the caring situation. The theories and world-views which guide our practice must be selected by practitioners and for practitioners, on the basis that they work for *them* in *their* practice. Ultimately the knowledge which guides practice must meet the needs of patients and clients, not the express needs of scholars and theorists. But here we must return to our title again, for in nursing there is no such thing as a practitioner in isolation. The practitioner is always in relation, is always in the context of nurse–patient. Therefore, when we speak of practitioner choice, it must always be practitioner and patient choice. The alternative is no less a tyranny than the expropriation of practice choices by those who are not practitioners.

Espousing a caring praxis

The position presented in this chapter rejects the argument that the two perspectives are mutually exclusive and incompatible. Conversely, it is argued that both aspects must come together and be integrated in a true praxis of nursing as a caring relation. An evidence-based, highly skilled and technically proficient nursing which is impersonal, lacks compassion and fails to view the whole person as opposed to a particular symptomatic configuration or health care problem is inadequate. But so too is a nursing which claims to care with compassion but which is lacking in evidence-based knowledge, technical skill and professional competence. Such a nursing lacks responsible caring in any true sense. It may even be adjudged, in the view of Gadow (*op. cit.*) and Noddings (1984) to be unethical. Nursing as a true caring praxis can only exist as compassionate *and* skilled caring within a health context.

It can be reasonably argued that our problem has never been with recognising and accepting the skill dimension. While the extent to which our skill and technology has been adequately evidence-based may be questioned, our acceptance of nursing as a skilled activity is unchallenged. It is in the dimension of compassionate caring that we encounter difficulties. It is seldom spoken of in our nursing curricula and some (for example, Powell, 1982) would argue that in the past it has been actively discouraged. Yet this is at the very core of what nursing is said to be. It is this capacity for compassionate caring which is at the heart of what is in fact nursing's 'social contract', what society recognises in and expects of its nurses. We ignore this social contract at our peril. In adopting a primarily technical and skilled role which excludes this dimension we are alienating ourselves not only from our own legacy but from the very society we came into existence to serve. The words of Mary Wolff-Salin (1989) inform us here:

> 'Refusal to choose the depths, the centre, the heart condemns one to wander forever in a domain of superficiality where both one's life with God and one's human relationships become only a fraction of what they could be.'

To address how we can confirm the humanity of our nursing relations we must first recognise what influences them and then consider how we must both envision and live them. Just as nursing in its enactment is in a social context, so too is it influenced by social factors.

SOCIAL CONSTRUCTIONS: FROM PAST TO FUTURE

Begging the question

There is a need to address the question of the extent to which one or other of the perspectives represented by 'The Two Cultures' does hold sway. This is important, because it indicates to us the nature of the nurse–patient relation as it exists in reality and as a reflection of and indeed a social construct of a particular culture. The culture which has been socially constructed within health care agencies and the ethos this culture emanates has a profound influence on the nature of relationships. An understanding of these social constructs is therefore fundamental to our understanding of nurse–patient relations and our capacity to develop these in the interests of those we serve.

The social forces

The forces which determine the cultural ethos for health can be seen to come from both within and outside of the health care system.

Internal forces

Within the health care system the social forces are predominantly four: the medical profession; the managers and administrators of health care; others who work within health care, of whom nurses are the major element; and those who partake of the services, who are variously described as patients, clients, users, consumers, customers (the choice of descriptor itself often giving an indication of the ethos that exists). It is widely recognised that traditionally the balance of internal power was strongly biased towards two of these entities, the medical profession and managers, and that all others within the health care system occupy relatively weaker positions.

Medicine

Since the inception of the National Health Service (NHS) in Britain the medical profession has been the most constant dominant force (Klein, 1989, 1995). Indeed, the NHS only came into existence in 1948 as a system of social welfare, free to all at the point of delivery, as a consequence of the government of the day agreeing to significant autonomy and favourable contractual arrangements pertaining to the medical profession. As an already powerful professional group with a social mandate as the monopoly provider of health care, and as the backbone of the new NHS, the medical profession was in a position to strongly influence health care. This situation has continued to the present day to a greater or lesser extent. In the words of Klein (1995), 'medical authority became synonymous with the service and was institutionalised in ways that enabled the profession to control management, through presenting definitions of issues that reinforced their own authority'. Such was this power and influence that Harrison and Pollitt (1994) have argued that the NHS was the result of an 'aggregate outcome of individual doctors' clinical decisions, rather than the result of decisions made by politicians, policy makers, planners or managers'.

This medical dominance had about it important characteristics, some of which had relevance far beyond the parameters of health care delivery. The profession, particularly in the post-Second World War period, with the increasing number of medical specialisms in this period, had strengthened its position as a dominant profession which advances itself on a scientific basis. The claim to specialised, monopolistic knowledge and a strong scientific base had far-reaching social influences.

First, what in earlier times may have been termed witchcraft, immoral behaviour or even criminality are now often labelled as illnesses. For an increasing number of problems medical labels are devised and medical solutions proposed. Therefore, many problems become viewed as health problems, in the domain of the doctor rather than the priest, lawyer or policeman. Those who in another age may have sought the confessional now seek the therapy couch. The normal trials and exhaustions of modern living are given medical labels and, in the very act of labelling, through self-fulfilling prophecy they take on the mantle of major illnesses. This trend of the increasing medicalisation of society has been well-documented by such authors as Szasz (1962), Zola (1972), and Illich (1976). Such trends within society strengthen the power of medicine within its health services.

Second, the scientific orientation within medicine derives clearly from the positivistic tradition of the natural sciences with their particular empirical perspective. This is predominantly an objective science that emphasises empirical observation, controlled clinical trials and experimentation. It views such sources as the only legitimate source of sound knowledge. It is a perspective very much aligned with that one of 'The Two Cultures' which Snow (1959) described as the scientific. It refutes knowledge from any source other than its recognised scientific paradigm and, therefore, expropriates health knowledge to fit with its own perspective and to meet its own ends.

Third, and not entirely unrelated to the latter phenomenon, it must be recognised that the power, in science in general *and* in medicine, is gender-biased. This means that in effect the dominant perspective in health care has traditionally been male. Most scientists and senior doctors are men. The very notion of acknowledging intuitive ways of knowing alongside empirical ways of knowing is nothing short of anathema within such a perspective. Indeed, intuitive knowing is often aligned with the notion of 'woman's intuition' and as such is considered an irrelevance in comparison to empirical knowledge. The work of Polanyi (1958, 1966) on intuitive and tacit knowledge, or of Dreyfus *et al.* (1986) and Benner (1984) on intuitive expertise are not to be found in the medical curriculum, and are virtually unknown in that discipline. The influence of this gender domination phenomenon on the nursing profession in particular has been notable. The traditional socialised role of the nurse is that of the doctor's assistant, someone who in the final analysis follows the instructions of a physician (Stacey, 1988). The term 'doctor's handmaiden' represents the denigratory labelling of this phenomenon. As a reaction to this status, and particularly in the latter half of the twentieth century, nursing attempted to establish itself as a profession on the same basis as medicine, law and the other esteemed professions. A significant trend in this quest was the espousing of that same objective, natural science paradigm which was the mark of the medical profession itself. This has often resulted in a rejection of alternative ways of knowing, despite the suggestions by Carper (1978), Kikuchi (1992) and Slevin (1995a) that scientific knowledge cannot be the only source of knowledge in a caring enterprise which centres so much on close personal relating.

The resulting trend has thus been a shift away from a handmaiden–nurturing role towards a technical–scientific role which follows the traditional medical model (Schulman, 1958, 1972; Davies, 1995). This drift has significant implications for the nurse–patient relationship, and has led to some health service policy-makers in the UK such as Caines (1993) suggesting greater efficiencies by restricting nursing to high-technology and supervisory roles while the business of general hands-on personal care would be provided by support workers. This notion has not disappeared in recent years but reemerges in a suggestion that in the future the majority of direct patient care may be provided by a generic worker (Clark, 1997).

Management
Until the 1970s, while managers held significant status within the NHS, they were nevertheless not a serious threat to medical supremacy. This situation shifted significantly in the 1980s and first half of the 1990s during which a Conservative government was in power. The underpinning philosophy of the New Right was an increasing emphasis on the primacy of the individual, free market forces and personal freedom. In line with the monetarist philosophies which accompanied these attitudes there was an increasing emphasis on privatisation, cost-effectiveness, efficiency and value for money. Changes to the NHS, culminating in the NHS and Community Care Act 1990 and a major report on *The Health of the Nation* (DoH, 1992) introduced a new ethos and a new managerialism into the NHS. The introduction of an internal market, within which providers (mainly NHS trusts, within which consultants and other hospital doctors were employed) had to compete for contracts from NHS purchasers (NHS health authorities and GP fundholders) presented the most significant challenge to the medical profession since the inception of the NHS.

However, this trend had other effects. Through the various NHS reorganisations, nursing management as a major voice in the old NHS consensus management era virtually disappeared and as a consequence nursing as well as medical leadership became weakened. The old medical model of treating the patient as a case, or as a medical condition or problem to be solved, was replaced to some extent by the new managerialism model which viewed the service user as a consumer or customer. The emphasis was on production of a quality product and a contractual obligation to the customer presented in various patient's and client's charters. However, this new managerialism was no less empirical and objective and no less gender-biased than the medical model. Its concern was with measurable needs and measurable outcomes, as expressed in performance indicators related to such issues as waiting lists and day-surgery turnover. The implanting of a new commitment to research and development strategies (Baker, 1996) is a further example. In themselves laudable, the strategies which emerged, while rightly emphasising multidisciplinary approaches and the empirical underpinning of service delivery and clinical effectiveness, also seemed to align themselves exclusively with the objective, natural science perspective.

There were claims to involvement of the customer and responding to demand. But there were also conflicting forces of allocation of scarce resources, income generation and profitability which in fact limited real choice except through recourse to private medicine and paid-for services. The dominant philosophy underpinning the new managerialism was driven by economics rather than welfare ideology. It rejected consensus and power-sharing and stated that to a large extent the manager (the general manager or more recently the chief executive) was the final arbiter. A scene emerged of rapid turnover, day surgery, closure of longer-stay facilities and local hospitals and clinics. Increasingly the provision was one of treatment rather than care, despite the liberal use of this term as new NHS trusts spoke to their populations of a caring service. In this situation the notion that patients might continue to be provided with a service, or have their stay in an in-patient facility, because they needed *care* but not *treatment* was quite literally unheard-of.

Nurses and their patients
It might indeed be reasonably argued that in such a scenario the position of the nurse and the patient was considerably weaker. It might also be argued that as the great forces of medicine and

management, with their male-orientated ways of thinking and acting, vied for position or reached compromise on power distribution within the new NHS, the position of nurses was further marginalised and weakened.

Within the new NHS structures, by the second half of the 1990s the presence of nursing at middle and senior management levels has virtually disappeared. With this there is a view that the issue of leadership in nursing had reached a state of crisis. Decisions relating to nursing services, and thus concerning how nursing care would be delivered, were increasingly taken by others who were not nurses. As Davies (1995) has stated:

'There is the sheer invisibility of nurses in debates about the future of the NHS and the absence of information about them which is collected and examined in a systematic way. There is the matter of the male yardstick, of men's lives as the template, the constant point of comparison against which women can rarely measure up.'

The patient may seek of the nurse solace, compassion and comfort as well as technical skill and expertise, all those things which are the hallmark of what we refer to as caring. But where is the concern for such issues in the modern NHS? Where, amidst the multimillion-pound clinical trials industry is there a single significant, counterpointing, publicly sponsored research project on the nature of caring and caring relationships, which should be at the very heart of our NHS? Where, within the nursing education system in the UK is there a single funded Chair in nursing ethics or philosophy? Were it not for the contribution of some non-governmental, non-NHS agencies, such as the Royal College of Nursing, through initiatives such as its Ward Nursing Leadership Project, the University of East London, with its European Centre for Professional Ethics, and the establishment of the Highland Centre for Human Caring at Inverness, there would be an almost total absence of institutional commitment to the perspective in the UK.

External forces

Policy shifts

There is of course a diversity of external influences on the internal working of the NHS. The most obvious of these, and those which have already been alluded to, are the influences of government and policy-makers. Of particular significance in the period following the NHS and Community Care Act 1990 has been the increasing commitment to the notion of a primary-led service with an emphasis on health promotion, prevention and care in the community. The adage that we should have a health service as opposed to the current *ill* health service is one which has literally crossed the generations without any real and significant change. However, there are now signs to suggest that the commitment to this aspiration is growing. While there may have been much criticism of the Conservative government's health policies, the identification of national targets for health and social well-being now challenges the purchasers and providers of health services to make real incursions. The identification of such targets challenge the traditional sources of power within the health services, particularly those centred upon acute services and their attendants, the hospital consultants.

With the change in government in the UK in mid-1997 it can be anticipated that policy shifts will influence the future shape of the NHS. The new Labour government's concerns about the costs and ethos of an internal market, and its commitment to a less individualistic and more pluralistic society is one significant indicator of a change in direction. The Labour emphasis on a commitment to cooperation and partnerships rather than competition and its commitment to a return to a welfare as opposed to market orientation, if carried forward, would also herald change. It has also been the Labour view that previous approaches to the involvement of those who partake of the service have been unsuccessful and there is within their policy a stated commitment to greater community involvement.

These aspirations are now being carried forward in the government's consultations on major changes in the NHS and the decisions arising from these (see, for example, DoH, 1997 and 1998; DHSS, 1998).

Social emancipation

However, not all external forces emanate from institutional sources. It must be recognised that there are other influences. Significant among these is a society of people who are generally more informed and better educated, and thus more capable of making demands from the health services and utilising them to greater effect. While it may be accepted that we still live in a highly medicalised society, this has shifted considerably from the situation described by Zola (1972), Illich (1976) and Szasz (1962). Society is now more tolerant of alternative life-styles and less likely to allow a medicalisation process whereby such lifestyles are deemed as illness or deviance. While at the beginning of the twentieth century young single mothers may have been incarcerated as moral defectives, now this is the preferred lifestyle for many. Also, while more people may now turn to therapy rather than religion for help, there is a greater disenchantment with conventional medicine and a virtual explosion of uptake of alternative and complementary therapies.

Professional maturity

A final external influence upon the caring situation is in one sense also an internal influence. This is the influence upon its members of the profession itself as a conscious social entity. In the UK context this includes the regulatory bodies – the United Kingdom Central Council for Nursing, Midwifery and Health Visiting (UKCC) and the National Boards for nursing, midwifery and health visiting in each of the four UK countries. It also includes the various staff organisations such as the Royal College of Nursing, the Community Practitioners' and Health Visitors' Association and the Royal College of Midwives.

The current regulatory bodies were established by the Nurses, Midwives and Health Visitors Act 1979, with subsequent statutory changes being consolidated in the Nurses, Midwives and Health Visitors Act 1997. While nursing has been regulated by statute since the early years of the twentieth century, the developments in regulation since the inception of the UKCC have been significant. Major UKCC-initiated changes in nursing education have moved the pre-registration and formal post-registration education of all nurses into the higher education sector, as has been the case with community nurses for a number of years. Nurses now receive a more holistic and advanced education, centred on evidence-based practice and health care. The establishment of a Code of Professional Conduct and guidance on how nurses can extend their scope of professional practice together with the major advances in education and training are establishing a new maturity and increasing confidence within the profession.

It is also clear that the professional staff organisations are contributing to this emancipation. Bodies such as the Royal College of Nursing in the UK and the American Nurses' Association and National League for Nursing in the USA are no longer merely staff representative bodies, but are at the cutting edge of extending the knowledge and practice of nursing. Such bodies play an increasingly important part in pioneering innovative developments in education, management, leadership and research. This has been of increasing importance in the decade preceding 1997, when within organised health services the internal forces have with only a few exceptions had a negative effect on such developments.

It might be suggested that while the balance of power still rests with doctors and managers and that the scientific orientations they adopt still hold sway, there are positive signs of significant shifts. Included in these are the aforementioned policy shifts occasioned by the coming to power of Labour, with its emphasis on a more collective approach to a health care system that is welfare-orientated and patient-empowering. There are also, as suggested above, signs of a coming of age within the nursing profession. A servile attitude no longer exists and nurses increasingly assert their equal membership in the health care team. In addition, nurses are questioning a restricted scientific knowledge base to their practice and more courageously establishing their contribution on a wider knowledge and care-orientated basis. The users of health services are also, as suggested above, becoming less subservient and more demanding of a say in the services provided.

IMPLICATIONS FOR THE CARING RELATION IN NURSING

Context

The social construction of the health care milieu as briefly outlined has a direct influence on the caring relation in nursing. The context as we have explored it above has a number of attributes. We can summarise the most significant of these in the following list:

- Nursing takes place mainly in the context of health care settings which remain dominated by a particular medical ethos and a medical model characterised by an objective, case-centred, disease-orientated approach founded on a rational–technical–scientific paradigm.
- The development of an internal market-orientated new managerialism is characterised by a similar rational–technical paradigm which also incorporates a health economics perspective. This emphasises measurable outcomes, performance indicators,

cost-effectiveness, efficiency, value for money and a rapid turn-over orientation.

- Both these influences are to an extent gender-specific in that they promote traditional male values of science and objectivity and devalue alternative ways of knowing and being. They are thus naturally in conflict with many nursing values which are by definition characteristic ways in which women know and are.

- In its quest for professional status there has been a tendency in nursing to espouse the objective–rational–scientific model as a means of advancing the profession. Where this trend is at its strongest nurses, who are mainly women, reject women's ways of intuitive, personal and ethical being and attempt to approach nursing care (often inappropriately) through perspectives which reject the subjective–humanistic–caring orientation.

- Previously the profession was characterised by those who adhered to a more servile role supportive to medicine and those who aspired to the latter more technical–rational role.

- The latter trends have led some to suggest that the occupation might be split, with nurses adopting more technical, highly skilled and supervisory roles while generic or basic caring functions would be carried out by less expensive support workers or generic carers.

- Nursing is now recognising its core value as centred in caring. Despite refutations of the approach by some who espouse the technical–rational–scientific model, a significant body of nursing literature emphasises the caring dimension as fundamental to nursing.

- The increasing emphasis on care in the community and the development of a primary-led service may have far-reaching implications. This may include significant shifts in power bases within the NHS, particularly as regards shifts away from hospital-based medicine. It may also have significant implications for GPs, community nurses and others who work in primary care.

- The major professional developments carried forward by the professional regulatory bodies and professional staff organisations have played a significant part in the continuing emancipation of nursing as a mature and assertive caring profession.

- The users of health services are as a whole becoming increasingly informed and educated, and more capable of demanding and utilising health services. The increase in utilisation of alternative and complementary therapies may indicate dissatisfaction with conventional health services and desires for greater control over health.

- The new UK Labour government may establish trends away from a valuing of market forces and individualism towards cooperation rather than competition and a more collective welfare ideology which incorporates more involvement and empowerment of health service users. Such developments would make further incursions on the power of the medical profession and new managerialism within the NHS.
- The consequence of the latter four trends may finally lead to a health as opposed to ill-health orientation within the NHS, with implications for the nature of nursing work and in particular the nature of community nurse–client relations.

The caring relation in community nursing

Caring in context

In the earlier sections of this chapter it was stated that the separation of nursing into two cultures detracted from a true sense of caring and the view was expressed that nursing must integrate both perspectives. That is, for true caring to exist in the nursing context there must be skill and competence, drawn to a significant extent from technical–rational science as an evidence base, *and* compassionate caring. In essence, it was argued, compassionate caring cannot exist without the former, as uninformed caring is in fact unethical and breaches that which was described as an ethic of care.

On the latter basis the nurse–patient relation becomes the space within which *skilled caring* is realised. But, as suggested above, this must be recognised as a relation which exists in a context. The context as it now exists is one in which the medical monopoly of power within the health service no longer exists to the extent it did previously and the traditional restrictive medical model of treatment is increasingly replaced by a broader caring orientation. The new managerialism also begins to lose its economics-driven cutting edge as both government and society demand a more responsive, welfare-orientated and caring service in which clients feel empowered and are involved at all stages in decision-making. The scientific dominance remains, and as an underpinning of evidence-based health care empirical science is an essential source of clinical effectiveness and professional competence. With the demand from society at large and from the political Left for a more compassionate service, the recognition of a broader knowledge and moral basis of care than that allowed by an *exclusively* narrow scientific orientation is recognised. Up until recently the dominant culture within nursing mirrored that within the health service and wider social context in terms of its technical, skills-orientated and scientific perspective. But there is within nursing a more extensive body of knowledge on the nature of compassionate and ethical caring than in any other professional group with the possible exception of the religious professions. Nursing is therefore in the strongest position not only to respond to the above demands, but to lead that response.

Health as the focus

We can illustrate the latter point by returning to our title and its emphasis on 'caring in the *health* context'. Our excursion through this title with its nurse, patient and health elements, when viewed in a socially constructed context, which in essence is the environment of care, is significant. Encapsulated here is the entirety of a nursing *metaparadigm*, a word which describes and defines the context, frame and core concepts of a phenomenon (in this case nursing). This was originally described by Fawcett (1984; 1995) as consisting of the interacting elements nursing, person, health and environment (see Figure 3.1).

Taking a different view, on the argument that a metaparadigm cannot include the phenomenon it describes, which in this case *is* nursing, Slevin (1995b) proposed a modification of the metaparadigm (see Figure 3.2).

The view here is that the metaparadigm is a conceptual frame which identifies the parameters of nursing work. Nursing cannot be

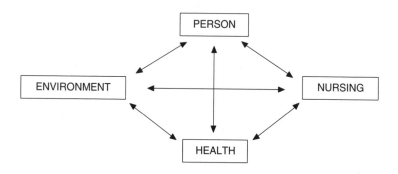

Figure 3.1   The nursing metaparadigm (Fawcett, 1995)

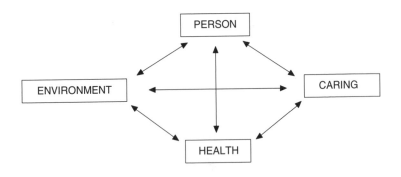

Figure 3.2 The nursing metaparadigm (Slevin, 1995b)

an element of the framework but is in effect described by that framework. Thus, Slevin (1995b) argues that the primary areas of concern to nursing and those which establish its parameters are person, environment, caring and health. The significant thing about both of the above postulations of the nursing metaparadigm, and indeed most others, is the recognition of *health* as a key concept (see Newman *et al.,* 1991; Parse, 1992, 1995; Kirby and Slevin, 1992).

The question begged here is what is meant by health. Just as we have argued that caring must be viewed in the wider context of health care and the forces which influence this, so too must we recognise that within the nursing metaparadigm and more specifically within the nursing relation, health as a concept must be contextualised. If the relation addresses health, it must do so on the basis of a shared understanding of the concept. It is for this reason that context or, to use a different expression, *environment* – both physical and social – is recognised both in the nursing metaparadigm *and* in the nurse–patient relation.

It must be understood that health, like so many other concepts in our rapidly changing health care system, is a notion which is in a constant state of flux. Traditionally, the notion of health was viewed simply, as the absence of ill health. Indeed, even recently, in a major survey of 9000 adults in England, Scotland and Wales, 30 per cent of respondents defined health in the latter way (Cox, 1987). This definition falls short of that adopted by the World Health Organisation (1948) at its inception, when health was defined as 'a state of complete physical, mental and social well-being and not merely the absence of disease and infirmity'. More recently it has become accepted that health is to a significant extent culturally determined and greatly influenced by individual interpretation. The interpretation of health by a young, vegetarian, jogging housewife in stockbroker-belt Surrey may differ greatly from that of an elderly male traveller living in a caravan on the rural outskirts of Glasgow.

Recognising the more complex conceptualisation of health in social and cultural contexts, the World Health Organisation (1984) more recently describes health in terms of:

> 'the extent to which an individual or group is able, on the one hand, to realise aspirations and satisfy needs and on the other hand, to change or cope with the environment. Health is therefore seen as a resource for everyday life, not an objective of living; it is a positive concept emphasising social and personal resources as well as physical capabilities.'

There are two significant aspects of this conceptualisation. The first is that health is embedded in social contexts and rests to a large extent on an individual's aspirations for quality of life. The second is that the capacity for change and willingness to make changes is fundamental to each person's evolving commitment to health. A recent study in the UK indicated that in their relations with health care professionals clients are generally satisfied with the quality of skilled intervention but feel they are insufficiently informed and involved in terms of diagnosis, treatment choices and care management (Baker *et al.,* 1997). This is also well-illustrated by Thorne (1993) in her study on negotiating health care in Canada. She found that patients were generally dissatisfied with the lack of information and the lack of a key person to coordinate their care and act as their advocate within the system. In the USA a major study of patients' experience of health care, the Picker/Commonwealth Program for Patient-Centered Care found similar patterns of dissatisfaction (Gerteis *et al.,* 1993). Across seven dimensions relevant to the promotion and maintenance of patient-centred care (respect for patients' values, preferences and expressed needs; coordination and integration of care; information, communication and education; physical comfort; emotional support and alleviation of fear and anxiety; involvement of family and friends; and transition and continuity) the researchers found that while some health facilities have a marked patient-centred focus and attempt to address the dimensions, many fail in this regard. It was further recognised by the researchers that:

'The nursing profession in particular contributes to every dimension of patient-centered care, working to enhance the personal aspects of caring and serving often as the personal link between patients and a seemingly impersonal institution.'

The indication from these various studies is that patients or clients require more than safe and competent management of their health or ill-health problems. They require other things, such as the seven dimensions identified by Gerteis *et al.* (1993), and they wish in particular to be informed, consulted and involved in their care management. This is entirely in line with the emerging conceptualisation of health as it is presented above. It emphasises in particular that health is intimately related to social norms, cultural values and personal choices. Notions of health cannot be imposed on individuals and changes in health can only be achieved through negotiation, empowerment and facilitation.

This is a realisation of major significance for the nurse–patient relation and caring. As these are placed in the health context, and health sets the parameters of nursing care as one of the main nursing metaparadigm components, caring must be viewed as involving partnership and negotiation. This orientation is of particular relevance in community nursing. In community nursing, much more so than any in any other branch of nursing, the nurse is thrust into the social context. This is a context of social and cultural influences. It is a context of family, friendship and community networks. And it is a context in which all those internal and external forces which map the social context of health care, as outlined above, interface with the patient or client and his or her community. The significant power of the community nurse–patient relation to influence health and well-being can not be overestimated. But this power can only fulfil its true potential if it is recognised that nurses and other health care workers can no longer impose definitions of health constructed in isolation from the social context of health and can no longer impose health care interventions without consultation and involvement. In all health care contexts, but particularly in the community nursing context, care can no longer be an imposition but becomes a negotiated order.

The framework for care

In the earlier sections of this chapter a case was made for the establishment of the nurse–patient relation on the basis of a coming together of two interlinked orientations, the integration of compassionate caring with technical skill and competence. In the latter section it is again noted that the orientation of nursing is health. But health is recognised as being socially and culturally embedded, and as involving personal choices. Improvements and changes in health can therefore only be achieved through partnership and negotiation. Within such an environment, care must by definition be established on a model which is essentially one of negotiated care. Taking this third orientation, a framework for caring in nursing may be presented as in Figure 3.3.

The nurse–patient relation: a model for nursing care

The model
Assuming that care can be based on the latter framework, there is then the need to consider the nature of the nurse–patient relationship which would be true to such a framework. The model proposed here is adapted from that proposed by Kirby and Slevin (1992) and described in Slevin (1995c). The approach has humanistic and philosophical influences, drawing on the work of nursing scholars such as Paterson and Zderad (1976), Watson (1985), Roach (1987) and Gadow (1989) and existential and hermeneutic philosophers, in particular Heidegger (1962), Sartre (1958), Buber (1958, 1988) and Gadamer (1975). But it also recognises the importance of evidence-based care, and the indivisibility of skill and competence from compassionate moral caring.

The orientation of the approach has already been touched upon in the Introduction to this chapter. The emphasis is upon an

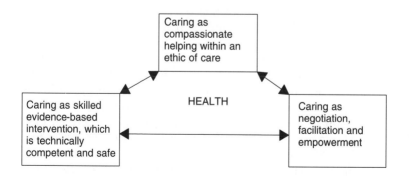

Figure 3.3   A framework for caring in nursing

authentic way of being with and for patients or clients in which *the elements of care* are enacted within *a caring relation*. The overall schema of the model is as presented in Figure 3.4.

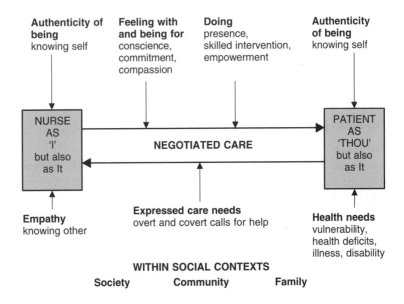

Figure 3.4   A relational model for care

The heart of the matter
At the centre of the relationship are the two people who are in relation. The model draws on Buber's (1958) work on human relating. Here Buber proposed that we may be in either an 'I–Thou' or an 'I–It' relation with the other. It may be argued that in the latter case the term 'regard' is more appropriate. We are in I–It regard to the other when, even if the other is a person, we regard this other as an object. We look to the person, we observe them, we experience that person as another. But even this experiencing is within ourselves, because we are sensing and perceiving *things* about the other–their eye colour, their responses to us, their perceived joy or pain. We are seeing a sum of connected parts; we are in fact *regarding* an 'it', or a 'he' or 'she'.

But in the I–Thou relation, we do not merely *regard,* we *relate* to the other as being to being. In I–Thou, unlike I–It, we are in true relation. We go out to the other with our whole being. There is no non-disclosure of a part of the self, so that what is presented to the other is a part which is limited to and delineated by a professional role. To connect in this latter fashion would be what as we noted earlier, Heidegger (1962) described as 'inauthentic being' and Sartre (1958) described as an act of 'bad faith.' This would also limit and withhold the therapeutic and healing capacity of the whole person, so succinctly described by Emmett (1966) and by Downie (1989) in his description of role versus person in the professional relationship. Furthermore, we go out to the other who is *also* a whole person, not simply as a medical condition or health care problem, or one whose only legitimate call upon us is through the window of a restricted sick role in which only certain issues may be addressed and others are excluded. Individuals so delimited become objects and so are called 'it.' But the whole person with whom in our fullest sense we are in communion is 'thou.'

This does not mean that by definition I–It is negative and I–Thou is positive. Buber (1988) states that we must always withdraw for a while, to observe, to reflect, to know and understand the other so that we can again move back into moments of being with the other. Of this rhythmic movement of relation, Kirby and Slevin (1995) have stated:

'It is of course necessary to move from the I–Thou to the I–It position to enable an objective appraisal of the patient's condition, and the use of skilled technical intervention. But it is also necessary to go back in again, to respond to the patient in the I–Thou mode, as whole person to whole person, and to journey with him through the "real presence" and meaning of his illness. There can be no true excellence in nursing which deals only in parts and ignores the patient as a whole self, who is more and different to the sum of these parts. True excellence in nursing can be viewed as this capacity for movement between I–Thou and I–It, of coming in to *be* and going out to *see*, as nursing proceeds with a majestic rhythm.'

The proposal for a nurse–patient relation which is person-*with*-person in this way as opposed to role-*to*-role is a fundamental shift. It may be argued that there is no room for such relations in a highly technical and objectivised health service. Indeed some may even question the professional propriety of such relations. However, the research cited earlier, by Baker *et al.* (1997) Thorne (1993) and Gerteis *et al.* (1993) suggests that patients or clients often do want

71

more from professionals than technical skill and being done *to* without being told *why* and participating *in*. And, as also suggested above, the trends within our health care systems are towards more client choice and more involvement. This brings to the heart of the relation a further property. That is, that it is a relation within a wider social and cultural context, involving people in relation who have freedom of choice. In such contexts caring must always take place through negotiation. Such negotiation contains within it the liberation and empowerment of clients and their full participation in the caring process.

The elements of care

The elements of care presented in the model illustrated in Figure 3.4 which inform and enliven the relation are not discrete and separate elements. They present with simultaneity and integrity a way of coming to and being in the nursing relation. There is, however, a sense of journeying to and through the relation. This first involves a process of arriving at a sense of authenticity of being as a caring person, which is a prerequisite for journeying out to the other and then engaging with that other in a relation which is in its essence therapeutic and healing. But in its unfolding the relation is multi-dimensional and multidirectional. It unfolds as nurse goes out to meet patient and patient goes out to meet nurse, as the almost rhythmical movement of each between the I–Thou and I–It allows for a negotiated process of caring. Within this relation the patient's requirements for skilled intervention, empowerment and choice, as well as compassionate presence and support, are realised in the mutual journey of the nurse–patient through health, illness, disability or perhaps even to death. The elements contribute as follows.

- *Authenticity of being* This authenticity requires that the nurse countenances and knows herself. If she is not fully conscious of her own 'self', but hides behinds a role, she will not have the capacity to relate with the other as a person, or to get a true sense of his being in the world.. She in fact would have made a decision not to enter the world of intentional caring as a person. This capacity to intentionally view oneself as a being in the world and to similarly confront the patient as a person in the fullest sense in all that they are, as opposed to a case or a type, presents the nurse with choices and possibilities. From this she can confront her own essence and limitations, and her capacity for care. From this she can make a determination to journey out as a caring person to others who are care-needing persons.

- *Empathy* The position of authenticity and intentional concern for self and other relates closely to the condition of empathy, which involves understanding the patient from his own subjective, lived experience. This involves going beyond an observation or knowing of the patient's condition in objective terms. As Solomon (1991) states:

> 'If I want to know what you're thinking right now, all I have to do is care more about what you're thinking than what I'm thinking . . . As soon as I care more about what you're thinking than what I'm thinking I will give up my thoughts and I will absorb yours, and I will understand you.'

- *Conscience* This element is more than moral reasoning or applied ethics. It is the attitude of being moral, of the will to help or do good as a way of being. In this sense it is not something which co-exists with care, but is a fundamental aspect of care. This is why Noddings (1984) pinpoints care in itself as being an ethical position, and why she argues for an ethic of care. In this sense, if we view ethics as being to do with what is right and good or what is bad and wrong, the presence of true caring can be the one overriding force. Because, if we really care, we can not intentionally do bad or wrong.
- *Commitment* This is more than meeting the other's needs through a sense of duty or obligation. It is a total will to help because not only does one want to help but it is the fundamental motive within the relation. It is a will to help because, quite literally, our total commitment to care allows us no other course.
- *Compassion* In the framework for care presented, compassionate caring was one of the triadic foundations. This is not merely a feeling of concern for the other but a valuing of that other, a shared sense of being with and for them, and a sense of humility and honour in being given the opportunity to help them. It requires commitment and it is a going out to the other in a sense of being totally for and with that other, without regard to self. Of this, Nouwen *et al.* (1982) stated that:

> 'Compassion asks us to go where it hurts, to enter into places of pain, to share in brokenness, fear, confusion and anguish. Compassion challenges us to cry out with those in misery,

mourn with those who are lonely, to weep with those in tears
... Compassion means full immersion in the condition of
being human.'

Many will of course argue that this is a dangerous calling, that
the nurse cannot indulge in this degree of personal contact and
that to do so leads to personal pain and destruction. Others will
argue that the opposite is true, that if we do not enter into the
patient's pain we become incomplete and alienated as persons.
They will argue that being open to the goodness of compassion is
not a weakness but the response to a calling, that it is this which
more than all else fulfils that social contract we referred to earlier,
whereby those we serve call to us as their angels of mercy, not
merely as their impersonal service providers. It can be argued
further that, rather than damaging us, this immersion in compassion is enlivening and fulfilling. It is seen here as the beauty and
specialness of nursing which complements the technical and
scientific. In the opening pages of Victor Hugo's (1862/1982)
existential novel *Les Misérables*, Monseigneur Myriel reflects on
what brings the light of goodness to the world and on how it is
variously described as truth, wisdom, providence, and so on. He
ends, with this most powerful of statements: 'but Solomon names
thee Compassion, which is the most beautiful of all thy names'. It
can be seen that compassion must be at the very heart of nursing,
that it is in one sense its source of power.

- *Presence* From the authenticity of being and the growing
  empathy for the other, and through conscience, commitment
  and compassion, we finally, in each caring moment, come into
  the presence of the other. All these are prerequisites for 'presence'. But in a sense they are also contained within it. We cannot
  be a presence to the other if we have not confronted our own self
  and come here prepared to meet the full self of the other. To come
  here as a role is at best to confront in a casual or limited way, so
  often the case when this nurse arrives with that patient, conducts
  a technical procedure, and leaves, sometimes with never a word
  spoken. In its true sense, presence is not simply being there, being
  an object in time and space, irrespective of our close proximity to
  the other. It carries with it a sense of being available to or at the
  disposal of the other. Its test is in the knowing of that other that
  you are truly *with* him or her, that you are there to expend
  yourself in their cause. Gabriel Marcel (1956/1991) speaks of this
  as follows:

'Presence is something which reveals itself in a look, a smile, an intonation or a handshake . . . It will perhaps make it clearer if I say that the person who is at my disposal is one who is capable of being with me with the whole of himself when I am in need; while the one who is not at my disposal seems merely to offer me a temporary loan raised on his resources. For the one I am a presence; for the other I am an object. Presence involves a reciprocity which is excluded from any relation of subject to object or of subject to subject–object.'

But for *presence* to exist, the patient must recognise it, he must be shown it, he must in fact experience your presence in him. Because presence is always from one to the other, it exists in the relation. Each must be present to the other. When we treat the patient or client as a case, as what Marcel terms a subject–object, that person is immediately cast into alienation, into an exclusion from being fully human. There is a need, most often shown within the acts of relation but sometimes also even needed to be said, to let this person know that you come with intentionality, with empathic understanding or an openness to it, with conscience, commitment and compassion. The other needs to know this, to quite literally know that you are there for him or her.

- *Skilled intervention* To the relation and the caring moments within it, the nurse brings gifts. Her presence alone is such a gift. But there are also those other gifts we have already mentioned. The greatest gift of all to those who suffer is perhaps the gift of a caring, committed and compassionate self, presented in listening, speech, gaze, touch, holding, and sometimes in mere silent presence. But we must always remember that nursing is caring in the health context. That which we bring, with commitment and compassion, is the competence and expertise to enhance health, support treatment, ease suffering, assist in a return to independence, perhaps even prepare for death. Behind all this is knowledge and skills of an evidence-based practice, the capacity to apply the technology and therapies of health care with proficiency and safety. As this is what is expected of us, as this is what we bring to the presence, all these other gifts of self, empathy, conscience, commitment, compassion would be, in its absence, a betrayal.

- *Empowerment* So, thus we come, into the presence, bearing gifts. In our old dispensations, of course, these gifts were bestowed sometimes as an offering, sometimes with mere askance. In the traditional sick role (Parsons, 1966) the patient dared not even ask, but swallowed the potion. No question was begged of the nature of the gifts, of whether the 'patient' wanted them, even of whether they served for this or that person a useful purpose. Those who questioned, and thus threatened the very fabric and social order of the imposed health system, were labelled bad or unpopular patients and medico-social pressures were immediately brought to bear (Stockwell, 1972). But, as we have seen in our scanning of the developing context of health care, this is now all changing. There is a call now from society for greater involvement in health care. The call within the proposed model of *caring-as-relating* presented here, which speaks of a relation between persons, must acknowledge the full personhood of the client as a thinking, feeling and choosing individual.

This recognition must commence with a recognition of the potential of the individual. Of this, Buber (1988), in his dialogue with Carl Rogers, has stated:

'Confirming means first of all, accepting the whole potential of the other . . . I can recognise in him, know in him, more or less the person he has been. And now I not only accept the other as he is, but I confirm him, in myself, and then in him, in relation to this potentiality that is meant by him, and it can now be developed, it can evolve, it can answer the reality of life.'

In recognising this potential there is a need to proceed through dialogue, or what is identified in the model as negotiated care, to facilitate the patient or client in arriving at his or her free choices in determining his or her progression through health or disease. Therefore, while the nurse comes bearing gifts, the greatest gift of all may be the freedom of the patient, in dialogue with the nurse, to make life choices. It is this liberation of the patient as a negotiating partner in determining his journey through health, disease, disability or death which we describe as empowerment. When this happens, there are two knowing carers in the relation – both nurse and patient. We must recognise also that, in the community nursing context, the patient or client has family, friendship and/or community ties. Indeed, the family, friendship group or community are often in effect 'the client'. In such circumstances the nurse's key skill may not be in the use of sophisticated technology but in her capacity to free up the wisdom and skills within the client and in so doing release that person's healing potential in the caring process.

This is perhaps most practically illustrated in Parse's (1992, 1995) theory of human becoming. This theoretical viewpoint is perhaps the most relevant of all nursing theories to the community nursing context. It finds its origins in studies into the health as opposed to ill health of persons and families. The theory draws on existential processes which address health as a lived experience within cultural, family and community contexts. It is existential in that it requires an intentional confronting and acceptance of the individual's circumstances and the possibilities within these for both nurse and patient. Within the theory the person is viewed as a free agent, whose search for meaning and arrival at health choices is facilitated but not controlled by the nurse or influenced by her in any way. The model presented in Figure 3.4 diverges from the Parse theory in that the nurse enters the relation as an 'expert', to negotiate and agree though not control the health choices of the patient or client.

SUMMARY AND CONCLUSION

In this chapter an attempt has been made to describe the nurse–patient relation as caring in the health context. It was noted that the relation has evolved within the context of health care services and agencies which influence and to an extent have conditioned the relation. The relevance of the society-wide existence of 'The Two Cultures', one established on an objective–rational–technical–scientific philosophy and the other on a subjective–humanistic philosophy, was noted. It was suggested that the former, by being the dominant philosophy within the medical profession which in turn dominated the health services, promoted a restricted relational role. This dominance and the subsequent rise of a new managerialism and market orientation within the health services served to further restrict the development of nursing to a technical role, particularly as in a series of health service reforms the position of nursing in management was eroded and the presence of nursing leadership became increasingly weakened. The outcome was a male-dominated, rational–technical philosophy which, while it may have given lip service to caring as a human process, yet devalued all that was not measurable and all that could not be cost–outcome-linked. Indeed, devaluing of human caring within the services may reflect the attitudes of some who argue for more technical and supervisory roles for nurses while the basic human caring needs would be met by other less qualified staff.

The chapter continued by suggesting that there is now evidence of a shift in thinking. With the change from Conservative to Labour government, evidence points to shifts away from a competitive market economy and medical and managerial dominance in health towards a more cooperative and communal, welfare-orientated service characterised by partnerships and collaboration between professionals, managers and clients or patients. The growing evidence of dissatisfaction with a service viewed as impersonal and uninformative and the turning of many to alternative therapies within which desires for freedom and choice can be met, similarly points to a more fundamental shift within society as a whole. It is suggested that the demand for a more personalised and caring service, which is more responsive to client needs and desire for empowered decision-making, lays the ground for an emancipation of nursing as a caring profession.

As a response to these developments, a framework for care which encompasses a triad of caring as skilled intervention, caring as compassion and caring as negotiation of health choices was identified. On this basis a model for a caring relationship was proposed. This, while relevant in all nursing contexts, is particularly relevant to community nursing, which in a future primary-led service will be at the cutting edge of health care provision.

In this chapter the social construction of our health services and wider social milieu was contemplated. There was an indication in all of this that old dispensations are being cast aside, that from within society and at least from some within our own profession there is a new call for a more personalised and compassionate approach. This is not an alternative to science and technology but combines with these to enhance evidence-based and informed caring. Community nurses, whose work thrusts them into the very heart of the web of social relations and social problems, must recognise this otherness that is now afoot. They must respond to the opportunity to develop nurse–patient relations which meet the individual's and the community's needs for expertise, compassion and empowerment in the total caring process.

Note: The contributor, editor and publishers are grateful to Stanley Thornes Publishers for permission to reproduce material in this chapter from *Theory and Practice of Nursing*, Batsford and Slevin, 1995.

References

Baker, M., Fardell, J. and Jones, B. (1997) *Disability and Rehabilitation–Survey of Education Needs of Health and Social Services Professionals*. London: Disability and Rehabilitation Open Learning Project.

Baker, M. E. (1996). Challenging ignorance. In M. Baker and S. Kirk (eds), *Research and Development for the NHS – Evidence, Evaluation and Effectiveness*. Oxford: Radcliffe Medical Press.

Barker, P. J., Reynolds, W. and Ward, T. (1995) The proper focus of nursing: a critique of the 'caring' ideology. *International Journal of Nursing Studies*, 12(4), pp. 386–97.

Beauchamp, T. L. (1994) The 'four-principles approach'. In R. Gillon (ed.), *Principles of Health Care Ethics*. Chichester: John Wiley & Sons.

Beauchamp, T. L. and Childress, J. F. (1979) *Principles of Biomedical Ethics*. New York: Oxford University Press.

Benner, P. (1984). *From Novice to Expert: Excellence and Power in Clinical Practice*. Menlo Park: Addison-Wesley.

Bevis, E. O. (ed.) (1981) *Caring: A Life Force*. Thorofare, NJ: Charles B. Stack.

Buber, M. (1958) *I and Thou*. Edinburgh: T. & T. Clark.

Buber, M. (1988) *The Knowledge of Man*. Atlantic Highlands, NJ: Humanities Press.

Caines, E. (1993) *Amputation is Crucial to the Nation's Health*. The Guardian, May 11 1993. Manchester, UK.

Carper, B. A. (1978) Fundamental patterns of knowing in nursing. *Advances in Nursing Science*, 1, pp. 13–23.

Carper, B. A. (1979) The ethics of caring. *Advances in Nursing Science*, 1(3), pp. 11–19.

Clark, J. (1997) Virginia Henderson memorial lecture. Unpublished keynote address. International Congress of Nurses, 21st Quadrennial Congress, Vancouver.

Collins Pub. Co. (1978) *Collins Concise Dictionary of the English Language*. Glasgow: Collins.

Cox, B. D. (1987) *The Health and Lifestyle Survey: Preliminary Report*. London: Health Promotion Research Trust.

Davies, C. (1995) *Gender and the Professional Predicament in Nursing*. Buckingham: Open University Press.

Department of Health (1992) *The Health of the Nation*. London: HMSO.

Department of Health (1997) *The New NHS – Modern, Dependable*. London; Department of Health.

Department of Health (1998) *A First Class Service: Quality in the New NHS*. London: Department of Health.

Department of Health and Social Services (NI) (1998) *Fit for the Future*. Belfast: Department of Health and Social Services.

Downie, R. S. (1989) *Roles and Values*. London: Methuen.

Dreyfus, H. L., Dreyfus, S. E. and Athanasiou, T. (1986) *Mind over Machine: The Power of Human Intuition and Expertise in the Era of the Computer*. New York: Free Press.

Emmett, D. (1966) *Rules, Roles and Relations*. New York: Macmillan.

Fawcett, J. (1984) The metaparadigm of nursing. *Image*, 16, pp. 84–7.

Fawcett, J. (1995) *Analysis and Evaluation of Conceptual Models of Nursing 3rd Edn*. Philadelphia, PA.: F. A. Davis.

Fox, M. (1990) *A Spirituality Named Compassion – and the Healing of the Global Village, Humpty Dumpty and Us*. San Francisco: Harper.

Gadamer, H. G. (1975) *Truth and Method* 2nd rev. edn., trans. J. Weinsheimer and D. G. Marshall. London: Sheed & Ward.

Gadow, S. (1989) The advocacy covenant: care as clinical subjectivity. In J. S. Stevenson and T. Tripp-Reimer (eds), *Knowledge about Care and Caring: State of the Art and Future Developments*. Mo.: American Academy of Nursing.

Gadow, S. (1996) Narrative and exploration: towards a poetics of knowledge in nursing. *Nursing Inquiry*, 2(4), pp. 1–4.

Gadow, S. (1996) Ethical narratives in practice. *Nursing Science Quarterly*, 9(1), pp. 8–9.

Gerteis, M., Edgman-Levitan, S., Daley, J. and Delbanco, T. (1993) *Through the Patient's Eyes*. San Francisco: Jossey-Bass..

Gillon, R. (1994) *Principles of Health Care Ethics*. Chichester: John Wiley & Sons.

Gilligan, C. (1982) *In a Different Voice*. Cambridge, Mass.: Harvard University Press.

Harrison, S. and Pollitt, C. (1994) *Controlling the Professionals*. Buckingham: Open University Press.

Heidegger, M. (1962) *Being and Time*. London: SCM Press.

Hugo, V. (1982/1862) *Les Misérables*. Harmondsworth: Penguin Books.

Illich, I. (1976) *Medical Nemesis: The Expropriation of Health*. New York: Pantheon.

Kikuchi, J. F. (1992) Nursing questions that science cannot answer. In J. F. Kikuchi and H. Simmons (eds), *Philosophic Inquiry in Nursing*. Newbury Park: Sage Publications.

Kirby, C. (1995) The world of nursing. In L. Basford and O. Slevin (eds), *Theory and Practice of Nursing: an Integrated Approach to Patient Care*. Edinburgh: Campion Press.

Kirby, C. and Slevin, O. (1992) A new curriculum for care. In O. Slevin and M. Buckenham (Eds.), *Project 2000: The Teachers Speak*. Edinburgh: Campion Press.

Kirby, C. and Slevin, O. (1995a) Commitment to care. In L. Basford and O. Slevin (eds), *Theory and Practice of Nursing: An Integrated Approach to Patient Care*. Edinburgh: Campion Press.

Kirby, C. and Slevin, O. (1995b) *Ethics*. In L. Basford and O. Slevin (eds) *Theory and Practice of Nursing: an Integrated Approach to Patient Care*. Edinburgh: Campion Press.

Klein, R. (1989) *The Politics of the NHS*. London: Longman.

Klein, R. (1995) *The New Politics of the NHS*. London: Longman.

Marcel, G. (1991/1956) *The Philosophy of Existentialism*. Secaucus, NJ: Citadel Press.

Newman, M. A., Sime, A. M. and Corcoran-Perry, A. S. (1991) The focus of the discipline of nursing. *Advances in Nursing Science*, 14(1), pp. 1–6.

Noddings, N. (1984) *Caring, a Feminine Approach to Ethics and Moral Education*. London: University of California Press.

Nouwen, H. J., McNeill, D. P. and Morrison, D. A. (1982) *Compassion*. London: Darton, Longman & Todd.

Parse, R. R. (1992) Human becoming: Parse's theory of nursing. *Nursing Science Quarterly, 5*(1), pp. 35–42.

Parse, R. R. (1995) The human becoming theory. In R. R. Parse (ed.), *Illuminations – The Human Becoming Theory in Practice and Research*. New York: National League for Nursing.

Parsons, T. (1966) On becoming a patient. In J. R. Folta and E. S. Deck (eds), *A Sociological Framework for Patient Care*. New York: John Wiley & Sons.

Paterson, J. G. and Zderad, L. T. (1976) *Humanistic Nursing*. New York: Wiley.

Peplau, H. (1952) *Interpersonal Relations in Nursing*. New York: Pitman.

Peplau, H. (1969) Professional closeness. *Nursing Forum*, 8, (4) pp. 342–59.

Polanyi, M. (1958) *Personal Knowledge: Towards a Post Critical Philosophy*. London: Routledge & Kegan Paul.

Polanyi, M. (1966) *The Tacit Dimension*. New York: Doubleday.

Powell, D. (1982) *Learning to Relate*. London: Royal College of Nursing.

Roach, M. S. (1987) *The Human Act of Caring*. Ottowa: Canadian Hospital Association.

Roach, M. S. (1991) The call to consciousness: compassion in today's health world. In D. A. Gaut and M. M. Leininger (eds), *Caring: The Compassionate Healer*. New York: National League for Nursing.

Sartre, J. P. (1958) *Being and Nothingness*. London: Methuen.

Schulman, S. (1958) Basic functional roles in nursing: mother surrogate and healer. In E. G. Jaco (ed.), *Patients, Physicians and Illness*. New York: Free Press.

Shulman, S. (1972) Mother surrogate–after a decade. In E. G. Jaco (ed.), *Patients, Physicians and Illness*, 2nd edn. London: Collier-Macmillan.

Slevin, O. (1995a) Knowledge and theory. In L. Basford and O. Slevin (eds), *Theory and Practice of Nursing: An Integrated Approach to Patient Care*. Edinburgh: Campion Press.

Slevin, O. (1995b) Theories and models. In L. Basford and O. Slevin (eds), *Theory and Practice of Nursing*. Edinburgh: Campion Press.

Slevin, O. (1995c) European nursing models. In L. Basford and O. Slevin (eds), *Theory and Practice of Nursing: An Integrated Approach to Patient Care*. Edinburgh: Campion Press.

Snow, C. P. (1959) *The Two Cultures and the Scientific Revolution*. Cambridge: Cambridge University Press.

Solomon, P. (1991) Paul Solomon speaks on spiritual roots and the journey to wholeness. *Human Potential Magazine*, 16(3), pp. 28–32.

Stacey, M. (1988) *The Sociology of Health and Healing*. London: Routledge.

Stockwell, F. (1972) *The Unpopular Patient*. London: Royal College of Nursing.

Szasz, T. (1962) *The Myth of Mental Illness*. London: Paladin.

Taylor, B. J. (1994) *Being Human: Ordinariness in Nursing*. Edinburgh: Churchill Livingstone.

Thorne, S (1993) *Negotiating Health Care*. Newbury Park: Sage.

Watson, J. (1985) *Nursing: Human Science and Human Care*. Norwalk, Conn.: Appleton-Century-Croft.

Watson, J. (1988) New dimensions of human caring theory. *Nursing Science Quarterly*, 1, pp. 175–81.

Watson, J (1990) Caring knowledge and informed moral passion. *Nursing Science Quarterly*, 13(1), pp. 15–24.

Watson, J. (1992) Window on theory of human caring. In M. O'Toole (ed.), *Miller-Keane Encyclopedia & Dictionary of Medicine, Nursing and Allied Health,* 5th edn. Philadelphia, PA.: W. B. Saunders.

Wilhelm, R. (1987) *The Pocket I Ching,* trans. C. F. Baynes. New York: Arkana.

World Health Organisation (1948) *Preamble of the Constitution of the WHO.* Geneva: WHO.

World Health Organisation (1984) *Report of the Working Group on Concepts and Principles of Health Promotion.* Copenhagen: WHO.

Wolff-Salin, M. (1989) *No Other Light: Points of Convergence in Psychology and Spirituality.* New York: Crossroads.

Zola, I. K. (1972) Medicine as an institution of social control: the medicalisation of society. *Sociological Review,* 20(4), pp. 487–504.

CHAPTER FOUR

Barriers to Communication

David Dickson

'We are all islands, shouting lies to one another across oceans of misunderstanding.'
(George Eliot)

INTRODUCTION

Communication is, without doubt, the great forte of *Homo sapiens*. As a species we are unrivalled in the sophistication of the system that we use to engage with others. By means of language we can discuss happenings at this point in time on the other side of the planet; we can speculate about things that might happen at some distant point in the future; we can debate events that took place in the dim and distant past; we can exercise our imagination over things that might never happen. No other species has the communicative wherewithal to allow members to do these things. Their communications are very much about the concrete reality of the here and now (Pinker, 1994).

That said, and as pointed out somewhat extremely in the above quotation by George Eliot, communicating is not necessarily something that we always do particularly well. At times it does seem that the process is wracked by uncertainty, confusion, indecision and doubt; that we fail to make ourselves known as we had intended; that others miss some seemingly simple point that we have put, refuse to concur with our reading of the situation, inexplicably do quite the opposite to what we thought had been agreed, take offence at our ostensibly 'innocent' comments, or maybe find it difficult to enter into a meaningful relationship with us. Perhaps surprisingly it is only quite recently that scholars of communication have focused, in a concerted fashion, on the problematic nature of communication and given it recognition as a topic worthy of study in its own right (Cupach and Spitzberg, 1994; Mortensen, 1997). Traditionally, the emphasis has been placed upon how the system works, rather than on its failures and imperfections.

Health care delivery is one area of application which depends upon communication working well between health worker and patient, health worker and family or carers, and amongst health workers themselves (Davis and Fallowfield, 1991). Unfortunately it would seem that high standards of practice do not always obtain. Pettegrew (1982, p. 1) proffered that perhaps it is the very fact that communication plays such a pervasive role in health care that has sadly led, all too often, to 'neglect and complacency by those who must rely on it so routinely'. This chapter will explore the barriers that from time to time stand in the way of successful communication. In doing so, some comment will be made about the phenomenon and a model of the process presented. Sources of interactive difficulty will be located within this conceptual framework. The role of communication in health care delivery will be outlined and some of the respects in which it seems to fail the recipient of the service illuminated. These areas of concern give clues to the actual barriers that can get in the way of effective communication that is appropriately open, direct, honest, comfortable and respectful. Such barriers are of different types and operate in contrasting ways, at various levels. They include the more obvious difficulties posed by bodily disability and environmental distractions, as well as those that can be loosely characterised as semantic, perceptual, emotional, relational, demographic, dispositional, organisational and cultural.

THE IMPORTANCE OF EFFECTIVE COMMUNICATION FOR QUALITY HEALTH CARE DELIVERY

The establishment of facilitative levels of communication enabling meaningful and trusting relationships with patients to be developed is now widely accepted as being at the heart of effective patient management and care. As put by Ruben (1990, p. 51), 'The relationship between human communication and health care is a very fundamental one.' There is now considerable research evidence linking health worker–patient communication with a range of patient outcome measures. While any attempt at a comprehensive review is well beyond the scope of this chapter, these measures can be categorised as psychological, behavioural and physical/clinical. As such, patients who enjoy good quality communication tend to be more satisfied with the care received, exercise greater adherence to agreed/recommended treatment regimens and courses of action, and seem to make more rapid recoveries with fewer complications. (See reviews by Ley, 1988; Kaplan *et al.*, 1989; Kenny, 1995; Ong *et al.*, 1995; Stewart, 1995; Dickson *et al.*, 1997.) In concluding her review, Stewart (1995, p. 1429) stated that:

> 'The studies reviewed . . . suggest that effective communication exerts a positive influence not only on the emotional health of the patient but also on symptom resolution, functional and physiological status and pain control.'

It would therefore be reasonable to assume that health professionals manifest particularly high levels of interpersonal skill. The facts unfortunately often fail to bear this out. Indeed this aspect of care has consistently been criticised by recipients of health services (Meredith, 1993). In the report *What Seems to be the Matter* (Audit Commission, 1993) into communication with hospitalised patients, the conclusion was reached (p. 1) that:

> 'As health care processes and organisations become increasingly more complex, so the need to communicate with patients clearly about the clinical and non-clinical aspects of their care grows. But provision has not kept up with the growing need, and lack of information and problems with health professionals usually come at the top of the patients' concerns.'

Similar criticisms extend to the community, although they seem to be less prevalent in that setting. A fairly consistent criticism of the community psychiatric nurse by both clients and family carers, nevertheless, is that not enough information is provided about such matters as the client's condition, medication and available community services (Munton, 1990; Allen, 1993).

The Health Services Commissioner's Annual Report has consistently identified poor or inadequate communication between patient and health professional as the source of many of the grievances dealt with. The Annual Report for 1994–95, for example, places this category of complaint joint highest of the 15 categories established (HMSO, 1995). When considered by professional grouping, nursing, midwifery and health visiting, taken together, recorded the second highest number of communication grievances upheld, of the eight service groups mentioned. Overall complaints to do with poor communication showed a slight rise from the previous year. The Health Services Commissioner's conclusion was that :

'A failure in communication can have serious and far reaching effects . . . I find it particularly hard to comprehend failure by members of the "caring professions" to communicate adequately with patients, especially those who are terminally ill.'
(HMSO, 1995, pp. 8–9)

This decidedly depressing picture is made worse by those who have focused directly upon the interpersonal competence of health professionals. The interpersonal skills of students who had just finished medical school were found to be disappointing in a study carried out by Sloan *et al.* (1994). Even experienced hospital doctors have been accused of showing a lack of interest in patients and failing to acknowledge their needs. As a consequence, psychosocial dimensions of cases were largely neglected (Maguire, 1981). Nurses whose conversations with patients have been studied have fared little better. MacLeod Clark (1985) summarised the findings by saying that, 'The overall picture was one of tactics that discourage communication rather than skills that encourage it' (p. 16). Furthermore, it seems that some nurses at least may be aware of a lack of skill in some of the more challengingly interpersonal aspects of their work (Noble, 1991; Greenwood, 1993).

Clearly the path of communication between carer and patient would seem to be decidedly barrier-strewn. In order to begin to appreciate their origins and where they cause obstruction, we need to take a closer look at the nature of the communicative process.

THE NATURE OF COMMUNICATION

Communication is at one and the same time commonplace yet mysterious, uncomplicated but forever eluding our best efforts at comprehension. Approached at the level of interpersonal activity, in 'the doing of it' as it were, it is ubiquitous and characteristically accomplished in a largely effortless, indeed essentially 'mindless' way. Langer *et al.* (1978) distinguished between mindful activity where 'people attend to their world and derive behavioural strategies based upon current incoming information' and 'mindlessness' where 'new information is not actually being processed. Instead prior scripts, written when similar information was once new, are stereotypically reenacted' (p. 636). We can probably think of occasions when we are acutely mindful, of 'thinking on our feet', as we try to formulate some sensible strategy for handling an awkward, threatening or unaccustomed situation. But these occasions contrast sharply with more familiar encounters, for example, engaged in relaxed and easy conversation with friends, when we have little awareness of what we are doing as we are doing it. The point is, communicating is something that is, for the most part, effected simply and straighforwardly. This does not presuppose, though, as we shall see in this chapter, that it is therefore done with unerring success. Perhaps it is this very 'mindless' quality that on those occasions makes it frequently fraught and periodically problematic.

It is at the level of contemplation rather than action, when we pause for a moment to step back from the activity to consider just what it is that we have managed to do in communicating with another, that the awsomeness of the accomplishment hits home. But when we try to fathom just how we do what we do, communication characteristically slips like a spectre behind a veil of mystery, always just beyond the grasp of our ability to fully view or completely comprehend it. As put by Shulman (1992, p. 20):

'When one considers how complicated even the most simple communications are, the number of points in the process when meanings can be distorted, it is a wonder that any communication is ever completed'.

Through communication, we propose and have affirmed or rejected definitions of ourselves and others, create social situations, negotiate relationships, develop intimacy, and ultimately construct some sort of meaningful interpretation of the world and our place in it (Goffman, 1959; Satir, 1976; Myers and Myers, 1985). But even if we strip away the layers of complexity to expose an elemental act of communication (for example, the sharing of a limited piece of factual information) and account for it in terms of one of the most basic message transmission models of the process, the achievement is still quite awe-inspiring. At the initial stage of encoding the message, words have to be selected to best represent what we have in mind. The fact that we can probably never quite make complete representation of this mental content has to be acknowledged. As put by Scharfstein (1993, p. 13):

'we are internally so complex and personal an environment for the creation of thoughts that the internal "attitudes" and "positions" cannot be stated quickly and cannot be fully stated at all.'

For the process to work though, those 'words' must not only meaningfully represent our understanding, but must also be assumed to be capable of being interpreted in a corresponding way by the other. We must therefore entertain presumptions about the other person's assumptions. In telling the patient, 'Take the oval tablet for "your water", and the round one for your pain', there is an obvious presupposition that the patient can recognise a tablet and differentiate between those that are round and those that are oval. More interestingly, there is a further implicit belief that the patient will appreciate that while both are 'for' his or her complaints, the one will act to *increase* 'water', the other *reduce* pain. Inference and implication are endemic in communication. There must always be a tacit recognition on the part of the speaker that more will be understood than is said; that the listener will realise that more was meant than was spoken (Hargie *et al.*, 1994).

Having decided how best to put thoughts into words with the greatest chance, once received, of reconstituting the original thoughts in the mind of the other, as it were, these 'words' (which at this stage are themselves mentalistic) must be formulated into physical symbols that can be transmitted. Additionally, to have the impact intended, they have to be said in a particular way, perhaps with a certain tone of voice, volume, speed, and so on. All this depends upon a vocal apparatus capable of effecting subtle perturbations in air pressure. Assuming that there is no external interference to mask or distort these, and that they ultimately cause vibrations on the tympanic membrane of the receiver, these minuscule movements, still in the form of physical energy, have to be relayed to the cochlea, to be converted into neural pulses to be further relayed to the relevant parts of the brain, passing through levels of sensory and perceptual filtration on the way.

But this is the simple bit. As we shall see, meanings are not in words, but in people, shaped by the unique life experiences of each. It is in attaching meaning to what is heard to constitute some reasonably accurate representation of the mental state of the sender, and successfully receive the message, that the near miraculous quality of what has taken place in the communicative act reveals itself. Small wonder that our best efforts to get our message across frequently result in only limited success. Summing up the situation, Mortensen (1997, p. 4) suggests that:

'Because we do not know all the complexities and complications that make it possible to engage in human communication in the first place, we cannot pretend to be able to understand other people completely – without flaw, error, mistake, or miscalculation. No personal idiom is infallible. There are no perfect translations, or flawless interpreters, of the human code.'

THE MULTIDIMENSIONALITY OF COMMUNICATION

Let us remind ourselves that the above analysis was based upon an example of one of the most simple forms of communication, relaying a piece of factual information from one person to another, and drew upon a very basic model of the process. But communication is inescapably multidimensional (Burgoon *et al.*, 1994). We communicate not only verbally but non-verbally and to a range of ends of which sharing substantive information is only one. There is another, although less conspicuous, side to the activity, involving such matters as identity projection together with relationship negotiation and how interactors define their association.

In the choice of topic for discussion (and topics avoided), particular words and forms of expression adopted, manicured accents, speed of speech and a whole dynamic of non-verbal behaviours and characteristics, including dress and appearance, interactors project social, personal and professional identities. Goffman (1959) suggested that, as social beings, we work at presenting a *face* – at what is sometimes called *self-presentation* or *impression management*. This has to do with publicly expressing one's self as a particular type of person. Some nurses in this way seem to nurture an habitually 'busy' image in an attempt, it has been suggested, to avoid communication with patients. Pollock (1987) reported that perceived busyness was one of the characteristics of the community psychiatric nurse that carers found less helpful.

Face is a statement of the positive value claimed for self. Goffman (1959) observed that people not only characteristically engage in self-focused facework but are careful not to invalidate the face being presented by those with whom they interact. In a seminal work, Brown and Levinson (1978) analysed how politeness operates as a strategy intended to reduce the likelihood of this eventuality. Illness, and the health care procedures and settings that embellish it, can pose particular risks to face for patients and constitute the foundation of some of the barriers to effective communication that we will consider later in the chapter.

Communication also serves relational ends in other ways by helping determine how participants define their association *vis-à-vis*, for instance, degree of affiliation, status relationship and the balance of power enjoyed. Status differences are often negotiated and maintained by subtle (and not so subtle) means. Power is also implicated. When people with relatively little social power, occupying inferior status positions, interact with those enjoying power over them, the former manifest their increased 'accessibility' by, among other things, being asked more questions, providing more self-disclosures, initiating fewer topics for discussion, being more hesitant in what they say, engaging in less eye contact while speaking, using politer forms of address, and being more likely to be touched than touching (Berger, 1995; Argyle, 1988). Sets of expectations are constructed around these parameters. It is not only the case that people with little power behave in these ways, there are norms or implicit expectations that they *should* do so. In an early study, Stein (1968) observed that it was unacceptable for nurses to offer doctors direct advice on treatment matters. They could, however, get their message across in a more veiled fashion by indirectly indicating their views. This relational dimension is one that has traditionally characterised the health worker–patient relationship with that between doctor and patient, in particular, being prone to significant inequities of power and control (Stewart and Roter, 1989). Once more, relational differences along these lines can place obstacles in the way of full, free and effective interchange.

These two communicative dimensions, substantive content and relationship, are complexly interwoven and interrelated. Wilmot (1987) proposed that every statement has a relational significance and that the orchestrating of relationships is typically achieved in this 'indirect' way. While the relationship may become the topic of conversation (that is, form the content of talk) this seldom happens. Chalmers and Luker (1991), for instance, found that the development of health visitor–client relationships was a feature of the ongoing interactional process rather than being in some way separate and distinct from it. Even when the relationship became problematic it was uncommon for this topic to become part of the substantive content of communication and be dealt with explicitly. It was not talked about.

Finally, interactors can, in part, create the social situation which they share in communicating. An assessment interview, for example, can take on the trappings of a relaxed, friendly chat or something approaching an interrogation depending upon, amongst other features, furniture arrangements, formality of dress and the amount and types of questioning featured (Dickson, 1995).

A MODEL OF THE COMMUNICATION PROCESS

The study of interpersonal communication has been approached from a number of perspectives and a variety of theories and models to account for the process are available, as outlined in Chapter 1. The particular position adopted here is that it can be usefully conceived of as a skilled activity and explained in keeping with broadly social cognitivist assumptions. This way of thinking, first popularised by Argyle (1972), has been subsequently extended and applied to health communication (Dickson *et al.*, 1997; Hargie *et al.*, 1993; Skipper, 1992), including nursing in hospital (McCann and McKenna, 1993) and community settings (Dickson, 1995; Crute, 1986). Since any meaningful discussion of barriers to interpersonal communication must be grounded in a set of assumptions about how communication operates, the model presented by Dickson *et al.* (1997) will be briefly outlined.

In essence the model depicts dyadic interactors as essentially purposeful information-processors, planners and decision-makers; influenced by their personal histories, attributes and characteristics including emotional states and predispositions; sensitive to each other, their social environment and the effects of their actions; and operating within a nesting of communicative contexts. In addition to the immediate personal–situational framework which shapes interaction, organisational and cultural contexts can be posited. While these do not necessarily exhaust the possibilities, they do seem to be particularly relevant to a consideration of communication barriers in health settings. Indeed, all of the various elements of the model presented in Figure 4.1 can be thought of as potential harbingers of communicative dysfunction. At each of these points the operation may falter.

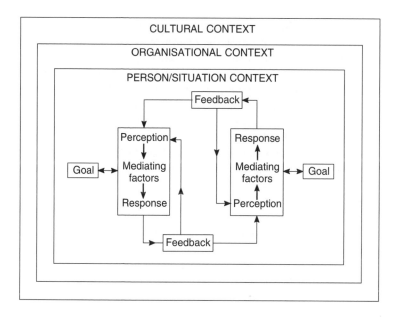

Figure 4.1   Contextualised model of interpersonal communication skill

Source: Dickson, D., Hargie, O. and Morrow, N. (1997) *Communication Skills Training for Health Professionals.* London: Chapman & Hall.

Goals

Communication is held to be essentially purposeful and goal-directed. A belief in the strategic nature of much of what happens is widely shared (Kellermann, 1992; Daly and Wiemann, 1994). This is not to deny the claim already made that it is also often largely 'mindless' (Langer *et al.*, 1978). Kellermann (1992) has no difficulty accepting that it can be both. It is possible, she argues, for intentional behaviour to be monitored outwith the ongoing stream of conscious awareness.

  Goals give direction to communicative activity and also contribute a more general energising effect (Dillard, 1990). They may be shared by interactors, be complementary or conflicting. Herein lies another configuration of possible obstacles to a successful interchange. Depending upon the patients' familiarity with the situation and circumstances, they may be unsure of their goals, leading to communication difficulties. Indeed the patient may be also unsure, in precise terms, of those of the health worker. Alternatively, the health worker may pursue his or her goals uncompromisingly to the neglect of those of the patient. This sometimes stems from insensitivity, overzealousness, time pressures, or may be a form of emotional defence. In the extreme this practice can lead to a pattern of interaction called 'pseudo-contingency', by Jones and Gerard (1967), with each talking past the other in their separate monologues. An important part of the initial contact with patients and clients, therefore, is the business of locating, clarifying and establishing appropriate sets of expectations (Saunders, 1986). This framework of common purpose Dinkmeyer (1971) referred to as 'goal alignment', and without it little of benefit can be achieved.

The importance in community health care nursing of promoting goals shared by both worker and patient/client is, not surprisingly, heavily stressed (Orr, 1992). More generally, Ashworth (1980) suggested four broad goals pursued by nurses through patient communication. They are:

1. To shape a facilitative relationship;
2. To establish patient needs and, if necessary, make the patient aware of them;
3. To assist the patient to use available resources, including their own, to help meet their needs; and
4. To provide information as a way of empowering the patient.

More recently, French (1994) observed that nurses engage in communication with patients in order to facilitate instrumental tasks (for example, carrying out various clinical procedures), provide social stimulation, give and receive information, control, facilitate patient self-expression, and alleviate negative emotion and stress thereby promoting recovery. Additionally, some communication has a role-related or ritualistic function.

For the most part, interactors pursue a multiplicity of goals during interaction, mirroring the different dimensions of interpersonal communication already mentioned. Traditionally nursing has placed a premium upon communication serving instrumental purposes (that is, communication entered into in order to accomplish some physical/clinical task). According to a hospital-based observational study by MacLeod Clark (1984) the majority of communicative episodes with patients were in the course of providing physical care.

Correspondingly, Morrison and Burnard (1989) reported that nurses seemed much more confident in their abilities to deal with clinical or community situations requiring essentially authoritative approaches such as informing, confronting or prescribing than with facilitative alternatives including supportive, catalytic or cathartic involvement. Paradoxically, it is just those approaches to care with which the nurse feels more comfortable that are regarded as often misapplied according to much contemporary thinking on community nursing practice (Orr, 1992).

Perception

How we perceive others is fundamental to skilful interaction yet is a profoundly precarious business. Despite naive assumptions, the belief that we perceive and observe other people in a correct, factual, unbiased, objective way is an exploded myth. Rather, what we observe typically owes as much, if not more, to ourselves in perceiving as it does to the other person in being perceived. As put by Wilmot (1995, p. 150):

> 'There is no "immutable reality" of the other person awaiting our discovery. We attribute qualities to the other based on the cues we have available, and the unique way we interpret them. Our perception of the other, while seeming certain, is grounded in permanent uncertainty.'

A consequence of the essentially selective and inferential nature of social perception and its heavy dependence upon the knowledge structures, expectations and attributional processes of the perceiver results, in many instances, in perceptual inaccuracy and hence miscommunication (Forgas, 1985; Hinton, 1993). Here we can locate a further potent source of barriers to quality communication between health worker and patient.

Mediating factors

Information stemming from perceptions of self, the situation, and the other interactor is processed in accordance with a complex of mediating factors. According to Berger (1995, p. 143):

'to understand the communication processes, it is not only necessary to study exchanges of symbols, but it is also crucial to understand the cognitive processes that subvert the interpretation and generation of these symbols.'

Some of the intrapersonal components of interpersonal communication which operate at this stage are discussed by Kreps (1988) in terms of the organising, processing and evaluation of information, decision-making and the selection of action strategies. Dickson *et al.* (1997) make reference to further cognitive and emotional factors involved. The resulting plan of action which is deemed to maximise opportunities for goal attainment, under the prevailing circumstances, will consequently determine action.

Given the inherent fluidity of unfolding events which constitute interaction and which social actors typically contend with, Berger (1995, p. 149) argued persuasively in favour of flexible planning since 'reducing the actions necessary to reach social goals to a rigid, script-like formula may produce relatively ineffective social action'. Unfortunately this is what sometimes characterises health worker–patient encounters where interactions become ossified to little more than repetitive, stereotyped rituals. Amongst the causes can be listed the tyranny of habit, the cynicism of familiarity and the emptiness of disillusionment.

Once more, a myriad of potential obstructions in the path of effective communication can be sourced amongst the processes that mediate between perception and action. Indeed this may be particularly so in a health care context where, as Barnlund (1976) noted, the complexities of problems faced often militate against the successful sharing of messages, without ambiguity or information loss. The health-care worker, client and family carer may differ in the concepts, language and knowledge base with which they respectively make sense of these matters.

Response

Regardless of the type of goal, in keeping with the model of skilled interaction presented in Figure 4.1, particular strategies of action are decided upon and operationalised in verbal and non-verbal responses (Argyle, 1983). But putting plans into action is seldom straightforward. Words are sometimes difficult to find when we need them most, often poorly chosen or not offered at all, while tones of voice and expressions escape our censorial clutches to mock our best intentions.

Feedback

By means of feedback, judgements can be made as to the extent to which messages have been successfully received and with what impact. Monitoring receiver reactions enables subsequent communications to be adapted and regulated to achieve a desired effect. Ultimately decisions about degree of goal achievement are taken on this basis. Haslett and Ogilvie (1988, p. 385) expressed it succinctly when they defined feedback, in the interpersonal setting, as:

> 'the response listeners give to others about their behaviour . . . Feedback from others enables us to understand how our behaviour affects them, and allows us to modify our behaviour to achieve our desired goals.'

As such, Gudykunst (1991) asserted that communicative success is directly proportional to the amount of feedback made available and acted upon. Convergence towards mutual understanding and shared meaning depends upon it. In any situation where one interactor provides insufficient or confusing feedback and/or the other does not pick up these cues and respond to them appropriately, an obstacle will be placed in the way of a successful interchange.

Adequate self-monitoring of performance seems to be an important component of feedback. High self-monitors are very much aware of their performance, controlling and adjusting their behaviour in purposeful ways (Snyder, 1987). Relatedly, the importance of nurse self-awareness has been stressed in promoting effective interpersonal interaction (Ashworth, 1985). As mentioned by Benicki and Leslie (1983), it is only through this means that the community learning disability nurse can avoid conveying, for instance, unintended messages of, perhaps, disgust in inappropriate non-verbal cues given off. There is some evidence, though, to suggest a certain lack of sensitivity in this regard amongst nursing staff (MacLeod Clark, 1984). Thompson (1990, p. 39), in her review of nurse–client interaction, wrote that nurses 'do not communicate as they profess they should nor as they think they do'.

Person/situation context

Communication is heavily context-bound, as represented in Figure 4.1. Interaction takes place within a person–situation context (Endler and Magnusson, 1976). Not only is what ensues a feature of personal characteristics such as the knowledge, beliefs, values, attitudes, stereotypes, emotions, expectations and predispositions of those involved but is co-determined by situational factors such as roles enacted and the rules which pertain. One need only look at this truncated list to appreciate how communication between health worker and patient can easily become distorted and dysfunctional. Hargie and Marshall (1986) also discussed the potential effect which physical aspects of the environment such as décor can exert upon the communicative process. Lack of privacy and issues of confidentiality are, in some cases, also attributable to the physical environment, and can be a very real obstacle to full and frank disclosure of deeply personal information in many health settings.

This situational component of the model in Figure 4.1 has, of course, particular significance for work in the community. Nursing in the client's home, for instance, brings with it an additional role not encountered in the hospital setting – that of guest (Baly *et al.,* 1987) – with possibilities of role conflict and confusion. Role uncertainty is one of the causes of difficulty in the relationship between health professional and patient, according to Northouse and Northouse (1992). They pointed out that neither role is always particularly clearly defined, leading to sets of expectations that do not always match. Those new to the role of patient may be unclear what is required of them. They will probably be even less certain what to expect from the variety of health workers encountered, leading to passivity, frustration, anxiety, and hesitation to raise other than physical concerns.

The acceptance of the role of guest is held by Trojan and Yonge (1993) to contribute to the initial phase of establishing a caring relationship when nursing older people in their own homes. There is some evidence that situations can arise where community health care nurses are very aware of a certain conflict between being 'a guest' and the more traditional, dominant role of nurse (McIntosh, 1981). Resolution depends, in part, on the particular circumstances which prevail. It seems that mostly the role of guest predominates save where, for instance, there is an evident inability of the informal family carer to cope adequately with the patient, resulting in possible neglect or harm.

Organisational context

In analysing the diversity of professional communication, and the factors that mould it, it is useful to think of individuals involved in varied situations within organisations. The organisation represents a framework of communication channels and structures, norms, expectations, opportunities (and barriers), which contribute to the creation of an identifiable climate. Here we can focus on, in the words of Ray and Miller (1993, p. 103):

'the dynamics within the organisation [that] enable the health-care providers to meet the needs of its patients in the best possible way. Thus we can look at communication processes within the organisation as they affect patient care'.

At a more macro level, therefore, the agency within which the nurse functions offers a broader multilayered context which shapes communication with its external public. Discussions can be found in the literature of organisational factors that create barriers to effective nurse–patient interaction (Lillie, 1985; May, 1990).

At the institutional level of the NHS, Tourish and Irving (1995) asserted that a quality service depends upon active steps being taken to audit the system and identify when, how and where communication functions to facilitate this aspiration and when, how and where it does not. Managers need information on, for instance:

'The amount of information overload or underload connected to major topics, sources and channels of information. The quality of information communicated from and to these sources . . . The identification of categories of positive and negative communication experiences and incidents.'
(Tourish and Irving, 1995, p. 9).

Cultural context

More broadly still, cultural and subcultural variables have a bearing on the different features of the communicative process depicted in Figure 4.1. Kreps and Thornton (1992, p. 157) defined culture as:

'the deposition of knowledge, experiences, beliefs, values, attitudes, meanings, hierarchies, religion, timing, roles, spatial relations, concepts of the universe and material objects and possessions acquired by large groups of people in the course of generations through individual and group striving.'

A subculture is held by a smaller group of people within the geographical boundaries of the dominant culture but which differs from it in identifiable ways with respect to beliefs, values or forms of expression.

Language is perhaps the most communicatively visible and frequently divisive manifestation of culture. In the context of intercultural contact, it can of course represent a formidable obstacle. But intercultural differences run much deeper, encompassing not only much of the non-verbal channels of communication but beyond to the underlying social order itself and the meanings and values that give it form. When a health worker and patient from radically different cultures come together, it is not that they are attempting to use different language codes to represent a shared world. Not only the codes but the social worlds differ – barriers indeed!

The influential relationship between communication and context is varyingly bidirectional. What transpires during interaction can bring about changes in the knowledge, beliefs, values, and so on, of those involved. Indeed effective health education and counselling depend upon it (Ewles and Simnett, 1992). Relationships are shaped and altered through unfolding interaction. Likewise situational factors can be redefined, within limits, by those taking part, as already mentioned. Furthermore, through intercultural communication, interactors can begin to appreciate and overcome cultural diversity which in turn can facilitate closer interaction between them.

COMMUNICATION DEFICITS IN HEALTH CARE

Further clues to the barriers that get in the way of effective interchange can be gleaned from the sorts of things that patients complain about in respect of their communication with health workers, or that have been noted by observations of practice. These seem to centre around five main areas of deficit.

1. *Gathering information* Badenoch (1986) highlighted this deficiency by relating the apocryphal story of the busy physician rapidly writing out the patient's history without looking up and

blithely unaware that the patient is deaf and his questions are being answered by the blind patient in the next bed! While this may be extreme, Newell (1994) made the comment that while done frequently, by and large health workers conduct interviews poorly. They often neglect important areas, interview in an overly practitioner-centred manner and collect detail in such a way that it is likely to be inaccurate or incomplete.

2. *Giving information* This frequently invites criticism either because the amount provided is inadequate or alternatively is delivered in an incomprehensible or insensitive way. The findings have been summarised by the Audit Commission (1993, p. 1) as follows: 'A common complaint is that there is not enough information. Equally, information often exists, but the quality is poor.' This chimes with more recent comments by the Health Services Commissioner who, in the report for 1994–95 already referred to, stated that:

'It is very easy to assume that information has been passed on, and understood, when that is in fact not the case. Individual responsibilities of staff need to be clearly defined and care taken to ensure that information given has been fully and correctly understood' (HMSO, 1995, p. 8).

3. *Poor listening* Health care personnel have been accused of taking little time to listen to what the patient wants to say (DiMatteo, 1994). Instead of 'saving time', which may sometimes be the motive, they frequently end up losing it!

4. *Neglect of psychosocial concerns* In a sense this is related to the last issue. Communication which does take place tends to be primarily factual, addressing physical aspects of the condition. As a consequence the psychosocial needs of patients are often overlooked. The professional's role in offering comfort and emotional support is thereby neglected. Male physicians would seem to be more negligent than their female colleagues in this respect (Roter *et al.,* 1991).

5. *Relationship work* Negotiating a mutually acceptable professional–patient relationship is an important communicative function (Ong *et al.,* 1995). It can lead to frustration and difficulty when the health professional insists on operating within the terms of the traditional paternalistic arrangement that has typified health care delivery, while the patient demands the right to a more egalitarian alternative in which a contribution to the decision-making process can be claimed. More mundanely, patients complain that health professionals often do not greet

them appropriately, introduce themselves, or explain what they intend to do.

CAUSES OF POOR COMMUNICATION

In this penultimate section of the chapter, some of the obstacles to full and open communication in health care delivery will be synthesised more precisely from what has already been said about the nature of communication, the fact that it often serves patients poorly as exercised by staff, and the broad areas of application where this seems to be particularly so. Barriers to communication have been discussed in the general literature on interpersonal communication (for example, Dimbleby and Burton, 1985; Burley-Allen, 1995; and Bolton, 1995) and to a lesser extent with particular reference to health (for example, Holli and Calabrese, 1991; DiMatteo, 1994; and French, 1994). These can be broadly grouped into categories of difficulty loosely described as physical, environmental, semantic, perceptual, emotional, demographic, relational, dispositional, organisational and cultural.

Disability

Perhaps the most conspicuous type of barrier to communication, although one which will not be pursued here in any great depth, occurs when the patient has some physical, neurological or psychological impairment that makes normal channels of communication difficult or impossible. Sensory disabilities such as deficits in hearing or seeing, and expressive deficits due to impaired speech and language, are obvious examples. Likewise, conditions such as Bell's palsy, stroke and Parkinson's disease can lead to varying degrees of facial paralysis, for instance, which may also have adverse effects on communication. In a study conducted by Pitcairn et al. (1990), observers watched videotapes of both Parkinsonian patients and a comparable group recovering from aeschemic heart disease. The former were more inclined to be seen as cold, withdrawn, unintelligent and moody, and as relating poorly to the interviewer.

Problems of memory, cognitive dysfunction, and most types of serious mental ill health can also be included under the present heading. Forms of communication including neologisms, word salad and thought-blocking that characterise schizophrenia come to mind as examples of the latter. Further difficulties of this sort are discussed by French (1994) as they affect the encoding, transmission and reception of messages.

Environmental barriers

The nature of the physical environment in terms of the layout of furniture and fittings, lighting, heating, colour, and so on, can have a distinct influence upon the behaviour of interactors (Dickson *et al.*, 1997). For example, people feel more comfortable and tend to disclose more about themselves in 'warm' environments with soft seats, concealed lighting and carpets. Furthermore, individuals feel more secure in their own homes than in unfamiliar locations. Doctors, health visitors and district nurses generally find patients more at ease during home visits as opposed to those at the health clinic. It could be that, 'The home setting may equalise role-related rights because the nurse is now a guest in the patient's home' (Abraham and Shanley, 1992, p. 126).

Hospitals can be particularly disturbing for some patients, owing to the nature of the ward environment, with little personal space or privacy, bright lights, intrusive noise and few personal possessions. In such situations, the patient is likely to feel a sense of loss of autonomy, and hence possible distress. That said, Canter (1984) claimed that areas of the ward or clinic are seen by patients to be more or less their 'territory', such that they may be more likely to engage with a nurse near their bed bay and less in the vicinity of the nursing station or office. Abraham and Shanley (1992) claimed that such territoriality can therefore inhibit communication.

Lack of privacy and threats to confidentiality are common in health care environments. Often the most personally intimate detail is requested of patients by health workers in hospital wards with only a curtain to contain the conversation from the person in the bed but a few feet away. The observation by a disillusioned patient that 'When you enter hospital you leave your modesty at the door', in part bears witness to the chagrin that can result. Such circumstances, of course, also obstruct patient-initiated disclosure of psycho-emotional concerns.

Semantic barriers

Problems here have to do broadly with information exchange and the sharing of meaning. Holli and Calabrese (1991, p. 33) estimated that some 90 per cent of the misunderstanding and breakdown that plagues communication can be laid at the door of the already stated principle that meanings are ultimately to be found in people, not in words.

Types of meaning

We need to distinguish between denotative and connotative meaning. The former is the word's objective, dictionary-based definition, deriving from the 'thing in the world' that it represents. Connotative meaning is the subjective nuances that the word conjures up for us, based upon our life experiences (DeVito, 1986). Some words may have little connotative meaning for us, others considerable. But the important point is that it is unlikely that a word will have precisely the same connotative meaning for any two people. Take the example of a young doctor telling the patient, 'Mrs Brown, your tests have shown up diabetes as the cause of the problems that you've been having.' Apart from what the word 'diabetes' denotes to each, imagine the different subjective images conjured up for the young woman whose mother finally succumbed to complications arising from the condition, after years of poor control and ill health, and for the young doctor with a special interest in diabetes and hopes of specialising in this area of medicine.

To sow further seeds of potential confusion, a word can, of course, have more than one possible denotation. Holli and Calabrese (1991) pointed out that the word 'fast' has fifteen! Given that the English language contains over two million words, most with multiple denotations and countless potential connotations, different subsets of which (or vocabularies) are available to different users, a picture begins to form of the vagaries of language.

Jargon

These two million and more words include those that have specialised technical, medical or scientific meaning and are therefore restricted in their usage to a select few. This is where jargon makes an entrance as an often-cited barrier to comprehensible exchange between patients and health workers. As mentioned, patients often complain that information is not provided or that they do not understand it when it is. All professional groups have their stock-in-trade of jargon. Indeed, in many respects it serves them well as a means of facilitating communication *within the group*, acting as a very conspicuous group identity marker, and denying access to information to non-group members (Kreps and Thornton, 1992) . Blocks to communication arise when what linguists call 'code switching' occurs and jargon forms part of the dialogue with those, such as patients, not privy to this lexicon. There is evidence that this is something that health workers do to a much greater extent than they seem to be aware of, or are prepared to admit to (Thompson, 1994).

When jargon is misused in this way, it creates multiple barriers to good communication. First, and most obvious, it serves to confuse. The patient is unable to successfully decode the words or interpret them accurately. Second, it leads to alienation. There can be fewer more convincing ways of proving to others that they are different, apart, and excluded than by demonstrating to them that they cannot even speak the language! On the other hand, and in keeping with speech accommodation theory (Giles, 1973), by adapting to the other's communicative characteristics, a greater desire for interpersonal affiliation can be conveyed. Third, jargon can serve to mystify. As an exercise in the misuse of power, it is sometimes used intentionally to draw a veil of secrecy over a topic that the health worker is not prepared to reveal or discuss with the patient (DiMatteo and Friedman, 1982).

Health and 'bilingualism'

More generally, it has be suggested that two languages can come to be used when health care staff and patients meet. Bourhis *et al.* (1989) observed that doctors and nurses are 'bilingual' in that they are privy to a highly specialised register, 'medical language' (ML), in addition to 'everyday language' (EL). Patients, on the other hand, have access only to EL. Notwithstanding, it was found that doctors typically persisted in using ML in medical settings with patients, while nurses switched from one register to the other as circumstances dictated. This often casts them in the role of 'communication broker' between patient and doctor.

Before leaving the point, though, it is important to acknowledge that even when health worker and patient use the same word, there is no guarantee that they are in fact using it in the same way, to refer to the same 'thing': the doctor can still be using ML and the patient EL. Samora *et al.* (1961) revealed that common words familiar to both, such as 'stomach' and 'palpitation', are often given a precise medical meaning by doctors, but a common lay meaning by patients. It is important for health staff, in an attempt to overcome this possible cause of miscommunication, to check what precisely the patient actually means by the word as they come to use it.

Mixed messages

Another form of barrier that, in a sense, has to do with meaning and is therefore relevant to this section (although operating at a different level from the previous discussion of semantic barriers) has to do with mixed messages. On occasion a message may be inherently contradictory. The community nurse may convey to the patient that, following a physical examination, everything is coming on fine, yet the patient may pick up a suggestion of grave concern. Sometimes the message sent verbally can be qualified non-verbally. At best this causes confusion and inappropriate action but often it compromises a climate of openness and undermines trust. If persisting within close relationships such as families, and particularly when centred around interpersonal attitudes and affects, it can take the form of 'double binds' and lead to emotional pathology (Bateson *et al.*, 1956). Here the recipient picks up two contradictory messages requiring incompatible responses. Whichever is pursued is bound to lead to failure and incur an emotional put-down.

Perceptual barriers

We look out on the world, and glean information about it, through a system of perceptual filters that invariably colour the impressions we form. As already mentioned, nowhere is this more prevalent than in our perceptions of other people. Here the judgements that we make are often focused through the lens of our own assumptions, expectations, needs and values leading to endemic distortions and inaccuracies (Zabrowitz, 1990). Once more, we have located a complex set of hazards on the road to successful communication.

Perceptual sensitivity

Based upon a review of research, Biley (1989) concluded that 'the results of the studies on nurse perception . . . show that nurses are not accurate in perceiving worry, anxiety, and stress in patients' (p. 576). Indeed, Johnson (1982) found that fellow patients were more accurate than staff in picking up patients' worries! Interestingly, nurses tended to err through overestimation of these concerns. On the other hand, they have also been accused of frequently failing to notice or misconstruing emotional cues (Faulkner and

Maguire, 1984). This led Hogstel (1987) to advocate that part of nurses' training should be explicitly concerned with sharpening their observation skills. Certainly the salience to the communication process of the community learning disability nurse being able to read 'the patient's individual body language; for example his facial expression, posture, and hand movements' has been stressed (Benicki and Leslie, 1983, p. 92).

Representational systems

According to proponents of neuro-linguistic programming (NLP), we use the same sensory-based systems to represent our experiences inwardly as we do to garner external information directly in the first instance (O'Connor and Seymour, 1990). Consequently mental content can be mainly represented visually, aurally or kinaesthetically. People commonly have a preferred or primary representational system, clues to which can be grasped partly from the sorts of expressions that characterise their speech. For instance, they may 'hear what you say' (auditory system), 'see what you mean' (visual system) or 'catch your drift' (kinaesthetic system). In a recent BBC Radio 4 broadcast, for example, Tony Benn MP mentioned that although he read considerably, he always had difficulty accessing information in this way and that he had learned much more, and with greater ease, listening to people. Forcing someone to rely upon a secondary system to assimilate information can put them at a disadvantage. Furthermore, NLP recommends conversationally switching to the primary representational system utilised by the other as a way of promoting rapport.

Attributional processes

A further feature of our perceptions which can get in the way of our relationships with others centres around the processes through which we attribute causes to the things that they do. According to attribution theory, how we perceive those with whom we come in contact depends upon whether we infer that significant actions committed by them were due to personal characteristics and qualities, on the one hand, or a reflection of situational circumstances, on the other (Heider, 1958). As such, a patient with AIDS who contracted the disease through contaminated blood products during the course of a hospital procedure is likely to be perceived quite differently from one who fell ill as a result of a debauched, promiscuous and drug-ridden, homosexual lifestyle. In a study by

Morrison (1990), nurses were more tolerant of violent behaviour by patients considered 'sick' (and therefore not responsible for this behaviour) than by those labelled 'bad' (who presumably were). Similarly, Olsen (1997) interviewed qualified nurses and those in training to establish if they reacted differently to those felt to have in some way been the cause of their illness. He concluded (p. 520) that:

> 'a substantial percentage of these nurses and nurses-to-be believe that their sense of caring, concern for patients, and thus the quality of their relationship with patients is influenced by the degree of responsibility they perceive the patient to have for the clinical condition.'

This particular barrier is likely to get in the way, for some, when nursing patients who have had abortions, taken drug overdoses, or been hurt in the course of some illegal or antisocial act – perhaps even injured through sport.

But we tend to apply attributions in quite distorted ways, which in turn skews our broader perceptions of others. These tendencies can be traced to both motivational and cognitive sources (Zebrowitz, 1990). For a start, we tend to favour attributions that are internal and dispositional over those that are external and situational. In other words, we are more inclined to believe that people do the things they do because they are the kinds of people they are, rather than the alternative explanation that they are the victims of circumstance. When it comes to accounting for our own actions, however, we are less blind to circumstantial effects, especially when we are less than proud of the behaviour under consideration. Furthermore, we tend to perceive others sharing our views, opinions and habits, to a greater extent than is strictly warrantable (Hinton, 1993).

Social categorisation and stereotyping

The important role of social categorisation, stereotyping and prejudice in further colouring interpersonal perception must not be overlooked (Oakes *et al.*, 1994). The following quotation from Jourard (1964, p. 135) is telling in this respect:

> 'There are nurses who cannot care for a patient who is known to be immoral. One of our students mentioned that with some

young mothers of illegitimate children who were having their babies in a local hospital she, the nurse, would stay a minimum length of time and get out of the room as fast as she could.'

However, since this topic is taken up in some detail in Chapter 7, it will not be developed further at this point.

Demographic barriers

A range of demographic attributes of interactors also exerts a significant influence on the communicative process and has at least the potential to spoil it. Only two will be briefly considered here, gender and age.

Gender

Differences in how males and females communicate non-verbally are well-documented (Knapp and Hall, 1992). Other things being equal, females, compared with males, typically interact at closer interpersonal distances and are more tolerant of spatial intrusion; make greater use of eye contact and touch; smile more and are more facially, gesticularly and vocally expressive; and at the end of the day are more adept at both encoding and decoding non-verbal messages (Burgoon, 1994). While this diversity does not necessarily constitute a barrier to inter-gender communication, it can do in some instances. In health care delivery, expressive touch (touch which conveys relational information) is commonly recognised as positive practice, indicating warmth and care. But it is not always received as such. Lane (1989) found that male surgical patients were more receptive to female nurse touch that were female patients. However, nurses felt that the latter reacted more positively and therefore the nurses appeared to be more comfortable touching female patients.

Interestingly, the results of an earlier piece of research were somewhat at variance with those cited above (Whitcher and Fisher, 1979). Here touch by the nursing staff at the preoperative stage produced a positive response to surgery amongst female but not male patients. As noted by Davidhizar *et al.* (1997), touch can suggest overfamiliarity and be seen as a demonstration of power and control. It is arguably more likely that status-conscious males will have heightened sensitivity to this possibility and this could explain the finding by Whitcher and Fisher (1979).

Males and females also express themselves differently using language. There is some evidence, reviewed by Ng and Bradac (1993) that male discourse, oral and written, is associated with higher ratings on dynamism, and female discourse with higher ratings on aesthetic quality and socio-intellectual status. These findings resonate with work published by Tannen (1995) who analysed how males and females typically respond to 'trouble talk' – being told about some personal problem or difficulty. When women disclose personal predicaments, they primarily expect (and tend to get from other women) a listening ear, confirmation of their concerns and an understanding reaction. Indeed this type of talk serves, in part, to strengthen interpersonal bonds between friends. Men, however, instinctively respond by tackling the problem head-on in an attempt to solve it through giving information or offering advice. Miscommunication is such that men see women wallowing in their problems rather than discussing practical steps to solve them, as men do. Women on the other hand, feel that men do not understand them and are not prepared to make the effort to do so. Frustration is shared equally.

Gender effects can also be located in the patterns of interaction adopted by health workers in engaging with patients. Based upon detailed analyses of 537 audiotaped consultations by 127 doctors, Roter et al. (1991) discovered that compared to their female colleagues, male doctors had shorter consultations in which they engaged in less positive talk, partnership-building, question-asking and information-giving. These differences also affected how patients reacted such that they offered more opinions and information and asked more questions of female doctors.

Age

Age differences can also get in the way of quality communication between patient and heath worker. The study of the particular ways in which communication is used by older people and issues surrounding inter-generation talk is something of a growth industry in the field, at the moment (for example, Coupland et al., 1991; and Nussbaum and Coupland, 1995). How these differences emerge in health settings and with what effects has also attracted attention (Giles et al., 1990). While acknowledging that there is probably more commonality than diversity in provider–patient health care delivery spanning adult age ranges, Beisecker and Thompson (1995) nevertheless accept that older people are not treated quite the same as those of more tender years. This is due, first, to the fact that they often have distinctive patterns of communication; second, that some health workers react differently to older people; and third, to an interaction between these two factors. In reviewing some of the research, it emerged that in consultations involving older compared to younger patients, doctors tended to be less egalitarian, engaged and patient; gave less information and support; spent less time; and were less prepared to address psychosocial concerns (Roter and Hall, 1992; Beisecker and Thompson, 1995). Generally the emotional climate of these interviews was thought to be more negative. On the other hand, with the 'old old', some contrasting evidence emerged that doctors reacted with greater warmth and courteousness to those over the age of 75.

Ageism is recognised by Ryan and Butler (1996) as at the root of some of these negative reactions to older people. Ageism is a stereotypical reaction to those of advanced years in keeping with a set of negative beliefs to do with eroded capacity and ultimately diminished worth, which creates 'distance between conversational partners and failure of the helper to identify with the client' (p. 192). It is acted out, for instance, in avoidance (that is, discussing the older person with a relative or carer, rather than with the patient directly), impatience, being overly controlling, using simplified speech or unnecessarily loud speech, being dismissively familiar, and employing 'secondary baby talk' (BT) (using a register similar to that used with small children). In working with institutionalised older people, BT has been found to feature largely by carers and often regardless of the level of personal competence of the receiver (Grainger, 1995). While recognising the positive affect message often intended, recipients themselves felt that BT was more appropriate for those with limited independence. No doubt this form of patronising speech, despite best intentions on the part of the carer, can be particularly unwelcome when addressing someone valiantly trying to preserve an identity in which some sense of autonomy and independence is central.

Emotional barriers

Negative emotion, either expressed or anticipated, can be found at the bottom of many of the instances where communication between health worker and patient goes wrong. It can intrude at different levels and operate dysfunctionally through the health care provider, the patient, or both.

Emotional defensiveness

At the most evident level, the direct expression of strong emotion, especially negative emotion and particularly when directed towards the carer, can get in the way of effective listening (Hargie *et al.* 1994). The fact that listening suffers under these circumstances can be due to the triggering of defence mechanisms on the part of the recipient to protect against feelings of threat or anxiety. Burley-Allen (1995, p. 59) explained that to 'reduce these feelings, we flee mentally from what is being said by tuning out what the talker is saying or by distorting it so we won't have to alter our perception, belief or opinion'. Of course we can also think of additional ego-defence mechanisms, such as projection and rationalisation, brought to light by Sigmund Freud, that represent obstacles on the path of open and inclusive discussion.

But it is not only hostility or emotional distress by the patient that can trigger threat and raise the provider's personal defences. Burley-Allen (1995) referred to the fact that seemingly innocent words, topics, or phrases can touch a 'hot button' that sends internal alarm bells ringing and calls for defensive measures. These topics that expose our vulnerability and that we find threatening could be to do with death, abortion, sex, or whatever. What they have in common is the ability to surface personal feelings and issues that we have not successfully resolved or come to terms with, and that therefore fizz with uncomfortable emotional effervescence.

Blocking tactics

There is ample evidence that providers actively use blocking tactics with patients to cut off lines of conversation found inconvenient or uncomfortable (MacLeod Clark, 1982; von Friederichs-Fitzwater *et al.*, 1991; Wilkinson, 1991). It would seem that the threat of having one's lack of knowledge exposed, amongst other triggers, can lead to impoverished nurse communication with patients (Crockford *et al.*, 1993). Other reasons suggested by Wilkinson (1991) include: preventing patients from unleashing such a powerful tide of emotion as to threaten the nurse's capacities to cope with the situation; fear of losing their composure in front of patients; and fears to do with their own mortality.

A range of blocking tactics are available to the interactor intent upon escaping the clutches of some present line of conversation, or its affective impact (Hargie *et al.*, 1994; Bolton, 1995). They include preempting the raising of an unwelcome matter or, once raised,

112

diverting the line of talk by introducing a rapid topic switch, as von Friederichs-Fitzwater *et al.* (1991) reported doctors frequently doing when confronted by patients' psycho-emotional concerns. In a study by Wilkinson (1991) amongst nurses caring for cancer patients, diverting was also a commonly recorded blocking technique. Another tactic is intellectualisation or using logical argument as a way of marginalising affect. Thompson (1994, p. 704) noted that health staff may 'resort to quasi-scientific explanations when emotional issues that they would rather evade are raised'. Further ways that nurses have of blocking communication include using normalising/stereotyped comments, inappropriate reassurance, poor questioning, 'passing the buck', jollying along, chit-chat and switching the conversational focus to another person present (Wilkinson, 1991).

Engagement and detachment

A more permanent way of attempting to regulate the demands placed upon the nurse is by adjusting the emotional distance within the relationship. Expectations about the degree of engagement present in the nurse–patient relationship have shifted over the years in keeping with broader conceptualisations of the nursing process. The trend has been away from an earlier task-centred and essentially functional approach towards one that demands a less affectively neutral stance. But not all nurses comply, nor do those who do, do so all the time, or with all patients. Kralik *et al.* (1997) describe the 'detached' type of nurse, in their research, as avoiding personal contact, appearing busy and efficient, and being insensitive, thereby creating an experience for patients of being treated as a number rather than a person, having little or no say in their care, being handled roughly by a person 'just doing a job', and being dealt with coldly and brusquely.

This type of distancing can serve as a coping mechanism for staff in emotionally demanding nursing environments (May 1990; Faulkner, 1992). The avoidance of all but the most superficial communication by nurses when dealing with patients may be a defensive strategy operating in the interests of preventing possible personal distress. This particular barrier may be a structure to shelter behind: a survival mechanism to avoid 'burn-out'. One-fifth of the nurses sampled by Seale (1992), who dealt specifically with terminal illness, felt that they did not receive adequate emotional support in their work. Improved support systems for staff under these circumstances are obviously required if patients are to benefit from better communication. Faulkner (1993) outlined ways in which health professionals can be facilitated in this regard. Greater improvements in communication skills were found by Faulkner and Maguire (1984) amongst nurses working with mastectomy patients in ward contexts where staff experienced group cohesion and support, compared to the community setting where nurses often had a strong feeling of working on their own.

Taboo, stigma and loss of face

So far we have looked at emotional experiences, or anticipated emotional experiences on the part of the health worker, that constitute obstacles to effective communication. The other side of this particular coin is the difficulty that patients may have in raising or discussing certain troublesome, awkward or threatening topics. Such avoidance may be on issues considered taboo and hence felt to be wrong or too uncomfortable to raise. In their exploration of clients' failure to expose material to therapists in long-term therapy, Hill *et al.* (1993) found that not only insecurity but also embarrassment and shame were reasons given by clients for not revealing childhood sexual abuse.

Embarrassment and shame can be explained in terms of what Goffman (1963) referred to as losing face. In order to avoid this possibility, stigmatising information has to be managed in such a way as not to unmask the individual as 'a discredited person facing an unaccepting world' (p. 31). As such, the stigmatised person has to make a strategic decision whether to disclose the troublesome information but at the expense of maybe being shunned and, in Goffman's terms, incurring a spoiled identity, or concealing the facts and running the risk of being exposed later, which could be even more compromising. The role of trust in this dilemma is pivotal and will be taken up in the following section. But trust can be betrayed in very subtle and unintentional ways. Hill *et al.* (1993) cautioned that 'therapists might reinforce this shame and insecurity about sexual issues as a result of their own discomfort in discussing sexual issues' (p. 286).

Relational barriers

A further characteristic of interpersonal communication is that it is transacted between individuals in a relationship. While such features may be constrained by role demands, there is usually scope for the individuals concerned to mark their association in more individualistic ways. Their relationship may be one of strangers, old friends, or sworn enemies, but each communicative act is shaped and interpreted within this historical context. Being prepared to disclose highly personal and perhaps potentially discrediting information in health care settings, for example, is heavily influenced by this factor. Indeed, it may be much easier to reveal such details to a perfect stranger, safe in the knowledge that their paths will never cross again, than to someone known (Hargie *et al.*, 1994). Having a sexually transmitted disease, for example, dealt with in the anonymity of a clinic, may be preferable to going to the family GP. Under these circumstances, therefore, the relationship shared can make it difficult to relate in a full and open way, and hence constitutes a barrier.

Community health care nursing, of course, involves providers and recipients in longer-term contact than is typically the case in the hospital setting. The relational context is, therefore, a further distinguishing feature of community nursing which has an effect upon the communicative process between nurse, clients and informal carers. Sharf (1993) pointed out, however, that little communication research in health has taken such a longitudinal perspective.

Trust

Trust is an important relational quality, operating at different levels, that can ameliorate the effects of perceived vulnerability through revealing prejudicial information about the self (Steel, 1991). At one level it may be reflected in having the confidence to expose a vulnerability, safe in the knowledge that the esteem and worth bestowed by the other will not be revoked. Northouse and Northouse (1992) drew attention to this very worry as a reason why patients sometimes find it difficult to open up to health workers. Furthermore, patients have a concern that not only the esteem in which they are held, but also levels of care received, could suffer as a result. At another level, trust means believing in the discretion of the other. According to Derlega *et al.* (1993, p. 69):

'trust in the other person's discretion is a critical factor, and when there is a high need to be open (e.g., to "get something off their chest"), people tend to be very tolerant of possible vulnerabilities.'

Returning to a point made earlier in the chapter, a further relational dimension that has been recognised in health settings, and that can stem the flow of communication, has to do with the distribution of power and control between provider and recipient. This is played out in often subtle ways. Influence can be claimed and maintained in the success with which topics for discussion are initiated and changed, requests are made, questions are asked and answers elicited and information given or withheld. Roter and Hall (1992) suggested that this task of negotiating control can lead to one of four outcomes that they called: default (low provider control – low patient control); consumerism (low provider control – high patient control); paternalism (high provider control – low patient control); and, mutuality (high provider control – high patient control).

Despite the benefits of mutuality which acknowledges the contributions and resources of both provider and recipient in a respectful arrangement of collaborative decision-making, the paternalism that has typified much of health care delivery, especially in medicine, still lives on. As such, it is the doctor's agenda that predominates and gives form to the consultation, often to the neglect of concerns that the patient might have. For instance, von Friederichs-Fitzwater *et al.* (1991) observed physicians frequently initiating topic changes, especially when patients introduced issues that were emotion-laden. Based upon a review of research in this area, Beisecker (1990) concluded that patients exercise little control over their encounters with doctors and have little active participation in the decision-making process surrounding their care. Indeed, lack of compliance with recommendations was suggested as a final defiant attempt by patients to assert their power and autonomy.

Nurses also wield considerable control over patients in their charge. In an illuminating study, Hewison (1997) used participant observation methodology to investigate the relationships and interactions between nurses and patients in a small hospital for the care of the older person. The results demonstrated quite convincingly that nurses do indeed exert extensive power through the language which they employ in caring. The conclusion reached was that:

'The fact that this is the "normal" situation and accepted by both staff and patients constitutes a barrier to nurse–patient communication. The emphasis on more "open" and collaborative relationships with patients, in current nursing practice, is constrained by this pre-existing power relationship.' (Hewison, 1997, p. 81).

Dispositional barriers

Under this subheading will be discussed several sorts of what can be perhaps best described as interpersonal stance that interactors sometimes adopt that jeopardise what happens between them.

Egocentricity

Here the individual is self-centred to the exclusion of any significant appreciation of needs, circumstances and experiences of the other. The fact that these may be radically different from his or her own, but still be perfectly valid – indeed the only reality that the other person has available and, therefore, the basis of their interpretations and ways of relating – is dismissed or neglected. There is an inability or unwillingness to accept that others may hold different sets of beliefs or values, have contrasting perspectives on issues, and lead their lives in different ways. A consequence of this narrowness of vision is that proper listening suffers and empathy is denied.

Various nuances of meaning have been brought out by those exploring the concept of empathy. At its heart is the ability to put yourself in the other's position, to think and feel yourself into his or her shoes, to experience the world as if you were him or her (without ever losing sight of the 'as if'), and to have the capacity to convey this level of understanding to the person empathised with (Lang and van der Molen, 1990). As such, it is at the core of skilled interpersonal involvement between health worker and patient. Northouse and Northouse (1992, pp. 21–2) stated that:

'Of all the variables used to explain health communication, empathy is regarded as one of the most essential and at the same time one of the most complex variables operating in the communication process . . . Without empathy, the communication between people lacks the essential quality of understanding.'

Patients benefit in experiencing a feeling of value, acceptance, understanding and attachment. There is research evidence that positive therapeutic outcomes can also result (Irving, 1995)

Judgementality

A related barrier to quality communication is erected by someone who deals with others in a characteristically judgemental manner (Bolton, 1995). This may be expressed in criticism, negative labelling or moralising. Indeed, Rogers (1961) asserted that this tendency to tell others that they are right or wrong (although not always in so many words), to approve or disapprove of what they do, is *the* major obstacle to communicating effectively. Holli and Calabrese (1991) explained how in situations where causes of ill health in the patient's lifestyle have to be confronted, a preferred strategy for the health professional is to 'describe rather than evaluate' (p. 23). Accordingly, the patient is made aware, in a non-threatening way that does not have to be defended against, of what they are doing, what negative consequences this might have, and the alternatives that could be considered.

Ego-states

Transactional analysis (TA), as a framework for thinking about interaction, has been applied to health care delivery by, for example, Elder (1978). Here someone who is habitually criticising and laying down the law can be thought to be in their Critical Parent ego-state (Berne, 1964). This is a way of relating borrowed from our own parents or significant authority figures. Elder points out that health workers often operate from this position as they tell patients what to do and not to do, as they praise and criticise. (We have already discussed collateral imbalances in power and control in the relationship.) As a consequence, and in order to sustain the interaction, patients are forced into a reciprocal Child ego-state, so called because it involves them replaying from their past, child-like ways of responding to those in authority. Not to comply in this Parent–Child arrangement would be to effect a 'crossed transaction', hence blocking the exchange and leading to communication breakdown. The alternative Adult–Adult arrangement, however, is often the preferred but under-used option offering greater opportunities for constructive, participative decision-making.

Organisational barriers

So far, all of the communication pitfalls that we have considered can be thought of as features of the communicators and the process which they share. But a variety of organisational and administrative factors which reflect present-day realities of the health service militate against good communication (May, 1990). As noted by Jones *et al.* (1997, p. 108), 'The organizational context of the relationship between staff and patients had profound effects on its character.' Reductions in budgets inevitably increase the pressures under which staff work. Clearly this has implications for the quality of interpersonal relationships formed not only with patients, but also with colleagues (McIntee and Firth, 1984). Faced with an ever increasing case-load and the necessity to prioritise, it is likely that the physical rather than psychosocial needs of patients will be tended to.

Time factors

Time available to talk with and listen to patients may well suffer as budgets are straitened. Meikle and Holley (1991, p. 158) observed that:

> 'It is often very difficult for professional staff to fulfil the communication needs of patients because staff shortages result in tremendous stress and often there is no time for a nurse, for example, to sit and just have a chat.'

Indeed, health workers in several studies have expressed a desire to spend longer with patients and their families, particularly when a counselling/support role is called for (Bergen, 1991; Seale, 1992).

However, it has been argued that health workers often grossly overestimate the additional time taken to accommodate a more patient-centred communicative style. Epstein *et al.* (1993) reported findings that patient-centred consultations take, on average, only one minute longer than physician-centred alternatives. The total amount of time spent with a patient could be actually reduced in the long run, in circumstances where good communicative practice prevails (DiMatteo, 1994).

Furthermore, Davis and Fallowfield (1991) voiced suspicions that in many instances health professionals use 'lack of time' as an excuse when they do not communicate properly with patients. One of the findings reported by Grainger (1995) from her work on nursing older people in residential care was that while nurses complained about not having enough time to talk to the residents, when they did appear to have spare time on their hands, they seemed to prefer to spend it chatting with other nurses. Additionally, Thompson (1994) reviewed some evidence to suggest that there is little correlation between time spent with the patient, per se, and quality of communication entered into.

While it would appear that time available to communicate with patients is not always used to best purposes, there can be no doubt that it is one of a number of organisational barriers detrimental to effective engagement with patients.

Cultural barriers

That cultural and subcultural differences can create fundamental barriers to interpersonal contact has already been mentioned and scarcely needs repeating. In a survey of doctor–patient communication in two large Californian hospitals (a state where 16 per cent of the population have no or only a limited command of English), 44 per cent of the doctors sampled indicated that the language barrier negatively affected patient care to either a significant or very significant extent (Chalabian and Dunnington, 1997).

Additionally, cultural influences permeate values, beliefs and cherished practices. Indeed so pervasive are cultural effects that they can be thought to shape the individual's understanding of the social world that he or she inhabits. A classic study conducted by Hofstede (1980) exposed four underlying dimensions along which a large sample of different national groups could be plotted in respect of fundamental values espoused. These dimensions were: (i) power distance – the amount of respect and deference displayed by those in different positions on a status hierarchy; (ii) individualism–collectivism – the extent to which one's identity is shaped by individual choices and achievements or a feature of the collective group to which one belongs; (iii) uncertainty avoidance – the degree to which life's uncertainties can be controlled through planning and foresight; and (iv) masculinity–femininity – this has to do with the relative focus upon competitive, task-centred achievement versus cooperation and harmonious relationships. It was found, for instance, that a group of mostly European and North American cultures scored high on individualism and low on power distance, while another group of largely Latin American and Asian countries were low on individualism but high on power distance. Such differences have significant implications for health-related beliefs and behaviours. Those from collectivist cultures are much less likely than their individualist equivalents to go to their doctor on account of affective, as opposed to somatic symptoms (Smith and Bond, 1993).

Rogers (1991) illustrated eight different constructions that can be placed upon illness, depending upon where in the world meanings are sampled. Not all of these accounts will be mentioned here, but two are the 'body as machine' and the 'body under siege'. Both of these are common in Western culture as 'man-in the-street' popularisations of scientific or medical theory and research findings. On the other hand, the 'God's power' explanation, once widespread in the Western world, is now much more prevalent in countries where fundamentalist religious beliefs hold sway. It can still be found in the UK though, in pockets of immigrant subculture and amongst older people in more marginal regions.

Further differences between Western countries have been noted when it comes to the emphasis placed on certain forms of sickness and how they should be cured. Payer (1988) posited that much of French medicine focuses upon diseases of the liver and stomach, while in Germany the emphasis is on the heart and circulatory system. Hypotension in Germany is more likely to be seen as a condition to be treated than, for example, in the UK. In France significantly fewer caesareans and hysterectomies are performed than in the USA. Diagnosis and treatment decisions, it was concluded, seem to be based as much upon cultural as scientific factors to the extent that treatment of choice in one country can be regarded as malpractice if carried out on the other side of the national border.

It can be seen, then, that cultural differences can lead to contrasting beliefs about what is ill health, what causes it and how it should be properly treated. These ways of thinking, in turn, can represent a formidable obstacle to communication between the health worker and the patient.

But barriers also exist at another level, in terms of the culturally prescribed norms that govern how people conduct themselves in interaction with others. These norms determine punctuality, interpersonal distance, touch, use of gestures, facial expressions, gaze patterns – indeed all the non-verbal codes (Knapp and Hall, 1992: Burgoon, 1994). Machismo in Hispanic cultures, for example, imposes display rules that forbids expressions of pain. In Muslim cultures there may be gender difficulties surrounding even instrumental touch by a male health worker in the course of a physical examination of a female patient. Kreps and Thornton (1992, p. 163) advised that 'Health professionals need to recognise many cultural factors as quickly as possible as they prepare to work with clients.' They go on to offer suggestions on how best to overcome obstacles in this area, including carrying out a cultural assessment in order to appreciate the patient's values, attitudes, beliefs and theories about what is right and wrong and how things can be improved, and to establish how he or she prefers to be engaged with. It may then be necessary to enter into 'cultural negotiation' as a way of arriving at a mutually satisfying arrangement for the delivery of health care.

CONCLUSION

Communication with others is at the same time a prosaic yet impressively intricate process. Despite the fact that we do it so often, success is by no means guaranteed. From the information available, this would seem to be particularly so in the field of health care delivery where standards of communication between doctors/ nurses and patients often invite negative comment. This chapter has presented a conceptual model of the interpersonal process as a framework for a discussion of barriers to effective dialogue. These barriers can be loosely categorised as physical, environmental, semantic, perceptual, demographic, emotional, relational, dispositional, organisational and cultural. Ultimately, attempts to improve levels of communication with patients are unlikely to be particularly successful unless each of these is acknowledged and steps taken to remove it. Quality health care delivery demands no less. At the risk of adulterating a communication metaphor made popular by Stewart (1995), barriers must be turned into bridges!

References

Abraham, C. and Shanley, E. (1992) *Social Psychology for Nurses*. London: Edward Arnold.

Allen, C. (1993) Clients' needs, views and wishes. *Community Psychiatric Nursing Journal*, 13, pp. 6–12.

Argyle, M. (1972) *The Psychology of Interpersonal Behaviour*, 2nd edn. Harmondsworth: Penguin.

Argyle, M. (1983) *The Psychology of Interpersonal Behaviour*, 4th edn. Harmondsworth: Penguin.

Argyle, M. (1988) *Bodily Communication*. London: Methuen.

Ashworth, P. (1980) *Care to Communicate*. London: Royal College of Nursing.

Ashworth, P. (1985) Interpersonal skill issues arising from intensive care nursing contexts. In C. Kagan (ed.), *Interpersonal Skills in Nursing: research and application*. London: Croom Helm.

Audit Commission (1993) *What Seems to be the Matter: Communication between Hospitals and Patients*. London: HMSO.

Badenoch, J. (1986) Communication skills in medicine: the role of communication in medical practice. *Journal of the Royal Society of Medicine*, 79, pp. 565–7.

Baly, M., Robottom, B. and Clark, J. (1987) *District Nursing*. London: Heinemann Nursing.

Barnlund, D. (1976) The mystification of meaning: doctor–patient encounters. *Journal of Medical Education*, 51, pp. 716–25.

Bateson, B. Jackson, D. Haley, J. and Weakland, J. (1956) Toward a theory of schizophrenia. *Behavioural Science*, 1, pp. 251–64.

Beisecker, A. (1990) Patient power in doctor–patient communication: what do we know? *Health Communication*, 1, pp. 105–22.

Beisecker, A. and Thompson, T. (1995) The elderly patient–physician interaction. In J. Nussbaum and J. Coupland (eds), *Handbook of Communication and Ageing Research*. Mahwah, NJ: Lawrence Erlbaum Associates.

Benicki, A. and Leslie, F. (1983) The mental handicap nurse's specialist role. In A. Tierney (ed.), *Nurses and the Mentally Handicapped*. Chichester: Wiley & Sons.

Bergen, A. (1991) Nurses caring for the terminally ill: a review of the literature. *International Journal of Nursing Studies*, 28, pp. 89–101.

Berger, C. (1995) A plan-based approach to strategic communication. In D. Hewes (ed.), *The Cognitive Bases of Interpersonal Communication*. Hillsdale, NJ: Lawrence Erlbaum Associates.

Berger, C. (1994) Power, dominance and social interaction. In M. Knapp and G. Miller (eds.), *Handbook of Interpersonal Communication*. Thousand Oaks, Cal.: Sage.

Berne, E. (1964) *Games People Play*. Harmondsworth: Penguin.

Biley, F. (1989) Nurses' perception of stress in preoperative surgical patients, *Journal of Advanced Nursing*, 14, 575–81.

Bolton, R. (1995) Barriers to communication. In J. Stewart (ed.), *Bridges not Walls: A Book About Interpersonal Communication*. New York: McGraw-Hill.

Bourhis, R., Roth, S. and MacQueen, G. (1989) Communication in the hospital setting: a survey of medical and everyday language use amongst patients, nurses and doctors. *Social Science and Medicine*, 28, pp. 339–89.

Brown, P. and Levinson, S. (1978) Universals in language usage: politeness phenomena, in E. Goody (ed.), *Questions and Politeness: Strategies in Social Interaction*. Cambridge: Cambridge University Press.

Burgoon, J. (1994). Nonverbal signals. In M. Knapp and G. Miller (eds), *Handbook of Interpersonal Communication*. Thousand Oaks, Calif.: Sage.

Burgoon, M., Hunsaker, F. and Dawson, E. (1994) *Human Communication*. Thousand Oaks, Calif.: Sage.

Burley-Allen, M. (1995) *Listening: The Forgotten Skill*. New York: Wiley & Sons.

Canter, D. (1984) The environmental context of nursing: looking beyond the ward. In S. Skevington (ed.), *Understanding Nursing: The Social Psychology of Nursing*. Chichester: Wiley & Sons.

Chalabian, J. and Dunnington, G. (1997) Impact of language barrier on quality of patient care, resident stress, and teaching. *Teaching and Learning in Medicine*, 9, pp. 84–90.

Chalmers, K. and Luker, K. (1991) The development of the health visitor–client relationship. *Scandinavian Journal of Caring Science*, 5, pp. 33–41.

Coupland, N., Coupland, J. and Giles, H. (1991) *Language, Society and the Elderly*. Oxford: Blackwell.

Crockford, E., Holloway, I. and Walker, J. (1993) Nurses' perceptions of patients' feelings about breast surgery. *Journal of Advanced Nursing*, 18, pp. 1710–18.

Crute, V. (1986) *Microtraining in health visitor education: an intensive examination of training outcomes, feedback processes and individual differences*. Unpublished DPhil thesis, University of Ulster.

Cupach, W. and Spitzberg, B. (1994) *The Dark Side of Interpersonal Communication*. Hillsdale, NJ: Lawrence Erlbaum Associates.

Daly, J. and Wiemann, J. (eds) (1994) *Strategic Interpersonal Communication*. Hillsdale, NJ: Lawrence Erlbaum Associates.

Davidhizar, R., Giger, F. and Giger, J. (1997) When touch is not the best approach. *Journal of Clinical Nursing*, 6, pp. 203–6.

Davis, H. and Fallowfield, L. (1991) Counselling and communication in health care: the current situation. In H. Davis and L. Fallowfield (eds), *Counselling and Communication in Health Care*. Chichester: Wiley & Sons.

Derlega, V., Metts, S., Petronio, S. and Margulis, S. (1993) *Self-disclosure*. Newbury Park: Sage.

DeVito, J. (1988) *The Interpersonal Communication Book*. New York: Harper & Row.

Dickson, D. (1995) Communication and interpersonal skills. In D. Sines (ed.), *Community Health Care Nursing*. Oxford: Blackwell Science.

Dickson, D., Hargie, O. and Morrow, N. (1997) *Communication Skills Taining for Health Professionals*. London: Chapman & Hall.

Dillard, J. (1990) The nature and substance of goals in tactical communication, in M. Cody and M. McLaughlin (eds), *The Psychology of Tactical Communication*. Cleveland, England: Multilingual Matters.

DiMatteo, M. (1994) The physician–patient relationship: effects on the quality of health care. *Clinical Obstetrics and Gynaecology*, 37, pp. 149–61.

DiMatteo, M. and Friedman, H. (1982) *Social Psychology and Medicine*. Cambridge, Mass.: Oelgeschlager, Gunn & Hain.

Dimbleby, R. and Burton, G. (1985) *More than Words: An Introduction to Communication*. London: Methuen.

Dinkmeyer, D. (1971) Contributions to teleoanalytic theory and techniques to school counselling, in C. Beck (ed.), *Philosophical Guidelines for Counselling*. Dubuque, Iowa: W. S. Brown.

Elder, J. (1978) *Transactional Analysis in Health Care*. Cambridge, Mass.: Addison-Wesley.

Endler, N. and Magnusson, D. (eds) (1976) *Interactional Psychology and Personality*. Washington, DC: Hemisphere.

Epstein, R., Campbell, C., Cohen-Cole, S., McWhinney, I. and Smilkstein, G. (1993) Perspectives on patient–doctor communication. *Journal of Family Practice*, 37, pp. 377–88.

Ewles, L. and Simnett, I. (1992) *Promoting Health: A Practical Guide to Health Education*, 2nd edn. Chichester: Wiley & Sons.

Faulkner, A. (1992) *Effective Interaction with Patients*. Edinburgh: Churchill Livingstone.

Faulkner, A. (1993) *Teaching Interactive Skills in Health Care*. London: Chapman & Hall.

Faulkner, A. and Maguire, P. (1984) Teaching assessment skills. In A. Faulkner (ed.), *Recent Advances in Nursing, 7, Communication*. Edinburgh: Churchill Livingstone.

Forgas, J. (1985) *Interpersonal Behaviour*. Oxford: Pergamon.

French, P. (1994) *Social Skills for Nursing Practice*, 2nd edn. London: Chapman & Hall.

Giles, H. (1973) Accent mobility: a model and some data. *Anthropological Linguistics*, 15, pp. 87–105.

Giles, H., Williams, A. and Coupland, N. (1990) Language, health and the elderly: frameworks, agenda and a model. In H. Giles, N. Coupland and J. Wiemann (eds), *Communication, Health and the Elderly*. Manchester: Manchester University Press.

Goffman, E. (1959) *The Presentation of Self in Everyday Life*. Harmondsworth: Penguin.

Goffman, E. (1963) *Stigma: Notes on the Management of Spoiled Identity*. Harmondsworth: Penguin.

Grainger, K. (1995) Communication and the institutionalised elderly. In J. Nussbaum and J. Coupland (eds), *Handbook of Communication and Ageing Research*. Mahwah, NJ: Lawrence Erlbaum Associates.

Greenwood, J. (1993) The apparent desensitisation of student nurses during their professional socialisation: a cognitive perspective. *Journal of Advanced Nursing*, 18, pp. 1471–9.

Gudykunst, W. (1991) *Bridging Differences: Effective Intergroup Communication*. Newbury Park: Sage.

Hargie, O. and Marshall, P. (1986) Interpersonal communication: a theoretical framework. In O. Hargie (ed.), *A Handbook of Social Skills*. London: Croom Helm.

Hargie, O., Morrow, N. and Woodman, C. (1993) *Looking Into Community Pharmacy: Identifying Effective Communication Skills In Pharmacist–Patient Consultations*. Jordanstown: University of Ulster.

Hargie, O., Saunders, C. and Dickson, D. (1994) *Social Skills in Interpersonal Communication*. London: Routledge.

Haslett, B. and Ogilvie, J. (1988) Feedback processes in small groups, R. Cathcart and L. Samovar (eds), *Small Group Communication*. Dubuque, Iowa: W. C. Brown.

Heider, F. (1958) *The Psychology of Interpersonal Relations*. New York: Wiley & Sons.

Hewison, A. (1997) Nurses' power in interactions with patients. *Journal of Advanced Nursing*, 21, pp. 75–82.

Hill, C., Thompson, B., Cogar, M. and Denman, D. (1993) Beneath the surface of long-term therapy: therapist and client report of their own and each other's covert processes. *Journal of Counselling Psychology*, 40, pp. 278–87.

Hinton, P. (1993) *The Psychology of Interpersonal Perception.* London: Routledge.

HMSO (1995) *Health Services Commissioner for England, for Scotland and for Wales, Annual Report for 1994–5.* London: HMSO.

Hofstede, G. (1980) *Culture's Consequences: International Differences in Work-related Values.* Beverly Hills, Calif.: Sage.

Hogstel, M. (1987) Teaching students observational skills. *Nursing Outlook*, 35, pp. 89–91.

Holli, B. and Calabrese, R. (1991) *Communication and Education Skills: The Dietician's Guide.* Philadelphia, Penn.: Lea & Febiger.

Irving, P. (1995) *A reconceptualisation of Rogerian core conditions of facilitative communication: implications for training.* Unpublished DPhil thesis, University of Ulster, Jordanstown.

Johnson, M. (1982) Recognition of patients' worries by nurses and by other patients. *British Journal of Clinical Psychology*, 21, pp. 255–61.

Jones, E. and Gerard, H. (1967) *Foundations of Social Psychology.* New York: Wiley.

Jones, M., O'Neill, P., Waterman, H. and Webb, C. (1997) Building a relationship: communications and relationships between staff and stroke patients on a rehabilitation ward. *Journal of Advanced Nursing*, 26, pp. 101–10.

Jourard, S. (1964) *The Transparent Self.* Princeton, NJ: Van Nostrand.

Kaplan, S., Greenfield, S. and Ware, J. (1989) Assessing the effects of physician–patient interactions on the outcomes of chronic disease. *Medical Care*, 27, pp. 110–27.

Kellermann, K.(1992) Communication: inherently strategic and primarily automatic. *Communication Monographs*, 59, pp. 288–300.

Kenny, D. (1995) Determinants of patient satisfaction with the medical consultation. *Psychology and Health*, 10, pp. 427–37.

Knapp, M. and Hall, J. (1992) *Nonverbal Communication in Human Interaction.* New York: Holt, Rinehart & Winston.

Kralik, D., Koch, T. and Wotton, K. (1997) Engagement and detachment: understanding patients' experiences with nurses. *Journal of Advanced Nursing*, 26, pp. 399–407.

Kreps, G. (1988) The pervasive role of information in health and health care: implications for health care policy. In J. Anderson (ed.), *Communication Yearbook 11.* Beverly Hills, Calif.: Sage.

Kreps, G. and Thornton, B. (1992) *Health Communication: Theory and Practice*. Prospect Heights, Ill.: Waveland Press.

Lane, P. (1989) Nurse–patient perceptions: the double standard of touch. *Issues of Mental Health Nursing*, 10, pp. 1–13.

Lang, G. and van der Molen, H. (1990) *Personal Conversations: Roles and Skills for Counsellors*. London: Routledge.

Langer, E., Blank, A. and Chanowitz, B. (1978) The mindlessness of ostensibly thoughtful action *Journal of Personality and Social Psychology*, 36, pp. 635–42.

Ley, P. (1988) *Communication with Patients: Improving Communication, Satisfaction and Compliance*. London: Croom Helm.

Lillie, F. (1985) The wider social context of interpersonal skills in nursing. In C. Kagan (ed.), *Interpersonal Skills in Nursing: Research and Application*. London: Croom Helm.

McCann, K. and McKenna, H. (1993) An examination of touch between nurses and elderly patients in a continuing care setting in Northern Ireland. *Journal of Advanced Nursing*, 18, pp. 838–946.

McIntee, J. and Firth, H. (1984) How to beat the burnout. *Health and Social Services Journal*, 9 February, pp. 166–8.

McIntosh, J. (1981) Communicating with patients in their own homes. In W. Briggs and J. MacLeod Clark (eds), *Communication in Nursing Care*. Aylesbury: HM&M.

MacLeod Clark, J. (1982) *Nurse–patient verbal interaction: an analysis of recorded conversations on selected surgical wards*. Unpublished PhD thesis, University of London.

MacLeod Clark, J. (1984) Verbal communication in nursing. In A. Faulkner (ed.), *Recent Advances in Nursing, 7, Communication*. Edinburgh: Churchill Livingstone.

MacLeod Clark, J. (1985) The development of research in interpersonal skills in nursing. In C. Kagan (ed.), *Interpersonal Skills in Nursing: Research and Application*. London: Croom Helm.

Maguire, P. (1981) Doctor–patient skills. In M. Argyle (ed.), *Social Skills and Health*. London: Methuen.

May, C. (1990) Research on nurse–patient relationships: problems of theory, problems of practice. *Journal of Advanced Nursing*, 15, pp. 307–15.

Meikle, M. and Holley, S. (1991) Communication with patients in residence. In M. Denham (ed.), *Care of the Long-stay Elderly Patient*. London: Chapman & Hall.

Meredith, P. (1993) Patient satisfaction with communication in general surgery. *Social Science and Medicine*, 37, pp. 591–602.

Morrison, E. (1990) Violent psychiatric inpatients in a public hospital. *Scholarly Inquiry for Nursing Practice*, 4, pp. 65–82.

Morrison, P. and Burnard, P. (1989) Students' and trained nurses' perceptions of their own interpersonal skills: a report and comparison, *Journal of Advanced Nursing*, 14, pp. 321–9.

Mortensen, C. (1997) *Miscommunication*. Thousand Oaks, Calif.: Sage.

Munton, R. (1990) Client satisfaction with community psychiatric nursing. In C. Brooker (ed.), *Community Psychiatric Nursing*. London: Chapman & Hall.

Myers, G. and Myers, M. (1985) *The Dynamics of Human Communication*. New York: McGraw-Hill.

Newell, R. (1994) *Interviewing Skills for Nurses and Other Health Care Professionals. A Structured Approach*. London: Routledge.

Ng, S. and Bradac, J. (1993) *Power in Language: Verbal Communication and Social Influence*. Newbury Park: Sage.

Noble, C. (1991) Are nurses good patient educators? *Journal of Advanced Nursing*, 16, pp. 1185–9.

Northouse, P. and Northouse, L. (1992) *Health Communication: Strategies for Health Professionals*. Norwalk, Conn.: Appleton & Lange.

Nussbaum, J. and Coupland, J. (eds) (1995) *Handbook of Communication and Ageing Research*. Mahwah, NJ: Lawrence Erlbaum Associates.

Oakes, P., Haslam, S. and Turner, J. (1994) *Stereotyping and Social Reality*. Oxford: Blackwell Press.

O'Connor, J. and Seymour, J. (1990) *Introducing Neuro-linguistic Programming: The New Psychology of Personal Excellence*. London: Mandala.

Olsen, D. (1997) When the patient causes the problem: the effect of patient responsibility on the nurse–patient relationship. *Journal of Advanced Nursing*, 26, pp. 515–22.

Ong, L., de Haes, J., Hoos, A. and Lammes, F. (1995) Doctor–patient communication: a review of the literature. *Social Science and Medicine*, 40, pp. 903–18.

Orr, J. (1992) The community dimension. In K. Luker and J. Orr, (1992) *Health Visiting: Towards Community Health Nursing*. Oxford: Blackwell Science.

Payer, L. (1988) *Medicine and Culture*. New York: Penguin.

Pettegrew, L. (1982) Some boundaries and assumptions in health care. In L. Pettegrew, P. Arnston, D. Bush and K. Zoppi (eds), *Straight Talk: Explorations in Provider and Patient Interaction*. Louisville, Humana.

Pinker, S. (1994) *The Language Instinct*. London: Penguin.

Pitcairn, T., Clemie, S., Gray, J. and Pentland, B. (1990) Non-verbal cues in the self-expression of Parkinsonian patients. *British Journal of Clinical Psychology*, 29, pp. 177–84.

Pollock, L. (1987) *Psychiatric nursing in the community: a study of a working situation*. Unpublished PhD thesis, Edinburgh University.

Ray, E. and Miller, K. (1993) Communication in health care organisations. In E. Ray and L. Donohew (eds), *Communication and Health: Systems and Applications*. Hillsdale, NY: Lawrence Erlbaum Associates.

Rogers, C. R. (1961) *On Becoming a Person: A Therapist's View of Psychotherapy*. Boston, Mass.: Houghton Mifflin.

Rogers, W. (1991) *Explaining Health and Illness*. New York: Harvester Wheatsheaf.

Roter, D. and Hall, J. (1992) *Doctors Talking with Patients/Patients Talking with Doctors: Improving Communication in Medical Visits*. Westport, Conn.: Auburn House.

Roter, D., Lipkin, M. and Korsgaard, A. (1991) Sex differences in patients' and physicians' communication during primary care medical visits. *Medical Care*, 29, pp. 1083–93.

Ruben, B. (1990) The health caregiver–patient relationship: pathology, aetiology, treatment. In E. Ray and L. Donohew (eds), *Communication and Health: Systems and Applications*. Hillsdale, NJ.: Lawrence Erlbaum.

Ryan, E. and Butler, R. (1996) Communication, ageing and health: towards understanding health provider relationships with older clients. *Health Communication*, 8, pp. 191–7.

Samora, J., Saunders, L. and Karson, R. (1961) Medical vocabulary knowledge among hospital patients. *Journal of Health and Human Behaviour*, 2, pp. 83-92.

Satir, V. (1976) *Peoplemaking*. Centre City, Minn.: Hazelden Foundation.

Saunders, C. (1986) Opening and closing. In O. Hargie (ed.), *A Handbook of Communication Skills*. London: Croom Helm.

Scharfstein, B. (1993) *Ineffability: The Failure of Words in Philosophy and Religion*. Albany: State University of New York.

Seale, C. (1992) Community nurses and the care of the dying. *Social Science and Medicine*, 34, pp. 375–82.

Sharf, B. (1993) Reading the vital signs: research in health care communication. *Communication Monographs*, 60, pp. 35–41.

Shulman, L. (1992) *The Skills of Helping Individuals, Families, and Groups*. Ithaca, Ill.: Peacock Publishers.

Skipper, M. (1992) *Communication processes and their effectiveness in the management and treatment of dysphagia*. Unpublished DPhil thesis, University of Ulster.

Sloan, D., Donnelly, M., Johnson, S., Schwartz, R. and Strodel, W.(1994) Assessing surgical residents' and medical students' interpersonal skills. *Journal of Surgical Research*, 57, pp. 613–18.

Smith, P. and Bond, M. (1993) *Social Psychology Across Cultures*. Hemel Hempstead: Harvester Wheatsheaf.

Snyder, M. (1987) *Public Appearances, Private Realities*. New York.: Freeman Press.

Steel, L. (1991) Interpersonal correlates of trust and self-disclosure. *Psychological Reports*, 68, pp. 1319–20.

Stein, L. (1968) The doctor/nurse game. *American Journal of Nursing*, 68, pp. 1–5.

Stewart, M. (1995) Effective physician–patient communication and health outcomes: a review. *Canadian Medical Association*, 152, pp. 1423–33.

Stewart, M. and Roter, D. (1989) Introduction. In M. Stewart and D. Roter (eds). *Communicating with Medical Patients*. Newbury Park, Calif.: Sage.

Tannen, D. (1995) Asymmetries: women and men talking at cross-purposes. In J. Stewart (ed.) *Bridges not Walls: A Book About Interpersonal Communication*. New York: McGraw-Hill.

Thompson, T. (1990) Patient health care: issues in interpersonal communication. In E. Ray and L. Donohew (eds), *Communication and Health: Systems and Applications*. Hillsdale, NJ.: Lawrence Erlbaum Associates.

Thompson, T. (1994) Interpersonal communication and health care. In M. Knapp and G. Miller (eds), *Handbook of Interpersonal Communication*. Thousand Oaks, Calif.: Sage.

Tourish, D. and Irving, P. (1995) Integrated communications perspectives and the practice of total quality management. *International Journal of Health Care Quality Assurance*, 8, pp. 7–14.

Trojan, L. and Yonge, O. (1993) Developing trusting, caring relationship: home care nurses and elderly clients. *Journal of Advanced Nursing*, 18, pp. 1903–10.

von Friederichs-Fitzwater, M., Callahan, E., Flynn, N., and Williams, J. (1991) Relational control in physician–patient encounters. *Health Communication*, 3, pp. 17–36.

Whitcher, S. and Fisher, J. (1979) Multi-dimensional reactions to therapeutic touch in a hospital setting. *Journal of Personality and Social Psychology*, 37, pp. 87–96.

Wilkinson, S. (1991) Factors which influence how nurses communicate with cancer patients. *Journal of Advanced Nursing*, 16, pp. 677–88.

Wilmot, W. (1987) *Dyadic Communication*. New York: Random House.

Wilmot, W. (1995) The transactional nature of person perception. In J. Stewart (ed.), *Bridges not Walls: A Book About Interpersonal Communication*. New York: McGraw-Hill.

Zebrowitz, L. (1990) *Social Perception*. Milton Keynes: Open University Press.

CHAPTER FIVE

Counselling for Effective Practice

Owen Barr

INTRODUCTION

Fundamental to successful nursing interventions is the community nurses' ability to communicate effectively with the people they come in contact with during the course of their work. Across all branches of community nursing, the knowledge and skills required to efficiently exchange information in an appropriate manner with clients, their families and other members of the interdisciplinary team are essential. Advanced skills in interaction, therefore, are crucial for the accurate understanding of information received from and provided to clients and their families. Moreover, successful communication exchanges facilitate the development and maintenance of trust and respect in the therapeutic relationship and during all stages of the caring process. Mutual trust between nurses, clients, families and other members of the interdisciplinary team, therefore, is an essential prerequisite for the development and delivery of a partnership approach when providing coordinated health and social services (Audit Commission 1989).

Community nurses have sustained contact with clients and their families, possibly over a period of weeks, months, or even years. The nature of their involvement usually brings them into close contact with most of the individual's carers, either directly by face-to-face interaction, or through finding out about other family members during discussions with the client. The increased level of involvement with family members and the need to acknowledge and work within complex family dynamics further highlight the importance of community nurses having effective interpersonal skills (Cain, 1995).

A central tenet within the current ethos of community nursing is the development of partnerships with clients and their families, encompassing the role of the community nurse in facilitating the empowerment of clients and their families. Although much debate exists about the precise nature of 'partnership' and its essential components (Cain, 1995; Dale, 1996), it is widely accepted that collegial partnerships are based on effective two-way communication. Recognition of the need for community nurses to have appropriate interpersonal skills has been well-documented (Dickson, 1995). This has been further emphasised by the introduction of specific learning outcomes for specialist nursing practice that highlight the importance of nurses developing and utilising appropriate interpersonal skills in their nursing practice (UKCC, 1994).

In addition to a well-developed knowledge of and ability to utilise interpersonal skills, community health care nurses are also expected to provide 'counselling and psychological support for individuals and their carers' (UKCC, 1994, p. 11). This requires community nurses to develop additional areas of knowledge and skills specific to understanding the nature of counselling and its use when working with clients and their families. Community nurses are frequently attributed with providing counselling for the people they visit, but this aspect of their role is usually very loosely defined and needs further clarification. This chapter is designed to focus on the nature of counselling and specific associated issues related to the role of community health care nurses. It is not a chapter on 'how to do counselling'. Rather, it seeks to clarify some of the misconceptions and vagueness that currently abound about this activity.

THE NATURE OF COUNSELLING

Interpersonal skills

Important distinctions as well as interrelationships that exist between interpersonal skills, helping skills, counselling skills and the provision of counselling have been outlined by some authors (Inskipp, 1996; Feltham, 1995; Burnard, 1994). These attempts to clarify distinctions are not supported by all the writers hence they remain a topic of much discussion and debate. However, they do raise issues that have implications for nurses and their ability to more fully understand their interpersonal actions.

It is possible to view interpersonal skills, helping skills, counselling skills and the provision of counselling at different levels on a communication continuum. At one end interpersonal skills form the *tools* necessary for effective communication and, at the other end, counselling involves specific *actions* to help people bring about change in their lives.

Interpersonal skills have been defined by Hargie (1986, p. 12) as:

'a set of goal directed, interrelated, situationally appropriate social behaviours (that can be learned and are under the control of the individual).'

This definition recognises the important match that exists between interpersonal skills used and the social context. Key interpersonal skills include: the ability to commence an interaction successfully; listening; communicating non-verbally; providing explanations; asking appropriate questions; giving and accepting praise and other forms of reinforcement; reflecting a person's thoughts and feelings; assertiveness; the ability to work effectively in groups; and to close interactions in a competent manner (Hargie *et al.*, 1994). So far it has been recognised that communicating with other people is a dynamic process that is influenced by a number of factors which arise from within the person and also from the environment in which the interaction is taking place (Hargie *et al.*, 1994). Further details on interpersonal skills have been discussed in Chapter 1.

Counselling has also been listed as an interpersonal skill by Burnard (1996). However, it is not a single category of skill. Counselling is a complex combination of several interrelated interpersonal skills. In essence effective interpersonal skills can be viewed as the foundation on which effective counselling is built. In other words they are the *tools* required for the successful delivery of counselling.

Nurses need to recognise the complexities inherent in interpersonal relationships and guard against the risk of viewing interactions in an oversimplified manner. All nurses have considerable experience in communicating with a diverse range of people across a large number of settings during the course of their work. This experience can be further advanced by paying careful attention to the internal and external factors that impact on their interpersonal communication at any given moment. Hence nurses should have the abilities to adapt their skills to increase communication effectiveness in relation to the goals of their interaction.

Helping skills

Community nurses regularly provide psychological support to the individuals and carers they work with across all branches of community nursing. The nature and degree of the support provided will be influenced by people's circumstances, their abilities and, to some extent, the needs of the nurse. Heron (1986) outlined the six-category intervention analysis that provides a communication framework consisting of three authoritative and three facilitative intervention categories. One or a possible variation of all six may be utilised depending on the level of psychological support to be provided by one person to another.

Within this framework nurses may be viewed as acting in authoritative ways by: offering advice (prescriptive); instructing or giving information (informative); or challenging aspects of a client's behaviour or thinking (confronting). Within the facilitative domain nurses may help individuals: express their feelings and anxieties more clearly (cathartic); encourage them to think about what they are doing and thinking in a manner that moves them into action (catalytic); or offer feedback, words of encouragement and personal recognition (supportive).

It is important to recognise that authoritative interventions, according to Heron, are not necessarily negative, nor are they always less desirable to use than facilitative interventions. The reverse is also true. The effectiveness of an intervention is more related to the match between the individuals involved, the situation they are in and the agreed goals of intervention. Nurses need to be able to recognise how their communication may fall into different categories from those they expected and later reflect upon the implications of this on their continuing relationship with clients and others involved. All categories of helping can be valuable when utilised appropriately, taking consideration of individuals' abilities and needs in their specific situations.

It has been reported that the most frequent intervention provided by nurses within the six-category analysis is the facilitative action of being supportive and providing encouragement (Burnard and Morrison, 1988, 1989). However, in these studies it was also found that nurses were more likely to act in the authoritative and directive modes of providing information and being prescriptive about advice than to utilise catalytic and cathartic interventions. Across the six categories nurses were most reluctant about acting in a confrontational manner (Burnard and Morrison, 1988, 1989). The findings of these studies are not surprising as they reflect the culture in which nurses currently work which stresses the importance of information provision, advice-giving, and the increasingly rapid 'treatment' of clients. This encourages the use of a directive focus in our work and at the same time discourages the use of facilitative interventions that are likely to be more time-consuming.

Despite this, nurses must recognise that all categories of helping can be valuable when utilised appropriately, giving due consideration to individuals' abilities and needs within the context of their specific situations. The above six-category interventions provide a communication framework for analysis of the nature and level of interventions. They may, therefore, involve the use of some counselling skills in the process. They do not, however, fully explain the nature of counselling.

Counselling skills

A reference to counselling is usually to be found among the listed roles of community nurses across all branches of community nursing. This is more prominent in areas that have strong association with offering psychological support such as community mental health and community learning disability nursing. District nurses often work closely with families in the provision of support for clients and in so doing they provide psychological support for both clients and carers. In health visiting psychological support is often provided to parents (predominantly mothers) and more recently psychological support is evident in the work of community children's nurses. Similarly, school nurses also provide support to teenagers. Occupational health nurses too provide psychological support, including the use of relaxation and stress management techniques for employees who use their service. Psychological support is also recognised as a component of the work of general practice nurses and is prominent within all nursing activities related to the provision of health promotion.

It is accepted that some nurses have undertaken additional education and training in counselling following their primary nursing qualification and this extra training should have prepared them more appropriately for a counselling role. For example, some counselling courses are designed in specific areas such as bereavement, abuse and coping with addictions. Other courses may be broad-based, focusing on a range of counselling techniques. However, despite the assertions that counselling is clearly a component of the nurse's role, the degree to which nurses actually *counsel* clients and carers in the course of their work remains open to question.

Betts (1995, p. 123) argues that:

'most nurses and midwives are not counsellors, but are professional helpers whose work includes to a greater or lesser degree providing psychological support to people who are experiencing a diversity of personally significant events.'

This position is supported by Burnard (1995, p. 261) who states:

'most nurses use counselling skills as part of their daily work; every time they sit down to talk something through with a patient . . . to act as a counsellor, however, is quite different.'

It has been argued that the use of counselling skills differs from both the use of listening skills alone and the provision of counselling (BAC, 1990). It is proposed that distinctions can be drawn according to the intention of the user and the perception of the client. The British Association of Counselling (1990) argues:

'what distinguishes the use of counselling skills from these other two activities [listening and counselling] are the intentions of the user, which is to enhance the performance of their functional role.'

For example, when nurses use skills such as listening, reflecting and questioning to increase the accuracy in their understanding of what clients are feeling or how they perceive their situation, then nurses are using counselling skills. Nurses may also use such skills in discussions with other members of the interdisciplinary team, for example, to help colleagues express how they are feeling during difficult or traumatic events in their work setting. In so doing they are using more than listening skills; *and yet they are not counselling their colleagues*. Using counselling skills can only become *pure counselling* when: 'the user and the recipient explicitly contract to enter a counselling relationship' (BAC, 1990). Contract in this sense does not always mean a written and formally agreed document (although it may take this form). It relates to the need for both parties involved to reach an agreement on roles, boundaries and the negotiation of objectives to be achieved during the period of counselling.

In essence counselling skills are a subsystem of interpersonal skills such as listening, questioning, reflection and empathy which are used for a particular purpose to offer psychological support. However, when nurses choose to use these 'counselling' activities to enhance their communication with clients without taking on the counselling role, then they are *only using counselling skills.*

Furthermore, when clients perceive nurses to be acting within their usual caring role (and not explicitly as counsellors) then once again it is argued that nurses are utilising counselling skills in the process (BAC, 1990).

As noted earlier some overlap does exist between the use of counselling skills and the provision of counselling. Nurses may pause here and reflect on their own actions and intentions and attempt to clarify for themselves if they are indeed counselling or merely using counselling skills. It is important to stress that the effective use of counselling skills can be a valuable activity if used competently; and as a by-product they may also help clients to move forward in their life.

However, there are some risks associated with using only counselling skills. In particular, clients may disclose some information relating to past traumas that nurses using counselling skills may find difficult to deal with in a brief situation. Therefore, it is essential for nurses who use counselling skills to think about what they would do if such information was presented to them unexpectedly. How might they, for example, ask clients' permission to refer them to a counsellor.

It is essential in relation to counselling also that when nurses are using counselling skills, they must operate within the *Guidelines for Professional Practice* (UKCC, 1996) and their *Code of Professional Conduct* (UKCC, 1992a), and give particular attention to personal responsibility for their actions, maintaining competence in their practice, careful management of their work, and client confidentiality (BAC, 1990).

The boundaries between the use of counselling skills and the provision of counselling remain somewhat blurred and have been challenged by some authors as imprecise and unhelpful (Burnard, 1996; Howard, 1996). It has been argued that the emphasis on the

139

distinction between counselling skills and counselling as an activity has more to do with serving the interests of those who wish to professionalise counselling and hence place restrictions on other professionals who can and do provide counselling, and less to do with interest in promoting the well-being of clients (Howard, 1996). A closer examination of the definition and nature of counselling may help clarify these issues further.

COUNSELLING

A considerable range of definitions that attempt to clarify the nature of counselling exist (see Box 5.1). Box 5.1 shows that some definitions focus on the aims of counselling, some highlight the role of the counsellor and what they attempt to do, and others summarise the features of a counselling relationship (Burnard, 1996). Implicit in most of the definitions is the message that counselling seeks to help clients help themselves. It aims to promote respect for the client's autonomy and seeks to promote healthy functioning largely through a problem-solving focus (Feltham, 1995).

In counselling, the intention is to facilitate client change, at their pace and in the direction they choose to move. This contrasts with the use of counselling skills, in which a key focus tends to be on increasing the functional role of the person by using counselling skills. If client change occurs as the result of this, it is likely to be a by-product and not a primary intention of the interactions.

Furthermore, counselling has been distinguished from the use of counselling skills by its use of the following criteria:

- the focus within counselling on facilitation;
- the negotiation of an agreement between the counsellor and counsellee on clear roles within the counselling situation;
- the ownership of personal and professional accountability;
- through knowledge of professional boundaries; and,
- the development of a clear understanding and competent application of psychological theories related to practice. (Feltham and Dryden, 1993; Bond, 1993).

Counsellors have to carefully suppress any personal desire to 'help' clients make decisions and/or to make decisions for them,

Box 5.1 Definitions of counselling

'Counseling is the "ing" word: it denotes an activity or series of activies in which the helper and client engage. The activity, however, has value only to the degree that it leads to valued outcome in the client's day to day life.'
(Egan, 1994, p. 7)

'the process of counselling is the means by which one person helps another to clarify his or her life situation and to decide further lines of action.'
(Burnard, 1994, p. 4)

'counselling is a principled relationship characterised by the application of one or more psychological theories and a recognised set of communication skills, modified by experience, intuition and other interpersonal factors, to client's intimate concerns, problems or aspirations. Its predominant ethos is one of facilition rather than advise giving or coercion . . . is more disciplined and confidential than friendship, and perhaps less stigmatising than helping offered in traditional medical or psychiatric settings.'
(Feltham and Dryden, 1993, p. 31)

'the skilled and principled use of relationships which develops self-knowledge, emotional acceptance, growth and personal resources. The overall aim is to live more fully and satisfyingly. The counsellor's role is to facilitate the client's work in ways that respect the client's values, personal resources and capacity for self-determination.'
(British Assocation of Counselling, 1990, p. 1)

'a process whose aim is to help clients who are mainly seen outside medical settings, to help themselves by making better choices and becoming better choosers. The helper's repertoire of skills includes those of forming an understanding relationship, as well as interventions focused on helping clients change spacific aspects of their feeling, thinking and acting.'
(Nelson-Jones, 1993, p. 4)

especially when clients are overtly signalling for them to do so. For example, clients may ask: 'What would you do, nurse?' They may also state: 'Whatever you think is best, nurse, that's what I'll do.' The emphasis embraced within counselling is on facilitating clients to become stronger and, therefore, more confident and personally skilled at making their own decisions. At times this is a long and ardous process, as opposed to a focus on getting decisions made as quickly as possible. Feltham and Dryden (1993) emphasise in their definition of counselling that the 'predominant ethos is one of facilitation rather than of advice giving or coercion' (p. 31).

The authors did recognise, however, that clients will be provided with information and may on occasions be challenged to support their beliefs or actions. However, the rationale for counsellors using these skills must be to facilitate clients' personal decision-making processes as well as their personal growth and development.

Fundamental within the counselling relationship is the belief that clients are awarded the central position. They are involved in negotiating all steps to be taken and outcomes to be reached. Both counsellor and counsellee agree on role boundaries and pace the process appropriately to match clients' needs.

Outcomes should be founded on clients' targets for achievement and not service-led priorities which are often based on the quantity of people visited by nurses and not on the quality of progress clients make.

Central to the success of counselling, and essential to the successful achievement of the agreed targets, is an understanding, by both the counsellor and counsellee, of what their roles and boundaries (often blurred) are. This does not require a formal signed contract, but necessitates that both the client and the counsellor agree to what is expected early in the initial counselling interview and decide what each person will be required to work through for the successful achievement of targets that have been set. The nature of the agreed roles may be influenced by a variety of personal and wider social factors, such as:

- clients' expectations of what counselling involves and their own role;
- their previous experience of counselling;
- their perception of the counsellor;
- their expectations of the counsellor (this in turn will be influenced by the title the counsellor may have, such as nurse);

- the reason for attending counselling; and
- the setting in which the session takes place.

Nurses who adopt a counselling role remain subject to the *Code of Professional Conduct* (UKCC, 1992a), *The Scope of Professional Practice* (UKCC, 1992b), and the *Guidelines for Professional Practice* (UKCC, 1996). These professional documents provide guidance on a broad range of issues relating to professional nursing practice and are also pertinent to nurses who provide counselling. In particular, cognisance must be taken of the need to act in the client's best interests, observe confidentiality, maintain competence (in counselling), obtain informed consent and work in a cooperative manner.

Further to the above UKCC documents, the British Association of Counselling has produced a *Code of Ethics and Practice* for people who provide counselling which has the stated aim of providing 'a framework for addressing ethical issues and encouraging optimum levels of practice' (BAC, 1990). This code provides specific guidance in relation to the key ethical and practice issues relating to:

- client safety (in particular, non-exploitation);
- accurate pre-counselling information;
- the need for clear contracts;
- maintaining competence;
- client autonomy;
- the safety of the counsellor;
- the counsellor's responsibility to other counsellors and members of the health care professions (being clear about what is and what is not being offered in counselling) and to the wider community; supervision of counsellors;
- advertising; and
- conducting research. (BAC, 1990)

Finally, and of utmost importance, counselling differs from interpersonal skills, helping skills and counselling skills in that counselling requires an understanding and competent integration of a range of counselling theories and frameworks with practice. Three key components of a theory exist; first, the assumptions of the theory; second, the definitions of terms and concepts; and third, the interrelationship between the concepts (Patterson, 1986). An examination of theories of counselling shows they provide a solid foundation for understanding why difficulties and growth blocks may occur within individuals. They also attempt to explain how people can be helped to overcome such growth blocks, change and move forward from their difficulties.

Several hundred individual therapies now exist in the counselling literature. However, the majority of these can be traced back to one of the four main psychological schools of thought, namely, psycho-analytic, behavioural, cognitive and humanistic approaches. The fifth grouping is that of combining a number of approaches to counselling to form an eclectic and integrative approach. It is recognised that valuable contributions to counselling have arisen from existential phenomenology, feminism, construct and systems theories. These approaches will not be covered in this chapter (see Woolfe and Dryden, 1996, for a detailed consideration of additional approaches). This chapter will continue by focusing on the four main approaches as an introduction to some main counselling theories.

COUNSELLING THEORIES

It is important to recognise that our understanding of people as individuals and their psychological processes is continuously being up-dated and new information is constantly being added to explain how and why people behave in particular ways. One theory tends to build on previous theories and ideas that have already existed hence they add new insights, often with a slightly different focus, but they also include areas of overlap. This pattern can be noted in the development and interrelationships between the theories now being examined relating to counselling. History shows a progression from the mainly psychoanalytic approaches through to cognitive ap-proaches. As you continue reading, consider which approach you might use when responding to a person who has anxiety-related problems.

Key differences can be distinguished across the four main approaches to counselling in relation to: the perspective on the person; the origins of the problems requiring counselling interven-tion; the aims and process of therapy; the role of the counsellor; and the role of the client (Corey, 1995).

The psychoanalytic approach to counselling

Within the psychoanalytic (or Freudian) approach, people's actions are viewed as being driven by internal unconscious forces that are striving to achieve personal desires (Patterson, 1986). These forces are strong and are viewed as having sexual and aggressive impulses that drive the person through the five stages of psychosexual development (Freud, 1974). During the process of development people establish their relationships with their parents and their own sexuality, and are socialised into what is perceived as socially acceptable behaviour. This often involves the need to temper strong unconscious impulses through the use of unconscious 'mental defence mechanisms'. Examples of these may be *repressing* one's feelings, *sublimating* antisocial behaviour into more socially acceptable channels, or *displacing* one's negative energies into other activities.

Early childhood experiences and the degree to which people have successfully managed to complete each psychosexual stage of development influences their adult personality and behaviour. Within the psychoanalytic approach, problems such as anxiety are viewed as arising in adulthood because of failure to successfully complete the earlier stages of development. According to Freud (1974), this results in unresolved internal conflicts which in turn cause anxiety and other difficulties related to functioning successfully as an adult. Due to the unconscious and repressed nature of these unresolved conflicts clients are unaware of the impact these earlier life experiences have had on their current behaviour.

Using the psychoanalytic approach the therapist works to establish a clear picture of the client's early development and life experiences and through this attempts to uncover previous repressed conflicts in the person's life. This involves clients talking freely about their early experiences and the therapist analysing the significance of this information for their early development. The therapist is very much in the role of *the expert* when using this approach and the client is passive in relation to gaining insight through uncovering their earlier, unresolved difficulties.

Much debate continues about the merits and limitations of Freudian theory that forms the foundation of the psychoanalytic approach to counselling. Indeed Freud's theory has been challenged on at least two counts; (1) it is impossible to replicate it; and (2) it has a limited scientific foundation (Masson, 1992). However, it has made a large impact on counselling and the theory is present in any approach that seeks to identify how painful experiences in early childhood may unconsciously influence adult behaviour.

The behavioural approach to counselling

The behavioural approach to counselling was, in many ways, a response to what was seen as the vagueness and biases inherent in the psychoanalytic approaches (Lazarus, 1971; Bandura, 1977; Wolpe, 1982). Behavioural approaches sought to develop a scientific approach to the provision of counselling and emphasised the need for objectivity. They rejected the personal analysis of early childhood experiences by therapists.

Within the behavioural approach, it was viewed that people had problems as the result of learning behaviour through past experiences, which were conscious as opposed to unconscious experiences. It is asserted that people learn through the process of reinforcement, in that those previous behaviours that have been positively reinforced by pleasant consequences will be repeated and over a period of time become part and parcel of people's repertoires of behaviour. On the other hand, those behaviours that have unpleasant consequences and, therefore, have been negatively reinforced, are less likely to be repeated and become established. This is known as operant conditioning (Skinner, 1974). Through this process people can learn adaptive behaviours that assist them in their successful functioning in society. Examples of adaptive coping mechanisms are problem-solving skills, effective interpersonal skills, how to resolve conflicts and how to manage stressful situations.

Equally, people may learn maladaptive behaviours that may have originally had 'positive consequences' and thus provided ways of coping. Examples of maladaptive mechanisms are: using aggression to get what they want; ignoring a problem in the hope that it will go away; investing all their time and energy into work (to the detriment of their family life) and outwardly believing this is the main way to achieve success.

Using the behavioural approach to counselling, the behaviour displayed when the person is anxious would be viewed as having an important role and function. Therefore, the consequences of this specific behaviour (or collection of behaviours) are in some way positive for the client. Attempts would be made, therefore, to assess in detail the antecedent to the behaviour, the behaviour and its consequences. Counselling continues with *teaching* clients new techniques and behaviours aimed at the more adaptive management of anxiety-provoking situations. This in turn, will reduce the need to use the previous maladaptive behaviours.

In the behavioural approach, the objective is to assist clients to learn new and more adaptive coping mechanisms and overt behaviours. The focus in therapy is on current behaviours and how the person can learn to function more effectively in their present environment. This is achieved through the identification of what triggers people to behave in a particular way, and what reinforces their behaviour. Clients are then set tasks by therapists that are designed to demonstrate to clients that their behaviours can change and alternative and more adaptive behaviours can be learned.

Although the therapist and the client work together to some degree to identify the behaviours to be learned and agree on targets to be achieved, the therapist is a type of 'teacher' directing the process. The behavioural approach permits therapists to objectively measure overt behaviours and to demonstrate the successful learning of new behaviours. Scientific data can be collated without the therapist ever knowing what is going on in the mind of the client. The behavioural approach is also biased towards clients taking action; it highlights that only through taking action (as opposed to talking about their difficulties) and monitoring consequences can clients learn.

However, the behavioural approach has been criticised because it has been viewed as treating merely symptoms, that is, the maladaptive behaviour, and possibly failing to address deeper causes of problems (Corey, 1995). Furthermore, the approach has been challenged due to the directive role of the therapist and the failure to adequately acknowledge cognitive processes in the learning of behaviours. Subsequent approaches, namely, person-centred and cognitive approaches, sought to correct these limitations.

The person-centred approach to counselling

Carl Rogers (1962) is probably the name most associated with counselling in the mind of the public. He popularised the person-centred approach to counselling as an alternative to what he viewed as the professionalised and expert-led approaches evident in psychoanalytic and behavioural approaches. As the name suggests, the focus within this approach is on perceiving clients as human beings who are 'pre-programmed' to move forward in life towards self-realisation, healing and recovery. Clients/persons, therefore, play a very active role in identifying the issues they wish to address in counselling as well as the targets they wish to achieve. Central to this approach is the belief that all human beings are inherently capable of becoming 'fully functioning' mature people, that is, human beings who are open to experience and are rational, who accept responsibility, and who value themselves and other people. Being human means acknowledging our dependence on others as well as accepting our independence and uniqueness. In addition, people value their own abilities and natural resources and possess a high degree of self-awareness (Rogers, 1962).

An examination of the person-centred perspective shows that problems arise for people when they become overly concerned about being evaluated by other people and by not living up to their expectations. Hence they set very high goals for themselves, goals they are rarely able to live up to. This may result in individuals denying or distorting reality and behaving in a way inconsistent with reality and, therefore, inconsistent with their self-concept. Examples of this may include: hiding feelings from friends and families; not paying attention to one's own feelings; not being true to oneself; and not valuing one's own abilities, needs and individuality.

This preoccupation with what they believe other people's perceptions of them to be can result in individuals always trying to please others and in so doing 'wearing different masks' to suit the occasion and appearing to be something they are not. The confusion and turmoil resulting from being overly concerned about what other people think and the heightened concern over being judged and evaluated by other people would be viewed as the origin of the client's anxiety.

Within person-centred therapy the focus is on the counsellor being warm, genuine and accepting of clients as valued individuals. The counsellor is required to have the ability to demonstrate empathy with clients in their life situations. The aim is not to change people by the use of techniques, or by setting tasks to be completed. Rather, this approach stresses that the counsellor should endeavour to accompany clients as they move through the process of self-discovery, recovery and healing. During the counselling process, clients' self-awareness is enhanced through the sharing of their life histories and their painful experiences. Great emphasis is placed on the need for counsellors to be open and sincere with clients and to refrain from taking on the persona of an expert.

Hence the interaction between therapist and client must always be a 'human with human' experience.

Counsellors using this approach may spend long periods of time in silence, listening attentively to clients and encouraging them to explore their situations and their own individuality. This is primarily encouraged through using skills of reflection of both *content* and more particularly of *feeling* back to clients for their consideration. Therapists using this approach should never try to interpret past experiences, nor give directions or behavioural-focused tasks to the client. Rather, agendas for action and responsibilities for taking action rest solely with clients.

Although the starting point for person-centred therapy is the presenting difficulties identified by the client, it aims to move beyond these 'symptoms' to facilitate clients to move towards becoming fully functioning people who are better prepared to cope with the ups and downs of their future lives. Therefore, this approach does not deal merely with discovering more effective ways of dealing with their current problems, it seeks to prepare people to cope with other aspects of their lives.

The person-centred approach continues to have a major influence on counselling and is present to some degree in all approaches that seek to involve clients in the decision-making process and strive to work with clients as valued people, capable of making their own decisions. A major contribution of this approach is the accessibility it created to counselling for both clients and professionals who wish to work as counsellors. Prior to this time the role of the counsellor had been constrained, mainly by the strong influence of the medical profession on counselling.

The person-centred approach does, however, appear to be over-represented in nursing textbooks with little consideration being given to the possibility of using other approaches. This restrictive representation of counselling is unhelpful as the other approaches, particularly the behavioural and cognitive approaches, are relevant to nursing practice, but tend to be confined to 'treatment' issues in mental health and not to the wider arena of nursing. Perhaps the focus on using the person-centred approach to counselling in nursing has been influenced by several erroneous assumptions such as that the person-centred approach is less technical, less demanding of people, and if wrongly implemented will not do clients any harm. It must be stressed that the person-centred approach arises from a theory as complex as any other approach and it is very specific about the qualities and actions required of counsellors. As with the other approaches it is capable of uncovering emotional distress in clients and dealing with this in an accepting manner requires much more than conversational skills. Indeed failure to resolve emotional distress could leave clients in more turmoil than ever.

The cognitive approach to counselling

Another major approach within the body of counselling is that which focuses on what people think. Although this was a component of psychoanalytic, behavioural and humanistic approaches none of them attempted to change how people thought. The psychoanalysts sought to analyse thoughts, the behaviourists focused on actions with little or no attention being given to internal thought processes, and the person-centred approach was particularly interested in how people felt.

The cognitive approach utilised some aspects of the previous approaches. It accepts that past experiences do influence adult behaviour; that behaviour is learned and, therefore, can be altered; and that the relationship with the client is important for effective counselling. Furthermore, the cognitive approach views people as active participants in their learning and believes that internal cognitive processes are a central aspect of this learning.

Using this perspective, it is considered that people who are anxious develop problems because of the negative way they think about other people, places or things. For example, individuals may have irrational beliefs such as: 'I must have love and approval from all the people I come into contact with. I must achieve perfection in all I do and, if I don't get what I want it will be terrible' (Ellis and Dryden, 1987) .

Alternatively, clients may have distorted thinking and faulty assumptions. For example, people may overgeneralise by thinking that a single negative incident will result in a catalogue of disasters or people feel and think they are a 'complete failure' due to the break-up of a relationship. Some view external events as always having a (usually negative) personal consequence: 'If I go on holiday by plane it will crash, just because I am on it.' This is 'negative self-talk' (Beck, 1976). The presence of negative self-talk results in an inaccurate assessment of reality which in turn leads to an expectation that things will go wrong which subsequently leads to further increased anxiety. Negative self-talk was further identified by Meichenbaum (1977) as a the major cognitive source of people's difficulties.

If individuals repeat this negative thinking over and over again, thus, for example, reinforcing the thought, 'I am fat and ugly', this can result in an gross amount of self-denigrating and self-defeating behaviours leading to an inability to 'psych' oneself up to perform difficult tasks. It is extremely difficult to break through the cycle of negative thinking and help change it if people had also been told they were 'fat and ugly' by others, particularly their parents or important others.

Considerable variation exists within cognitive-based approaches to counselling about how thought processes are affected and how these may be modified to assist clients more effectively. Generally, the counsellor works with clients to assess their beliefs and thought processes. This involves a detailed examination of how clients perceive life events that have occurred to them. The counsellor encourages clients to think about what they believe about the things they do.

Approaches may differ slightly. For example, within rational emotive behavioural therapy (Ellis and Dryden, 1977), the counsellor may be directly confrontational with clients and insist they examine their 'irrational' beliefs and at a later stage test these out in reality. Meichenbaum (1977), on the other hand, focuses on the language people use and on their 'defeatist self-talk'. Beck (1976), alternatively, examines the accuracy of conclusions that people reach and their underlying beliefs about these conclusions. He suggests counsellors should focus on helping clients realise that their beliefs are often too absolute and too rigid to live comfortable lives.

The boundaries between cognitive and behavioural approaches are particularly blurred. Many cognitive therapists, for example, also utilise behavioural techniques. They will set tasks and 'homeworks' to be completed inside and outside counselling sessions and use methods of reinforcement to enhance learning.

The common thread embroidered within all of these specific cognitive approaches is the goal of changing how people act and also how people think about their current and future situations. Hence the aim is to develop more positive patterns of thinking. The counsellor is in many ways a 'teacher' and clients, therefore, are 'students' who are learning new ways to think and to examine their perceptions of other people, places and situations (Corey, 1995).

COMBINED APPROACHES TO COUNSELLING

The reality of day-to-day practice in counselling is that the majority of therapists appear to combine different approaches as opposed to strictly adhering to one specific approach. It is argued that this enables them to be more flexible and responsive to clients as individuals (Nelson-Jones, 1993). Counsellors' choice of predominant approach will be influenced by their personal and professional perspectives on the nature of people, perceived origins of problems, and the desired aims of therapy.

Initially this means that counsellors have to combine various components of different approaches and in so doing develop a broad knowledge base and a variety of skills and techniques. After all this training the counsellor then chooses the counselling strategy that is most appropriate to match a particular situation with a specific individual. This strategy has been described as using an 'eclectic' approach to counselling (Nelson-Jones, 1993). Opponents of this approach have portrayed it as a fragmented approach that attempts to bring together divergent knowledge, skills and techniques from conflicting theoretical backgrounds. For example, the need for warmth, genuineness and empathy may be extrapolated from a person-centred approach and combined with some challenging techniques drawn from the cognitive approaches. It has been suggested that such a strategy could, in turn, result in a confused, inconsistent and ineffective approach that lacks an adequate theoretical underpinning, as opposed to an individualised flexible approach (Clarkson, 1996).

An eclectic approach to counselling has been distinguished from an 'integrative' approach that focuses on combining convergent components of other approaches in such a manner as to unify these components. Hence a new variant or approach to counselling may be created which includes drawing from an adapted theoretical base, resulting in a less fragmented collection of knowledge and techniques (Norcross and Grencavage, 1990).

By definition it is not possible to have a single integrative or eclectic approach that all counsellors will follow precisely. Their development occurs as the result of individualised variables relating in many ways to each counsellor's values and beliefs, the specific issues presented by the client and the physical and contextual factors that exist within the counselling environment. The ultimate goal to be achieved as a result of counselling must also be taken into account when choosing elements from a specific school of counselling.

However, an increasing number of eclectic and integrative frameworks have been developed and these act as maps to guide counsellors and clients through specific stages within the counselling process. Frameworks highlight the importance of the client and the counsellor moving through the process of problem-solving in a step-by-step manner. This helps to reduce the risk of counselling becoming a series of repeated conversations between the client and the counsellor with no movement towards a resolution of the difficulties that resulted in the person needing to come into the counselling situation (Betts, 1995).

The stages of three combined approaches to counselling that have become widely utilised within health and social care settings during the 1990s are outlined in Box 5.2. It is important to note that despite considerable variation among the combined approaches it is possible to identify some common characteristics within all three of them, namely:

- the focus is on the present situation the client is in;
- a good working relationship between the therapist and the client is viewed as valuable (if not essential) to bring about change;
- the clients' abilities and individuality should influence the type of techniques utilised; and
- the pace, direction and eventual outcomes of counselling should be influenced by and negotiated with the client who is active in decision-making during counselling.

Furthermore, the role of the counsellor is viewed as dynamic, selecting techniques to match the 'here and now' situation while clients reflect on and develop the combined use of affective, behavioural and cognitive techniques. The integrative approach also aims to move clients on from their present situation to a situation where they can function more effectively and it does this through a series of defined stages in the counselling process.

In essence, the frameworks combine components from the four main schools of thought and weave them into a structured approach to assist clients. The initial stages of the combined frameworks concentrate on establishing an honest and effective relationship with clients, which is reflective of the person-centred approaches. The importance of developing a therapeutic relationship prior to further progess in counselling is emphasised and the need to develop trust and to convey respect highlighted.

Box 5.2   An overview of the stages outlined in three
counselling frameworks

The skilled helper model

1. *Identifying and clarifying problem situations and unused development opportunities*: by the client telling her story, the identification and challenging of blind spots, the search for leverage to bring about change.
2. *Developing a preferred scenario*: through generating preferred scenario possibilities, creating viable agendas, focusing on choice and commitment.
3. *Formatting strategies and plans to achieve the preferred scenario*: by considering and selecting strategies into action, client selecting the best stategies, turning stategies into plans and deciding on action steps.

Source: Egan (1994)

Eight-stage map of the counselling relationship

1. Meeting the client.
2. Discussion of surface issues.
3. Revelation of deeper issues.
4. Ownership of feelings and possibly emotional release.
5. Generation of insight – the client's life is viewed by them in a different light.
6. Problem-solving and future planning.
7. Action by the client.
8. Disengagement from the counselling relationship by the client.

Source: Burnard (1994)

The DASIE model

- Develop the relationship, identify and clarify problem(s)
- Assess problem(s) and redefine them in skills terms
- State working goals and plan interventions
- Intervene to develop self-defining skills
- End and consolidate self-helping skills

Source: Nelson-Jones (1993)

As the relationship becomes established clients are encouraged to 'tell their stories' and gradually the full picture of their situation, as they view it, becomes clear. This may include the sharing of experiences from the distant as well as the recent past, and could span obstacles or growth blocks that have impacted on clients' progress through the earlier stages of personal development. Repressed trauma may also be uncovered in the process of counselling.

Although clients are encouraged to focus on their present feelings, thoughts, behaviours and perceived difficulties, elements of psychodynamic, behavioural and cognitive approaches are noticeable. The bias towards clients taking action and reviewing their perception of their situations within the latter stages of the combined frameworks illustrates behavioural and cognitive components. Clear evidence of the person-centred approach is noted throughout the framework in stressing the importance of client involvement in all decisions about the objectives to be set and targets to be achieved. The piecing together of a clear overview of the clients' position is often a slower process than anticipated as the first presenting difficulties outlined by clients may not be the most crucial ones. More issues and problems usually surface after clients feel comfortable enough to share them with the counsellor. This means that clients must come to trust the counsellor and learning to trust takes time. However, given time, the overall picture as the client perceives it will emerge (Corey, 1995).

At one level, the placing together of a range of values and techniques into an organised and structured approach appears to provide a straightforward way to proceed. Some might argue that combining approaches leads to a 'hotchpotch' of perspectives which may give rise to possible conflicts between the different components inherent in each. Indeed this is one of the key criticisms of counselling as an activity.

SOME KEY CRITICISMS OF COUNSELLING AS AN ACTIVITY

Counselling as an activity, with the myriad of issues relating to individual approaches as well as those attributed to specific therapists has not developed smoothly. Indeed it is not without its critics. It is helpful, therefore, to consider the key challenges as they provide some indication of how counselling skills and counselling may be more effectively utilised in nursing. For the purpose of this chapter criticisms examined will be grouped under three main headings: first, issues concerning theoretical underpinnings; second, questions relating to the need for counselling at all; and third, the quality of the counselling available.

Issues concerning theoretical underpinnings

It is evident that the range of counselling theories is diverse and it could be argued that this reflects the true individuality of people. However, an alternative line of argument may be that there is a lack of consensus about what the 'pure' components of counselling are. Furthermore, the conflict and contradictions that exist between theories means that counselling does not have a sound theoretical foundation (Howard, 1996).

In particular, the sparsity of research into counselling practice which empirically identifies specific evidence-based elements of counselling interactions that are consistently matched with successful outcomes supports this argument. It is interesting that improvements reported by clients, as a result of counselling, have more to do with non-specific factors relating to counsellors and the counselling environment than with any particular testable theoretical basis. Although research has identified a range of attributes of successful counsellors (Box 5.3) these are wide-ranging and not specific to any single theoretical approach (Feltham, 1995). An examination of the list shows it is clear that the attributes of an effective counsellor are targets which community nurses might strive to achieve in their personal and professional development if they are to work as counsellors.

Considerable research also exists about the difficulties inherent in measuring the effectiveness of counselling provided. Although the nature of these difficulties may vary to some degree within different approaches to counselling, essentially the crucial obstacle to be overcome is to establish valid and reliable measures of counselling success. This is particularly difficult given the fact that both clients and counsellors will have different views and perceptions as to what is entailed in any particular successful outcome. Conflict exists, therefore, as to which measures should be used (McLeod, 1993).

It has been argued that the lack of theoretical underpinnings encourages the development of 'gurus' in counselling and the evolution of a mythical quality to counselling. Smail (1987, p. 110) asserted that:

Box 5.3   Attributes of an effective counsellor

1. Well-developed interpersonal skills.
2. Personal attitudes and beliefs that value other people.
3. Respect for the individual's self-determination.
4. Ability to view the world from the client's viewpoint.
5. Ability to appreciate the influences of their own client's.
6. The conceptual ability to grasp the meaning of what the client is experiencing/saying.
7. An understanding of the principles of applied developmental, behavioural, cognitive and abnormal psychology.
8. An applied understanding of a range of approaches/models of counselling.
9. An understanding of the roles, functioning and interrelationships amoung the helping 'professionals' (across the statutory, voluntary and private sectors).
10. The ability to recognise the relevance of different approaches to counselling in assisting the client.
11. Personal soundness reflected in a well-developed self-awareness and recognition of one's abilities and limitations
12. Willingness to appear as real people, and not hide behind a professional image.
13. Openness to change, and ability to admit and learn from mistakes.
14. A mastery of a range of techniques.
15. The ability to understand and work within social systems.

Source: Adapted from Corey (1995) and McLeod (1993).

'as soon as people abandon their experience of themselves in favour of the dogma of 'experts' then the process of mystification becomes complete.'

Questions relating to the need for counselling at all

The second key area relates to the fact that counselling has become readily available through statutory, voluntary and private services.

It is considered to be a strategy for the management of personal difficulties and increasingly it may be presented as an alternative to the use of medical treatments. Consider why this transition has happened and ask yourself if this change of focus is really necessary.

Concerns have been expressed that the role of counselling may be to attempt 'to paper over the cracks' of major social problems by enabling people to 'adjust' and fit in with the desires of an unhealthy and greedy society. Masson (1992) argues that counselling cannot resolve difficulties that have their origins in wider social problems and highlights disadvantages such as poverty and discrimination.

In addition, it has been argued that people may become dependent on seeing their therapist as opposed to becoming more independent (Masson, 1992). At a wider level increased reliance on counselling is developing as the nature and combination of social networks alter, resulting in people having less contact with their families and local neighbourhood support systems. In some ways feelings of isolation are augmented through the development of a non-threatening counselling relationship and by 'friendships' that are maintained at a superficial level (Howard, 1996).

The quality of counselling available

Counselling has been challenged on the grounds that it has no agreed and mandatory accreditation and registration framework. There are no absolute criteria laid down which highlight 'essential' curriculum and course content or the necessary competencies required by students to prepare them to be counsellors. Indeed, it is not necessary to undertake any course at all. Some people have set themselves up in lucrative counselling businesses without any counselling qualifications. This leads to the development of a range of very diverse approaches being offered, all under the name of counselling. Currently there is no compulsory regulatory framework to challenge ineffective, incompetent or unscrupulous counsellors and, more importantly, to protect members of the public.

The emotional, financial and sexual exploitation of clients is a real concern for those who challenge the credibility of counselling. They present considerable evidence to support their concerns (Masson, 1992; Howard, 1996; Russell, 1996; Spinelli, 1996). All nurses should reflect on their own competencies. They need to be sure that they have the essential competencies required to undertake counselling activities with clients and consult the *Scope of Professional Practice* document when making their decisions (UKCC,

1992b). Nurses who undertake a counselling role remain clearly accountable to clients under the professional guidance outlined in the *Code of Professional Conduct* (UKCC, 1992a) and *Guidelines for Professional Practice* (UKCC, 1996).

The theoretical basis and the delivery of counselling are not beyond question, and this 'treatment', like any other treatment available, necessitates attention being given to actively seeking the informed consent of clients. The effectiveness of approaches used must be monitored and opportunities for redress should be readily available if difficulties arise with the service provided. This highlights the need for all nurses, both those who are involved in using counselling skills and those providing counselling, to be clear about: their role; the boundaries; the theoretical frameworks they use; and, finally, monitoring the effectiveness of their interventions in terms of client-based outcomes.

SOME KEY CONSIDERATIONS FOR DEVELOPING EFFECTIVE COUNSELLING PRACTICE IN COMMUNITY NURSING

Integral to effective nursing interventions is the ability to communicate effectively with clients, their families and other members of the interdisciplinary team (Cain, 1995; UKCC, 1992a, 1996). The author of this chapter has argued that most nurses utilise counselling skills in their daily work. It has further been suggested that only a few community nurses actively provide counselling within their nursing role.

There is no doubt that with the increasing emphasis being placed on the provision of counselling within primary care the demand for this service will increase. Consequently, more nurses will be expected to provide counselling for clients and their carers (Waskett, 1996; Curtis-Jenkins and Einzig, 1996; Robert, 1995). An expectation that community nurses will provide counselling is also evident within the learning outcomes for specialist practitioner courses (UKCC, 1994), where competencies in counselling are highlighted. The provision of counselling and psychological support are often identified in job descriptions for all branches of community nursing.

In the final section of the chapter some broad key issues are outlined for nurses who already view counselling as a current or future part of their role. These issues should be considered by nurses when they make the decision to provide counselling and during all stages of the counselling process. They should be reviewed in the light of the complex dynamics involved in the development and maintenance of a therapeutic nurse/client relationship (see Chapters 2 and 3 of this volume; Long, 1995; Cain, 1995).

It is important that nurses actively reflect on what is involved in their role when they work as counsellors and do not simply and without discussion drift towards what they term the provision of counselling. Similar to all other skilled nursing interventions, counselling requires a broad knowledge base and competence in its inherent skills. Being interested and willing to help clients is an important starting point but it is not adequate for effective practice. Competence is required in:

> 'the ability to give attention, listen, reflect, paraphrase, and summarise . . . these have become the bedrock on which counselling rests – if you can't do that you can't counsel.'
> (Inskipp, 1996, p. 1).

The principles highlighted within the *Scope of Professional Practice* (UKCC, 1992b) emphasise the requirement to ensure that nursing interventions are always directed in a coordinated (unfragmented) manner to meet identified needs and to serve the best interests of clients. This guidance also highlights the need to 'honestly acknowledge any limits of personal knowledge and skill and take steps to remedy deficits' and to avoid any inappropriate delegation to others which may compromise the interests of clients.

These principles apply equally to counselling as they do to any other nursing activity, such as giving an unfamiliar medication. Counselling should not be considered as always safe and free from harm. If it is inappropriately practised it can have negative consequences. Clients may end up feeling more distressed or angry than ever, with the additional problems of a reduction in any self-confidence they may previously have had as well as loss of privacy and dignity.

As a professional group community health care nurses must be clear about the expectations and boundaries around their professional role and be cognisant of job descriptions and local guidance/policies on the provision of counselling. Therefore, community nurses should clarify if they have the support of professional and local managers when they are providing counselling or if they should refer clients elsewhere (with their consent).

Having clarified the wider professional and local procedural guidelines, nurses must make several personal decisions about individual clients. Following the completion of a holistic nursing assessment of an individual's abilities and needs, community nurses should make decisions about the level and nature of nursing interventions they feel are appropriate to be 'prescribed' for the person. It may be the judgement of the nurse that a particular client would benefit from counselling to assist them build on their abilities and overcome some of the difficulties they are experiencing. The provision of counselling requires a rationale that is based on the assessment of the individual. It should not be provided simply 'because it seems like a good thing to do'.

The following questions may be asked prior to the commencement of counselling:

1. Am I the appropriate person to provide the counselling?
2. Am I aware of the client's abilities and needs?
3. Have I the necessary knowledge and am I competent in the essential skills to provide counsellling to this person?
4. Do I have the personal attributes and qualities to co-travel with this person on their journey of recovery?
5. Am I aware of my own abilities and needs and do I have adequate professional support from colleagues, other team members and managers?
6. Have I time to counsel (am I able to provide an adequate commitment to the specific counselling of this client over and above other interventions I may be undertaking)?
7. Is the client aware of the time constraints on the counselling that may be necessary from the outset?
8. Have I the client's informed permission and have steps been taken to enable the client to make an informed decision? (This includes an outline of what and who will be involved in counselling, the approach to be used and a sound rationale for its use).
9. Where will the counselling take place? (What facilities are available at the necessary times, how well do these suit an interaction that requires time, privacy and the possibility that the client may become upset?)
10. From whom do I obtain support and supervision? (The nurse should consider the need for professional and personal support.) (Adapted from Burnard, 1994)

Following the inital assessment the nurse negotiates with the client to agree on the proposed counselling intervention (Dryden and Feltham, 1994; McLeod, 1993). Details that clearly outline the reasons why counselling has been suggested as the most appropriate intervention to meet the objectives to be achieved can then be formalised in a nursing care plan. The approach to be followed and expected actions to be taken by the nurse and the client and any other people involved must also be recorded. Selection of the counselling approach from a range of approaches requires the counsellor (nurse) to have the knowledge and skills relating to several possible approaches. The individual identification of a specific approach that is matched to an individual client and counsellor has been reported to be more successful than applying the same or similar approaches to all clients (Inskipp, 1996). Each approach to counselling has its own view of people.

Seven principles of counselling have been outlined by Burnard (1994) (see Box 5.4). The principles broadly span the major approaches to counselling (although they largely relate to a person-centred approach) and provide some direction for negotiating objectives and providing counselling. A time-scale for evaluation of progress should be incorporated into the 'care plan' (or negotiated contract) in order to maintain a forward-moving momentum and reduce the chance of the counselling becoming a circular conversation (Betts, 1995).

Box 5.4   Seven principles proposed for counselling

1. The client knows what is best for him/herself.
2. Interpretation by the counsellor is likely to be inaccurate and is best to be avoided.
3. Advice is rarely helpful (in a counselling context).
4. The client occupies a different personal world from that of the counsellor and the reverse is also true.
5. Listening is the basis of the counselling relationship.
6. Counselling techniques should not be overused.
7. Counselling can be learned.

Source: Burnard (1994)

Confidential records of each interaction should accurately reflect what has taken place, progress made towards meeting the identified goals and need for any modifications to be made in the process. Nurses who are new to their role as counsellors, like other people new to the role, will have to grapple with a range of conflicting emotions and difficulties regarding their role and boundaries. Some of these difficulties are highlighted in Box 5.5. Experience and supervision offers opportunities to enhance practice and work in a manner that is personally and professionally effective.

Evaluation of the success of counselling interventions requires attention to qualitative and quantitative data. The latter may consist of the number of appointments attended or missed, the degree to which clients have worked towards their goals outside of sessions, any evidence of recordable behavioural changes and possibly some indicators of instruments used to measure anxiety and general perceptions of health. Such data may be complemented by qualitative information elicited from clients on their perceptions of how they 'feel' in 'the here and now' situation and of how they have resolved their initial difficulties (Barkham, 1996; McLeod, 1996; Barkham and Barker, 1996).

Box 5.5   Difficulties for beginner counsellors

1.   Dealing with personal and professional anxieties.
2.   Being and disclosing ourselves.
3.   Avoiding perfectionism.
4.   Being honest about our limitations.
5.   Understanding silence.
6.   Dealing with demanding clients.
7.   Dealing with uncommitted clients.
8.   Accepting slow results.
9.   Avoiding self-deception.
10. Avoiding losing ourselves in our clients.
11. Developing a sense of humour.
12. Establishing realistic goals.
13. Declining to give advise.
14. Developing a personal counselling style.

Source: Corey (1995)

Nurses must recognise that possible bias may arise due to the emphasis on market forces within the provision of current health and social care services. The quantitative evaluation of counselling may be viewed as more important within contemporary agenda. For example, nurses may be asked to prove counselling is effective because there has been a reduction in the need for medication or visits to the general practitioners. This is in opposition to gathering rich, qualitative data on the degree to which clients feel more able to live resourceful and satisfying lives as one of the consequences of counselling. The accurate evaluation of the effects of the provision of counselling on clients' health and social well-being is difficult but nevertheless it is achievable through an increasing array of methodological approaches and scientific instruments (Woolfe and Dryden, 1996; Mellor-Clark and Barkham, 1996; McLeod, 1993).

Failure to audit and implement agreed quality standards for the provision of counselling within primary health care services has been highlighted as a significant difficulty in recent times (Thomas, 1996; Robert, 1995). Although difficult, it is also essential, for it is largely through evaluating clients' perceptions of health gains and supervisors' feedback regarding professional practice that nurses and other counsellors gain insight into the quality of service they offer. The next few years will see an increased focus on the contribution of counselling to client care with attention being given to the contribution nurses will make to this area. Currently, nurses are not trained as counsellors in their pre-registration education, therefore they need to invest time in this area of study at post-registration level. It can be a long and difficult journey at times and it usually stirs up many personal and professional conflicts that need to be resolved (Primmer, 1996). Consequently, nurses need to be prepared to invest their time, energy and humanness into this area if they are to consider becoming effective counsellors.

References

Audit Commission (1989) *Making a Reality of Community Care.* London: HMSO.

BAC (British Association of Counselling) (1990) *Code of Ethics and Practice for Counselling Skills.* Rugby: BAC.

Bandura, A. (1977) *Social Learning Theory.* Englewood Cliffs, NJ: Prentice-Hall.

Barkham, M. (1996) Quantitative research on psychotherapeutic interventions: methodological issues and substantive findings across three research generations. In R. Woolfe and D. Dryden (eds), *Handbook of Counselling Psychology*. Sage: London, pp. 23–64.

Barkham, M. and Barker, C. (1996) Evaluating counselling psychology practice. In R. Woolfe and D. Dryden (eds), *Handbook of Counselling Psychology*. Sage: London, pp. 87–110.

Beck, A. (1976) *Cognitive Therapy and Emotional Disorders*. New York: New American Library.

Betts A. (1995) The counselling relationship. In R. B Ellis, R. Gates, and N. Kenworthy (eds), *Interpersonal Communication in Nursing. Theory and Practice*. Edinburgh: Churchill Livingstone.

Bond T. (1993) Counselling, counselling skills and professionals. In R. Bayne, P. Nicolson (eds), *Counselling and Psychology for Health Professionals*. London: Chapman & Hall, pp. 1–17.

Burnard P. (1994) *Counselling Skills for Health Professionals*, 2nd edn. London: Chapman & Hall.

Burnard, P. (1995) Counselling, or becoming a counsellor. *Professional Nurse*, 10(4) pp. 261–2.

Burnard, P. (1996) *Acquiring Interpersonal Skills. A Handbook of Experiential Learning for Health Professionals*, 2nd edn. London: Chapman & Hall.

Burnard, P. and Morrison, P. (1988) Nurses' perceptions of their interpersonal skills: a descriptive study using Six Category Intervention Analysis. *Nurse Education Today*, 8(5), pp. 266–72.

Burnard, P. and Morrison, P. (1989) Counselling attitudes in community psychiatric nurses. *Community Psychiatric Nursing Journal*, 9(5), pp. 26–9.

Cain, P. (1995) Community nurse – client relations. In P. Cain, V. Hyde and E. Howkins (eds), *Community Nursing. Dimensions and Dilemmas*. London: Arnold, pp. 27–41.

Clarkson, P. (1996) The eclectic and integrative paradigm: between the Scylla of confluence and the Charydbis of confusion. In Woolfe, R. and D. Dryden, (eds) *Handbook of Counselling Psychology*. Sage: London, pp. 258–84.

Corey, G. (1995) *Theory and Practice of Counselling and Psychotherapy*, 5th edn. Pacific Grove, Calif.: Brooks Cole.

Curtis-Jenkins, G. and Einzig, H. (1996), Counselling in primary care. In R. Bayne, I. Horton and J. Bimrose (eds), *New Directions in Counselling*. London: Routledge, pp. 97–108.

Dale, N. (1996) *Working with Families of Children with Special Needs*. London: Routledge.

Dickson, D. (1995) Communication and interpersonal skills. In D. Sines, (ed.) *Community Health Care Nursing*. Oxford: Blackwell Science, pp. 62–88.

Dryden, W. and Feltham, C. (1994) *Developing the Practice of Counselling*. London: Sage.

Egan G. (1994) *The Skilled Helper, a problem-management Approach to Helping*, 5th edn. Pacific Grove, Calif.: Brooks Cole.

Ellis, A. and Dryden, W. (1987) *The Practice of Rational–Emotive Therapy*. Secaucus, NJ: Lyle Stuart.

Feltham, C. (1995) *What is Counselling?* London. Sage.

Feltham, C. and Dryden, W. (1993) *Dictionary of Counselling*. London: Whurr.

Freud, S. (1974) *The Standard Edition of the Complete Psychological works of Sigmund Freud, Vol. 5, 1–24*, ed. J. Strachey. London: Hogarth Press.

Hargie, O. (1986) *A Handbook of Communication Skills*. London: Croom Helm.

Hargie, O. Saunders, C. and Dickson, D. (1994) *Social Skills in Interpersonal Communication*, 3rd edn. London: Routledge.

Heron, J. (1986) *Six Category Intervention Analysis*, 2nd edn. Guilford: Human Potential Research Project, University of Surrey.

Howard, A. (1996) *Challenges to Counselling and Psychotherapy*. London: Macmillan.

Inskipp, F. (1996) *Skills Training for Counselling*. London: Cassell.

Lazarus, A. (1971) *Behavior Therapy and Beyond*. New York: McGraw- Hill.

Long, A. (1995) Community mental health nursing. In D. Sines, (ed.), *Community Health Care Nursing*. Oxford: Blackwell Science, (pp. 249–87).

McLeod, J. (1993) *An Introduction to Counselling*. Buckingham: Open University Press.

McLeod, J. (1996) Qualitative research methods in counselling psychology. In R. Woolfe and D. Dryden (eds), *Handbook of Counselling Psychology*. London: Sage, p. 65–86.

Masson, J. (1992) *Against Therapy*, rev. edn. London: Fontana.

Meichenbaum, D. (1977) *Cognitive-Behavior Modification: An Integrative Approach*. New York: Plenum.

Mellor-Clark, J. and Barkham, M. (1996) Evaluating counselling. In R. Bayne, I. Horton and J. Bimrose (eds), *New Directions in Counselling*. London: Routledge, pp. 79–96.

Nelson-Jones, R. (1993) *Practical Counselling and Helping Skills: how to use the lifeskills helping model.* London: Cassell.

Norcross, J. and Grencavage, L. (1990) Eclecticism and integration in counselling and psychotherapy: major themes and obstacles. In W. Dryden and J. Norcross (eds), *Eclecticism and Integration in Counselling and Psychotherapy.* Loughton, Essex: Gale Centre, pp. 1–33.

Patterson, C. H. (1986) *Theories of Counselling and Psychotherapy,* 4th edn. London: HarperCollins.

Primmer, M. (1996) It is a rough road that leads to heights of greatness: a trainee counsellor's survey of the road to becoming a counsellor. *Counselling Psychology Quarterly,* 9(3), pp. 213–19.

Robert, G. (1995) *Counsellors in Primary Care.* Bristol: South West Regional Health Authority.

Rogers, C. (1962) *On Becoming a Person.* Boston, Mass.: Houghton Mifflin.

Russell, J. (1996) Sexual exploitation in counselling. In R. Bayne, I. Horton and J. Bimrose (eds), *New Directions in Counselling.* London: Routledge, pp. 65–78.

Skinner, B. F. (1974) *About Behaviorism,* New York: Knopf.

Smail, J. (1987) *Taking Care: An Alternative to Therapy.* London: Dent.

Spinelli, E. (1996) Do therapists know what they are doing? *Professional Therapeutic Titles: Myths and Realities.* British Psychological Society, Division of Counselling Psychology. London, pp. 55–61.

Thomas, A. (1996) Clinical audit: setting professional standards for counselling services. *Counselling Psychology Quarterly,* 9(1), pp. 25–36.

United Kingdom Central Council for Nursing, Midwifery and Health Visiting (UKCC) (1992a) *Code of Professional Conduct,* 3rd edn. London: UKCC.

United Kingdom Central Council for Nursing, Midwifery and Health Visiting (UKCC) (1992b) *The Scope for Professional Practice.* London: UKCC.

United Kingdom Central Council for Nursing, Midwifery and Health Visiting (UKCC) (1994) *Standards for Post-Registration Education.* London: UKCC.

United Kingdom Central Council for Nursing, Midwifery and Health Visiting (UKCC) (1996) *Guidelines for Professional Practice.* London: UKCC.

Waskett, C. (1996) Multidisciplinary teamwork in primary care: the role of the counsellor. *Counselling Psychology Quarterly,* 9(3), pp. 243–60.

Wolpe, J. (1982) *The Practice of Behavior Therapy.* New York: Pergamon Press.

Woolfe, R. and Dryden, D. (1996) *Handbook of Counselling Psychology.* London: Sage.

CHAPTER SIX

Secrets and Lies: Ethical Communication

Rosario Baxter

INTRODUCTION

The mental and physical health status of individuals is widely perceived to be a product of the degree to which people are valued and respected by themselves and others. As an essential component of any therapeutic relationship, the benefits of effective communication in the healing process are considered paramount (Ford and Urban, 1963). Radwin (1996) suggests that 'knowing patients' is one facet of caring that signifies expertise in nursing (Benner *et al.*, 1992). Knowing patients is said to include being open to learning patients' 'thoughts, concerns, fears and hopes' (Alexander, 1990, p. 66).

Opportunities for nurses to establish a close enough relationship with patients to allow us to know them as people have declined with the changing nature of health care delivery. Nurses are expected to convert and move with the rapidly mutating ethos underpinning the provision of health care. The development of the new speciality of 'nurse informaticist' demonstrates one response to the expansion of information technology in patient care (McAlindon, 1997). The growth of day surgery, shorter hospital in-patient stays, the advent of televisual or 'distance' health care and the pace of activity forced upon staff in hospital and community all conspire to reduce the time available for us to engage meaningfully with the people we care for.

Early studies (Johnson *et al.*, 1978; Ashworth, 1980; Bond, 1982) began identifying the role of communication skills in the prevention of post-operative complications in hospital patients, and in decreasing anxiety in patients being nursed in critical care situations. There is a dearth of research activity targeting the patients' perspective or contribution to the communication process (Wilkinson, 1991). Studies are often related to specific client groups, concentrating on the goal of completing nursing tasks. Critics of research on communication argue that this approach fails to explore the meanings, contributions and perceptions of the people involved as well as the social context of communication (May, 1990; Byrne and Heyman, 1997).

In community nursing, it is acknowledged that clients have a high regard for the benefits they receive from effective communication and having an empathetic listener (Poulton, 1995). Whilst, as nurses, we have progressed a long way in developing our technical skills in all aspects of communication, there remains a lack of professional accountability in respect of ethical facets of communicating with patients. For example, it has been demonstrated that there is a paucity of open and informative communication (Bond, 1982). In addition to communication skills, the quality of nurse–patient interaction is influenced by a myriad of factors, including institutional and professional demands and the cultural context of practice.

This chapter explores the proposition that there exists a profound and complex dimension to communication which is concerned primarily with the principle of truth-telling, or the 'wholesomeness' of our engagement with patients. The author asserts that it is impossible to separate the technical aspects of information exchange from the ethical responsibilities with which they are inextricably bound. The chapter continues with demonstrating that it is unrealistic to dissect 'parcels' of communication which reveal that decisions on information-giving are the responsibility of one professional and not of another. Interestingly, Lanceley (1985) suggests that patients who are involved in emotional disclosure are more likely to exercise control over the interaction than the professional. It is argued that the qualitative aspects of nursing work cannot readily be compartmentalised. They are, accordingly, less amenable to scrutiny. It is important, therefore, that the many valued aspects of nursing, of which communication is central, are not lost in the scientific pursuit of the advancement of technological nursing practice (Hall and Dornan, 1988).

NURSE EDUCATION AND PRACTICE

Most nurses support the view that the art of communication is an essential prerequisite for, and component of, effective nursing care. Contemporary nurse education programmes emphasise the competency-based aspects of communication skills and the rudimentary nature of communicating effectively with clients/patients. This is particularly so with the introduction of the Project 2000 curricula. Not everyone, however, welcomes the arrival of a thinking and critical practitioner as envisaged in this new preparation for practice (Hunt, 1995). Nevertheless, the potential scope of communication as a tool that may be utilised to enhance patients' health and social well-being is increasingly being recognised (Ley, 1988).

Poor communication has been identified as a contributory factor in a number of studies of medical accidents (Vincent, 1989; Barrett and Jarvis, 1990; Woodyard, 1990). In practice, ill-prepared professionals continue to be inappropriately directed to take care of perhaps some of the most delicate aspects of communicating with patients. This may be demonstrated with the following 'real life' experiences.

Vignette: the bad news

A lecturer was facilitating a teaching session with a group of community nursing students, all of whom are registered nurses. The session began with exploring the ethical aspects of conveying 'bad news' to patients. During the course of the session a discussion took place about the question of *who* in the health care team is best placed to communicate 'bad news' to patients and their families. After much debate, the consensus of opinion emerged that only a doctor (irrespective of rank or experience) should impart 'bad news' as it is part of *the doctor's job*. Following further discussion, it became increasingly difficult to establish the basis for the group's decision.

The ensuing themes and concepts provoked much discussion within the group. Some students argued that perhaps the professional qualification of the health care worker should be the only criterion used to decide who should be involved in this aspect of communicating with patients and their families. Others maintained that the kind of relationship the person (nurse or doctor) has established with the family, the length of time they have been in contact with the family, and the practitioner's skills in communicating should be included as more relevant criteria in decision-making than merely a qualification-based criterion. The room went quiet. What at first seemed quite a straightforward matter began to emerge as being very complicated. A final decision did not materialise.

An examination of this short vignette highlights a number of vital points. It illustrates the power of traditional role boundaries as they perfuse and confuse clinical work. Despite claims to utilise 'evidence-based practice' (the tensions that co-exist with such a claim will be considered later in this chapter), one fundamental question remains unanswered: why do nurses refrain from challenging the notion that the responsibility for certain areas of communicating with patients is, or should be, allocated into professional pigeon-holes? Further, the possibility of a multi-professional approach to solving the dilemma was largely ignored amid the debate about role boundaries and responsibilities. The concept that information should be regarded as the 'property' of a particular professional group was also left uncontested.

Although the responsibility for delivering bad news is currently often left to our medical colleagues, further analysis might suggest that we could do more to tailor this aspect of care to meet each individual's needs. Who may be considered best suited for the task of conveying bad news to a particular patient? A doctor with sensitivity and appropriate communication skills may indeed be the best person to deal with this situation. The oncology specialist nurse practitioners, perhaps? Their knowledge of the patient may intimate that they are comfortable enough to convey the information. District nurses who have been in daily close contact with the family during some of the most stressful moments of their lives may have a relationship with the family that would be of immense value at a critical time. Perhaps more than one professional may be involved in this process. Who would you prefer to communicate with you in a situation such as that outlined above?

Furthermore, there may be specific aspects of technical and medical knowledge that are outside the scope of community nursing. Aspects of information that are unique to one profession may be addressed at a later time when patients are ready to absorb those particular facts. Respecting the patient's autonomy may demand that professional boundaries converge in order to communicate ethically.

HONESTY AND SENSITIVITY

A consistent and clear approach to communicating with clients is necessary to avoid ambiguity and uncertainty. This method of communicating increases the reliability of information exchange within the context of care delivery. There are many other aspects of practice which confront nurses and doctors, creating huge repercussions on the delivery of quality care. Changing approaches may threaten even the most basic attempts to communicate effectively with patients. Moreover, lack of resources has been condemned as a contrary influence on the relationship-building that is required in the rehabilitation process (Jones et al., 1997). It is in the context of this reality that 'ethical communication', as an essential ingredient for enhancing the quality of the enterprise of community nursing, will now be explored.

The pledge to behave in a professional manner in our work spans the entire scope of professional nursing (UKCC, 1989, 1992a; 1992b, 1994). More specifically, elements of honesty and sensitivity embody and provide the cornerstone of a professional commitment to ethical communication. These key elements or concepts are central to a system of communication that aspires to address some of the tensions that currently exist in health care.

A chasm appears to be widening between the personal and professional responsibility which aims to reconcile the duty to minimise harm (non-maleficence) to patients while simultaneously promoting respect for patients (patient autonomy) in the light of shrinking resources. Caplan (1995, p. 42) attributes this and other sources of irritation for patients to the simple fact that nurses and doctors are far too busy, and work therefore in a situation that 'creates an environment that is as caustic to human feelings as cancer is to the human body'.

What about the hundreds of daily encounters that we, as nurses, probably forgot the moment the exchange with the patient had taken place? No matter how mundane patients' requests may seem to nurses, it is important for them to know that both their personhood and their communication are valued. Caplan (1995, p. 42) describes the frustrations that apparently trivial events can cause to patients – when the nurse's promises to 'be back in a minute' to do something for a patient 'were followed by mysterious unexplained disappearances that stretched into hours and left many a family member seething'. How many times have I implicitly promised to call back to visit clients in their homes and then forgotten to keep that promise in the bustle of bomb scares and traffic jams? How many patients are there today who remember, and may or may not have forgiven, the professional omissions in their past experiences of nursing care?

I recall visiting a friend who had been involved in a road traffic accident. As a result he had quadriplegia and was being nursed in a long-term care facility. He had learned to drink piping hot tea! Without the use of his limbs, he had learned that he got only one opportunity to drink the tea before either the nurse disappeared, or the cup was whisked away.

Nurses may argue that these illustrations depict patients as rather unforgiving if we are to be damned for such apparently minor transgressions. Yet nurses subscribe to the notion of individualised care through the use of tools such as the nursing process and models of nursing. Nurses claim that it is precisely such detail, the tailoring of care to meet the person's individual needs, that we aspire to provide (Sundeen *et al.*, 1994).

Seedhouse (1991, p. 65) accuses nurses of being at times 'almost obsessed with models of nursing'. He continues with suggesting that when medical analysis reaches maturity, it will also require models to guide practice. Interestingly, one type of model of medical practice proposed by Seedhouse (p. 71) is the 'caring' doctor whom he suggests will share many of the attributes 'commonly associated with the nursing profession'.

The belief that medical and nursing colleagues can continue to work alongside yet independent of one another becomes more difficult to justify in terms of serving the patient's best interests.

PRACTISING ETHICAL COMMUNICATION IN COMMUNITY NURSING

A conflict of interests

The following event occurred during my first week as a community children's nurse. A social worker telephoned requesting that I should go and visit Mrs Butterfly and her three-year-old daughter who were living in a block of flats in my area of practice. The social worker knew that the caretaker of the flats had previously been incarcerated for child sexual abuse. I was asked to visit this mother and try to illicit information from her regarding this man's behaviours.

How might you deal with this situation?

1. Had the social worker the right to request me to carry out this task?
2. Now that I owned this information, had I the right to say 'no' and dismiss the fact that I now knew this man's background?
3. Had I the right to use my professional visit to try to glean information from the mother in an undercover way?
4. As my primary duty was to make decisions based on what was 'the best interests of the child', had I the right to impart this knowledge to the mother I was visiting or to withhold it from her?
5. Had anyone a duty to inform this man's employer?
6. If you were Mrs Butterfly would you like to be given this information?
7. When does the professional confidentiality of community nursing end and the moral and personal responsibility to the public, as a citizen, begin?

I was later informed that it was not considered to be my duty to tell Mrs Butterfly the truth. This dictate served only to illustrate how little the professionals involved in this scenario, on reflection, understood about the nature of ethical communication. In the final analysis, my decisions had to be made on what I knew was morally right, for me. This experience highlights pragmatic issues.

Further, Roth and Meisel (1977) claimed that professionals are not capable of accurately predicting dangerousness. The best known predictor of dangerousness is past dangerous acts, yet the police and prisons are not held liable when they release dangerous individuals without warning to the public. Where is the threshold at which community nurses may warn possible victims about the fact that a known perpetrator of child sexual abuse lives next door to them? If the professional withholds this information and something untoward happens to the child then parents could possibly sue the professionals. Alternatively, if people are informed and nothing happens to the children in the area, then the person who has served his sentence and has subsequently been released may file suit against the professional for breach of confidentiality. An important exception to confidentiality was embodied in the 1971 *Tarasoff* decision of the California Supreme Court. They based their findings on the caveat that the privilege of confidentiality and individual protection ends when public peril begins.

Coercion, collusion or real care?

Jimmy was a thirteen-year-old child with cancer who was referred to me to be nursed at home. He was given about six months to live. His parents believed that he should not be told the truth about his prognosis and the professionals responsible for his care colluded with them in this respect. I was a newly qualified community children's nurse who visited Jimmy twice weekly initially and Jimmy and I became close. Needless to say he began asking me embarrassing questions about his future. I began to feel that I was practising a lie and that the collusion with this cloak of secrecy acted as a barrier between Jimmy and myself which further prevented me from being myself and being openly receptive to Jimmy. I was not practising in a way that permitted me to be open to learning and accepting Jimmy's thoughts, fears, concerns, dreams and ambitions. Indeed, the collusion barrier prevented me from offering Jimmy the 'best possible' therapeutic care. I also knew that my non-verbal communication, when questions were asked, did not synchronise in harmony with my spoken words. It became exceedingly difficult when the parents booked a family holiday abroad and began buying Jimmy new clothes for the trip he would not be alive to go on. I was continuously informed that it was not 'my duty' to disclose the truth to Jimmy.

This experience emphasises the importance of respecting the autonomy of patients who entrust their lives to professionals (Wardhaugh and Wilding, 1983), and the consequences of withholding the truth which 'cuts across patient autonomy' (Hawley, 1990, p. 11). Concepts of patient autonomy and professional autonomy sometimes assume a remoteness, which may make it difficult to articulate one's sense of despair about a patient's predicament. How devastating the impact of badly chosen words or words left unsaid can be upon people who depend upon our professional sensitivity to help them to face the most critical moments in their lives. The potentially valuable opportunity to respect the patient's autonomy is lost, and even if another meeting occurs, it cannot replace the original: as Lyotard, cited in Taylor (1993, p. 44), states 'one never puts a foot twice in the same river'.

Jimmy died about five months later. The paternalistic decision to withhold the truth from Jimmy was not subjected to discussion and negotiation; a situation referred to by Gillett (1989, p. 109) as 'a convenient smokescreen to hide our medical inexpertise in the face of the profound challenge posed by terminal patients'.

Utilising the principle of non-maleficence has been employed as the justification for being economical with the truth or manipulating language to disguise distressing facts. Jimmy was perceived in some way to have benefited from having the truth withheld from him, that is, harm was supposedly minimised to him. Caplan (1995) suggests that the jargon utilised in professional language reflects a moral and emotional ambivalence to patients and our work which he considers to be at 'epidemic' levels. The language used in professional vocabulary is considered a powerful element in the social stereotyping and subsequent judgements made by nurses and doctors, which directly affects quality of care and communication (Byrne and Heyman, 1997, p. 94). This ambivalence is reflected in the gradual adoption of 'affective neutrality'; an emotional distancing that is consciously or subconsciously a response to some of the most distressing aspects of health care work. The commitment to telling the truth in a kind and sensitive way does not need to compromise the principle of truth-telling in practice.

Professional relationships

The present health care system endorses and feeds the hierarchical nature of professional relationships which can prevent the development of meaningful working relationships (Levine, 1995). Traditional boundaries of professional practice often mitigate against realising the aspiration to perform honestly and sensitively as a team working together, with and for the patient (Campbell, 1988). Whilst the literature stresses the need for teamwork (Øvretveit, 1990), respect (Carlisle, 1990) and effective communication (Sinclair, 1988), Sweet and Norman (1995) state that such prescriptions are 'rarely supported with evidence of successful and satisfying relationships in practice'.

Despite many attempts by social scientists to define, catalogue and characterise the work of professionals, and to demarcate their work from non-professionals, there appears only a small number of core elements about which researchers agree. Claims to trustworthiness, confidentiality, impartiality and altruism are repeatedly cited as characteristics of the conscientious professional in 'personal service' work (Halmos, 1965). These attributes feature repeatedly in nursing and medical professional codes of practice and related documents (GMC, 1993, UKCC, 1989, 1992a, 1992b, 1994), despite claims that professional organisational goals are mostly interested in spreading the gospel of self importance (Titmuss, cited in Campbell, 1988).

The tensions that exist between caring and scientific rigour, nursing and medicine, and the distribution of power within professional groupings are only too evident in Mrs Butterfly's and Jimmy's circumstances. Such tensions are visible in the writings of nursing leaders as a response to changes in society at large, and are more concerned with the acquisition of political power than enhancement of interpersonal relationships. Stein *et al.*, (1990) estimate that the game playing which is enacted by doctors and nurses, observed by Pickering as far back as 1978, and reflecting a professional power gradient in health care, is less prevalent in the 1990s. This they attribute to a deterioration in public esteem for doctors and increasing acknowledgement of their fallibility, coupled with a greater regard for nurses as practitioners in their own right.

The importance of gender ideologies in the caring professions and the notion that 'care' itself is an extension of the female role, less worthy in status and reflecting the class distinctions between medicine and nursing, is well-documented and remarkably resilient to change (Navarro, 1978). Poor or dishonest relationships between doctors and nurses continue to act as a barrier to improving interactions with patients, creating resentment and conflict (Valentine, 1995). This situation reveals a disquiet that must have profound implications for the way in which we care for one another and our subsequent ability to care for others. The dissonance between prescription and practice remains a source of dissatisfaction for the professional trying to engage in a helping relationship (Ratcliffe, 1996).

HUMANISM IN A SCIENTIFIC WORLD

The notion that human beings should explain, control and predict is fundamental to the development of empirical science as the basis for expanding knowledge. Galileo stated that this new approach was designed to 'Measure what can be measured and make measurable what cannot be measured' (cited in Gaarder, 1991, p. 157). To some extent the notion that perception should overrule reason has prevailed since that time. This relatively singular approach to expanding the boundaries of knowledge has also provided one of the greatest barriers to the development of a humanistic approach to health care, one that respects the non-quantifiable nature of our work. The current appetite for measurement in initiatives, such as 'standards', 'audit', 'quality enhancement' and 'evidence-based practice', reflects the current trend to neglect the qualitative, human or process aspects of care (DoH, 1989).

Whilst reductionism has a powerful role to play in the physical sciences, it is increasingly challenged for failing to recognise other sources of knowledge as valid (Carper, 1978; Gortner, 1993), sanctifying the belief that the only reality is that which is expressible in a positivist model of empirical science (Gaarder, 1991). Gortner (1993, p. 52) considers this to be a 'useless opposition of science and humanism'. In a practice-oriented discipline, a paradigm that reflects a spectrum of reality which encompasses mind and body must expand to accommodate multiple modes of enquiry, knowledge and theory. The 'lens' of enquiry must be capable of focusing on the reality. Kuhn (1970) introduced a paradigmatic conception of science, as a recognition of the at least partial failure of deductive methods in the human sciences. Cody (1995) suggests that nursing has only two paradigms or world-views (totality and simultaneity) through which nursing knowledge is organised. The tendency to diminish the contribution of qualities such as intuition, commonly considered an unscientific (female) trait (Munhall and Oiler, 1986), in favour of evidence-based practice is prevalent, yet it is done 'at the peril of the nursing profession' (King and Appleton, 1997, p. 201).

Wimpenny (1993) points to the difficulties in changing to a new humanistic paradigm from the traditional dominance of a natural science paradigm within the educational framework of nursing whist acknowledging the opportunities that exist for enhancing nursing theory development and practice. Nursing theorists are beginning to realise the limitations of existing models in their application to practice (Meleis, 1987), and some have transplanted essential humanistic concepts into frameworks for nursing that recognise the value of human beings as being more than the sum of their parts (Parse *et al.*, 1985; Benner *et al.*, 1992). A high recognition of the value of these conditions has been included in approaches to the management of vulnerable families (Cody, 1996; Long, 1997). The therapist responds as his or her real self, without the use of gimmickry that denotes a false 'image'. This facilitates honesty or congruence between a person's experiencing and his or her thoughts and behaviour.

In medical practice, the limitations of statistics in predicting cure rates are only recently acknowledged. Concepts such as QALYs (quality adjusted life years) and decision analysis trees (Bradley, 1993) are now being introduced as tools which attempt to account for the 'human factor' in scientific enquiry. A professional knowledge base is considered incomplete without 'a deepening self-consciousness and an enriching of the perception of ordinary human relationships'. (Downie and Telfer, 1980, p. 141).

Nurses have been forced to explore the qualitative aspects of our work in response to the overwhelming need to understand the patient's perspective on health and illness, and the desire to improve the quality of care. This has thrust nursing research into the realms of qualitative research, utilising techniques that have been developed to specifically address phenomenological problems in health care that relate to beliefs, values and experiences. Studies have utilised ethnography (Schraeder and Fischer, 1987) to describe experiences, actions, rationales, and consequences of neonatal nurses' activity. Byrne and Heyman (1997) have employed a grounded theory approach to discover the influence of meaning and perception on the communication behaviours of nurses. These and related approaches such as hermeneutics are increasingly recognised as valued tools in helping nurses to touch and unravel the most challenging areas of practice.

THEORETICAL PERSPECTIVES

Most theorists in counselling and psychotherapy, irrespective of emphasis, methods or approaches to treatment, have proposed common core conditions which are widely considered to be at least necessary and sometimes sufficient conditions of engaging in a helping relationship (Rogers *et al.*, 1967; Carkhuff and Berenson, 1967). The therapist 'reads' the client's communication and meaning as it seems to the client, experiencing empathy with the client. The therapist also values and accepts the client for what he or she is, a term described by Rogers (1957, cited in Rogers *et al.*, 1967) as 'unconditional positive regard'. These therapeutic conditions,

Rogers argued, are necessary antecedents to change. Research conducted in the Wisconsin (Rogers *et al.*, 1967) study attempted to apply (and to some extent to bridge the gap between) empirical scientific methodology and humanism. The results yielded important data which suggests that the quality of the interpersonal relationship between the client (patient) and therapist (nurse) is more predictive of a positive outcome than either the nature of the client's condition, or the 'professional' expertise of the therapist. The so-called clients in the study, using the tools of measurement available at that time, were considered to have a much higher degree of perception in relation to the reality of the relationship than the therapists. The findings of Rogers' *et al.*, (1967) study indicate that qualities of genuineness, empathy and unconditional positive regard are core elements of any helping relationship. This model has subsequently been developed by Carkhuff who adds facilitative conditions such as 'concreteness', which he says are valuable in all interpersonal processes. The knowledge of self is a prerequisite to the establishment of a helping relationship, in determination of self-respect and confidence. Ellis (1952) adds that an individual's motivation for maintenance and enhancement of the self and personal life experiences can substantially impact upon the quality of interpersonal relationships. Although originating in studies where the respondents were people labelled as mentally ill, the same core conditions of empathetic relationships are found to be essential in helping relationships wherever they exist. According to Rogers *et al.*, (1967), clients will be in possession of the most accurate perceptions as to what they might realistically expect from relationships with particular nurses or doctors. In practice, in tandem with research into counselling and psychotherapy, experiential learning is respected as a legitimate route to develop models of practice.

COMMUNICATING FOR ADVOCACY

Nurses are expected to extend to patients a level of professional accountability that incorporates being entirely trustworthy, non-discriminatory and confidential. Wilding (cited in Campbell, 1988, p. 2) has an alternative view of the role of codes of practice which he describes as 'campaign documents in the battle for privilege and power'. All nurses face the conflict of adopting a value-free position from which we are expected to treat patients, whilst remaining faithful to our personal values; to provide individualised care, yet work within the limitations of resources that are mostly dictated externally.

Nurses are not a homogenous group; each individual brings to the profession a unique knowledge, intuition, skills and attitudinal base, irrespective of research, protocol or policy (King and Appleton, 1997). Patients or clients are considered to be doubly disadvantaged. They often possess a vulnerability that follows fear at the possibility of pain, usually the unknown, and sometimes even death. This fear is exacerbated by ignorance of the medical and nursing establishment. The emphasis which nurses place upon telling patients the truth and engaging in ethical communication will rest to some extent on the individual practitioner's motivation to respect the patient's right to self-determination.

Historically, nurses have perceived a major aspect of their role in communicating with patients as reinforcing information already relayed by the doctor. Apart from the obvious dangers associated with a 'Chinese whisper' approach to communication, such a stance fails to tackle the process of communication from the perspective of the professional accountability of both doctor and nurse.

Caplan (1995, p. 42) suggests that ill patients should have someone of their choosing, perhaps a friend or relative, present with them at all times in hospital to act as 'advocate, gofer, and confidant'. In fact he regards the health care system with so much trepidation that he argues that patients should 'never, ever' go to hospital alone. The health care system that is supposed to be designed to return people to health now demands that patients need some form of protection from the system itself (Copp, 1986).

It has been suggested that the power differential in professional work which traditionally disadvantaged nurses is a sound basis for justifying a role as advocate. Winslow (1984, p. 36) states: 'Nurses and patients should make obvious allies since both groups have often suffered the indignities of powerlessness in the modern health care system.' The understanding of ethical communication and its relationship with advocacy, particularly in respect of *who* is best placed to be an advocate, like that of the conveyor of bad news, are as yet to be scrutinised in terms of their potential benefit to patients. Mallik (1997) advises that support systems for patient representatives or advocates, particularly within institutions, are inadequate, with the result that formal advocacy roles are 'risky' (p. 130), and should remain the moral choice of individual nurses.

CONCLUSION

All health professionals are faced daily with the issue of deciding who should get what care, and at what cost (Wall, 1995, p. 59). Ethical communication may not be considered high on the list of priorities in a model of care that is primarily concerned with containing costs. The aim to promote communication within this model is, therefore, all the more challenging. As Caplan (1995, p. 420) notes:

'Backbreaking work loads . . . can go a long way towards defeating the best of intentions and the most indomitable of spirits. As we begin the task of reforming our health care system, we owe it to patients to make one that is not only more cost-effective but a lot more user-friendly.'

Theological doctrines attempt to explain the seemingly endless struggle for supremacy between good and evil. The presence of a mental or physical profound or life-limiting disease can provoke feelings of despair that are interrupted by only an occasional moment of hope. Compartmentalisation and the division of labour, control of resources, including knowledge, and the perceived boundaries of professional practice are some of the elements that combine to stifle the potential to promote effective communication (Daft, 1986). The devaluation or absence of caring (which Jaconi (1993) suggests is a euphemism for loving) for other people, is evidenced partly in the demonstration of caring activities and attitudes. The profession endorses the devaluing of caring skills ('basic' nursing care), whilst promoting the development of skills that are traditionally outside of the nursing domain, through initiatives such as the *Scope of Professional Practice* (UKCC, 1992b). Devaluing the role of ethical communication in such circumstances serves only to demonstrate a lack of respect for clients and their experiences, and for the relationship of client and nurse. The idea of nursing as a vocation has been long since replaced with trendier concepts, as it conjured up an image of a nurse who may have been dedicated, but was probably also ill-educated. The term 'vocation' could instead be used to describe aspects of nursing work that relate to caring, sensitivity, being in the service of clients, and striving for a humane system as legitimate pursuits in the best interests of patients. As Wigram (1957, cited in Patterson, 1980, p. 9) states:

'There is nothing more delightful and lovable on earth than one's neighbour. Love does not think about doing work, it finds joy in people.'

Frankl's philosophy (1952, cited in Patterson, 1980) generated partly through his personal experiences in Auschwitz and Dachau, has immense appeal due to the emphasis he places upon love as the highest and ultimate goal of human beings. He suggests that the meaning of life is unique to each individual and that by finding each person's latent value, one can help people to be answerable for their own lives. In this way, he argues, meaning and the opportunity for growth can be found, even in suffering. Whilst criticised for being vague in its approach and underdeveloped in techniques, Frankl (1952) uses examples from prison life to demonstrate that even in times of extreme stress, 'spiritual' freedom enables people to make choices, as long as they have some hope or faith in the future, no matter how short the future might be.

Emerging from this analysis is the need to develop a philosophy of ethical communication that puts individual patients' needs above other considerations, including perceived professional role boundaries. Only a commitment based upon a foundation of inter-professional alliance between medical and nursing staff will create the necessary conditions for ethical communication. Professional roles are mediated by personal experiences, and acknowledge the equality of partnership between the nurse and the person in need of help. The partnership should recognise the contribution of client and helper, and potentially enrich the scope for human interaction as a more appropriate vehicle for delivering care than current models can offer.

References

Alexander, L. (1990) Explication of the meaning of clinical judgment in nursing practice using Ricoeurean hermeneutics. *Dissertation Abstracts International* B52/02, 744 (University Microfilms No. AAC 9119796).

Ashworth, P. (1980) *Care to Communicate*. London: Royal College of Nursing.

Barrett, J. F. and Jarvis, G. J. (1990) Inconsistencies in clinical decisions in obstetrics. *The Lancet,* 336, pp. 549–51.

Benner, P., Tanner, C. and Chesla, C. (1992) From beginner to expert: gaining a differentiated clinical world in critical care nursing. *Advances in Nursing Science,* 14(3), pp. 13–28.

Bond, S. (1982) Communication in cancer nursing. In M. C. Cahoon (ed.), *Recent Advances in Nursing 3: Cancer Nursing.* Churchill Livingstone: Edinburgh, pp. 3–30.

Bradley, G. W. (1993) *Disease, Diagnosis and Decisions.* Chichester: John Wiley & Sons.

Byrne, G. and Heyman, R. (1997) Understanding nurses' communication with patients in accident and emergency departments using a symbolic interactionist perspective. *Journal of Advanced Nursing,* 26, pp. 93–100.

Campbell, A. V. (1988) Profession and vocation. In G. Fairbairn and S. Fairbairn (eds), *Ethical Issues in Caring.* Aldershot: Avebury, pp. 1–10.

Caplan, A. (1995) *Moral Matters.* Chichester: John Wiley & Sons.

Carkhuff, R. R. and Berenson, B. G. (1967) *Beyond Counselling and Therapy.* London: Holt, Rinehart & Winston.

Carlisle, D. (1990) The call of duty. *Nursing Times,* 86(20), pp. 54–5.

Carper, B. A. (1978) Fundamental patterns of knowing in nursing *Advances in Nursing Science,* 1(1), pp. 13–23.

Cody, A. (1996) Helping the vulnerable or condoning control within the family: where is nursing? *Journal of Advanced Nursing,* 23, pp. 882–6.

Cody, W. K. (1995) About all those paradigms: many in the universe, two in nursing. *Science Quarterly*, 8(4), pp. 144–7.

Copp, L. A. (1986) The nurse as advocate for vulnerable persons. *Journal of Advanced Nursing,* 11(3), pp. 255–63.

Daft, R. L. (1986) *Organization Theory and Design.* St Paul, NJ: West.

Department of Health (1989) *Caring for People: Community Care in the Next Decade and Beyond,* Cmnd 849. London: HMSO.

Downie, R. S. and Telfer, E. (1980) *Caring and Curing.* London: Methuen.

Ellis, A. (1952) *Reason and Emotion in Psychotherapy.* New York: Lyle Stuart.

Ford, D. H. and Urban, H. B. (1963) *Systems of Psychotherapy.* New York: Wiley.

Gaarder, J.(1991) *Sophie's World.* London: Phoenix House.

General Medical Council (1993) *Professional Conduct and Fitness to Practise (Blue Book).* London: GMC.

Gillett, G. (1989) *Reasonable Care*. Bristol: The Bristol Press.

Gortner, S. R. (1993) Nursing's syntax revisited: a critique of philosophies said to influence nursing theories. *International Journal of Nursing Studies,* 30, pp. 477–88.

Hall, J. A. and Dornan, M. C. (1988) What patients like about their medical care and how often they are asked: a meta analysis of the satisfaction literature. *Social Science Medicine,* 27(9), pp. 935–9.

Halmos, P. (1965) *The Faith of the Counsellors*. London: Constable.

Hawley, A. (1990) Morality and patient care. In D. Evans (ed.) *Why Should We Care?* London: Macmillan, pp. 10–17.

Hunt, G. (1995) *Whistleblowing in the Health Service*. London: Edward Arnold.

Jaconi, B. (1993) Caring is loving. *Journal of Advanced Nursing*, 18, pp. 192–4.

Johnson, J. E., Rice, V. E., Fuller, S. S. and Endress, M. P. (1978) Sensory information, instruction in a coping strategy and recovery from surgery. *Research in Nursing and Health*, 1(1), pp. 4–7.

Jones, M., O'Neill, P., Waterman, H. and Webb, C. (1997) Building a relationship: communications and relationships between staff and stroke patients on a rehabilitation ward. *Journal of Advanced Nursing,* 26, pp. 101–10.

King, L. and Appleton, J. V. (1997) Intuition: a critical review of the research and rhetoric. *Journal of Advanced Nursing,* 26, pp. 194–202.

Kuhn, T. (1970) *The Structure of Scientific Revolutions,* 2nd edn. Chicago, Ill.: University of Chicago Press.

Lanceley, A. (1985) Use of controlling language in the care of the elderly. *Journal of Advanced Nursing* 10, pp. 125–35.

Levine, M. E. (1995) The rhetoric of nursing theory. *Image: Journal of Nursing Scholarship,* 27(1), pp. 11–14.

Ley, P. (1988) *Communicating with Patients: Improving Communication, Satisfaction and Compliance,* Psychology and Medicine series. Cambridge: Croom Helm.

Long, A. (1997) Avoiding abuse amongst vulnerable groups in the community. Cited in C. Mason (ed.), *Achieving Quality in Community Health Care Nursing*. London: Macmillan.

McAlindon, M. N. (1997) Nurse informaticists: who are they, what do they do, and what challenges do they face? In, J. C. McCloskey and H. K. Grace, (eds), *Current Issues in Nursing,* 5th edn. St Louis, New Orleans: Mosby.

Mallik, M. (1997) Advocacy in nursing – a review of the literature. *Journal of Advanced Nursing,* 25, pp. 130–8.

May, C. (1990) Research on nurse–patient relationships: problems of theory, problems of practice. *Journal of Advanced Nursing,* 15, pp. 307–15.

Meleis, A. I. (1987) Revisions in knowledge development: a passion for substance. *Scholarly Inquiry in Nursing Practice,* 1(1), pp. 5–19.

Munhall, P. L. and Oiler, C. J. (1986) *Nursing Research.* Conn.: Appleton-Century-Crofts.

Navarro, V. (1978) *Class Struggle: The State and Medicine.* London: Martin Robertson.

Øvretveit, J. (1990) Making the team work. *Professional Nurse,* 5(6), pp. 284–8.

Parse, R. R., Coyne, A. B. and Smith, M. J. (1985) *Nursing Research: Qualitative Methods.* Bowie, Md: Brady.

Patterson, C. H. (ed.) (1980) *Theories of Counselling and Psychotherapy.* Cambridge: Harper & Row.

Poulton, B. C. (1995) Keeping the customer satisfied. *Primary Health Care,* 5(4), pp. 16–19.

Radwin, L. E. (1996) 'Knowing the patient': a review of research on an emerging concept. *Journal of Advanced Nursing,* 23, pp. 1142–6.

Ratcliffe, P. (1996) Gender differences in career progress in nursing: towards a non-essentialist structural theory. *Journal of Advanced Nursing,* 23, pp. 389–95.

Rogers, C. R., Gendlin, E. J., Kiesler, D. J. and Truax, C. (1967) *The Therapeutic Relationship and its Impact: a study of psychotherapy with schizophrenics.* Madison, WI: University of Winconsin Press.

Roth, L. H. and Meisel, A.(1977) Dangerousness, confidentiality and the duty to warn. *American Journal of Psychiatry,* 134, pp. 508–11.

Schraeder, B. and Fischer, D. (1987) Using intuitive knowledge in the neonatal intensive care nursery. *Holistic Nursing Practice,* 1(3), pp. 45–51.

Seedhouse, D. (1991) *Liberating Medicine.* Chichester: John Wiley & Sons.

Sinclair, F. (1988) Communication and the health care team. *Nursing,* 3(27), pp. 993–5.

Stein, L., Watts, D. T. and Howell, T. (1990) The doctor–nurse game revisited. *New England Journal of Medicine,* 322(8), pp. 546–49.

Sundeen, S. J., Stewart, G. W., Rankin, E. A. and Cohen, S. A. (1994) *Nurse–client Interaction. Implementing the Nursing Process*, 5th edn. St Louis, New Orleans: C.V. Mosby.

Sweet, S. J. and Norman, I. J. (1995) The nurse–doctor relationship: a selective literature review. *Journal of Advanced Nursing, 22*, pp. 165–70.

Taylor, M. (1993) The nurse–patient relationship. *Senior Nurse,* 13(5), pp. 14–18.

Titmuss, R. (1988) cited in A. V. Campbell, Profession and vocation. In G. Fairbairn and S. Fairbairn (eds), *Ethical Issues in Caring*. Aldershot: Avebury, pp. 1–10.

United Kingdom Central Council for Nursing, Midwifery and Health Visiting (UKCC) (1989) *Exercising Accountability*. London: UKCC.

United Kingdom Central Council for Nursing, Midwifery and Health Visiting (UKCC) (1992a) *Code of Professional Conduct.* London: UKCC.

United Kingdom Central Council for Nursing, Midwifery and Health Visiting (UKCC) (1992b) *The scope of professional practice*. London: UKCC.

United Kingdom Central Council for Nursing, Midwifery and Health Visiting (UKCC) (1994) *The Future of Professional Practice – the Council's Standards for Education and Practice Following Registration.* London: UKCC.

Valentine, P. E. (1995) Management of conflict: do nurses/women handle it differently? *Journal of Advanced Nursing, 22*, pp. 142–9.

Vincent, C. (1989) Research into medical accidents: a case of negligence? *British Medical Journal, 299*, pp. 1150–3.

Wall, A. (1995) Ethical and resource issues in health and social care. In P. Owens, J. Carrier and J. Horder (eds), *Interprofessional Issues in Community and Primary Health Care. London*: Macmillan.

Wardhaugh, J. and Wilding, P. (1983) Towards an explanation of the corruption of care. *Critical Social Policy, 37*, pp. 4–31.

Wilding, P. (1988) Cited in A. V. Campbell, Profession and vocation. In G. Fairbairn and S. Fairbairn (eds), *Ethical Issues in Caring*. Aldershot: Avebury, pp. 1–10.

Wilkinson, S. (1991) Factors which influence how nurses communicate with cancer patients. *Journal of Advanced Nursing, 16*, pp. 677–88.

Wimpenny, P. (1993) The paradox of Parse's theory. *Senior Nurse,* 13(5), pp. 10–13.

Winslow, G. R. (1984) From loyalty to advocacy: a new metaphor for nursing. *The Hastings Center Report,* June, pp. 32–40.

Woodyard, J. (1990) Facing up to errors. *Health Service Journal,* 29 March, pp. 468–9.

CHAPTER SEVEN

Communicating Beyond Individual Bias

Dennis Tourish

'The thing with Aborigines, and this is very well known now in Australia, is that post mortems show they definitely have smaller brains than white people.'
(*Author interview with Australian builder, 1997*)

'praise God for AIDS!' AIDS is wiping out the undesirables . . . it's taking out blacks by the thousands; before long it'll· completely depopulate Africa. You know they're over there, they're living like savages . . . the government says they're equal to the white man. And I don't believe that, there's no way that could be possible.'
(*Dave Holland, a leader of the Southern White Knights of the Ku Klux Klan, cited in Ezekiel, 1995, p. 93*)

INTRODUCTION

When we communicate with other people from a standpoint of individual bias, it means that we are failing to recognise the other person as the unique human being he or she is – with all the positive and negative qualities which constitute their own individual personality. Instead, we are viewing them as representative of a broader social category possessed of certain qualities which we dislike, and which we assume are shared by most or all members of that particular social group. In short, we have stereotyped the person concerned ('he or she must be stupid') on the basis of the category to which we have assigned them (he or she may be a nurse, but primarily 'he or she is black') and on to which we have projected a number of critical assumptions (such as 'all black people are stupid').

There is some evidence that a number of traditional intergroup prejudices have declined in the latter half of the twentieth century – for example, that white prejudices against blacks and Jews have moderated (Wilson, 1996). However, it is also possible that although blatant prejudice has declined its more subtle manifestations remain intact. Pettigrew and Meertens (1995) define the former as open, direct and hot, and the latter as cool, distant and indirect. Their research suggests that people who score high in tests measuring blatant prejudice want to restrict immigrants' rights further, send them back to what is defined as their home country and do little or nothing to improve immigrant–native relationships. Those who score highly on subtle indices of prejudice merely reject minorities in more socially acceptable ways. Thus, they do not wish to repatriate all immigrants, but would dispatch those against whom an ostensibly non-prejudicial justification for such action can be found. They do not support forceful methods for improving race relations, but would support 'soft' measures that place the burden on others and require little action from themselves. This suggests that stereotypes, whatever their character, reinforce the underlying habit of deindividuating people into distinct social groups rather than seeing them as individuals, and hence facilitates the development of prejudice.

The threefold purpose of this chapter is to discuss (1) the extent to which most of us are vulnerable to such biases (blatant and subtle); (2) how they come into being; and (3) to identify the communication skills most likely to help us communicate beyond individual bias. Therefore, we will begin by defining what we mean by prejudice, and explore how the stereotypes which guide biased communication transactions are formed and maintained. Given that the term 'bias' may itself be little more than a subtle and hence more socially acceptable version of the word 'prejudice' we will use the two terms interchangeably. We will also examine theories which claim to show how prejudice can be reduced, and the associated communication strategies which they suggest should enable us to eliminate prejudice from human communication. In the process, the reader is invited to consider the extent to which bias forms part of his or her own outlook. Box 7.1 contains an exploratory exercise designed to stimulate thinking on this topic.

Box 7.1   Measuring interpersonal attitudes

Examine the following general assumptions carefully. Rate each statement on a scale of 1 to 5 in terms of how strongly you agree with it, with 1 representing strong disagreement and 5 representing strong agreement. Then turn to the scoring system at the end of this chapter.

1. Nurses are caring and possess a vocation.
2. Irish people love Guinness and fighting and believe in 'the Little People.'
3. Academics are absent-minded.
4. Jewish/ Scottish people are mean.
5. Americans are loud-mouthed. Texans are the loudest of them all.
6. Men love football.
7. Politicians are in it for the money. They don't have any principles.
8. Women drivers are terrible.
9. Black people are thick, violent and work-shy.
10. Sex is the price women pay for marriage, while marriage is the price men pay for sex.
11. Parisians are invariably rude to visitors.
12. Gay men are more likely than heterosexual men to seduce little boys.
13. People with glasses are more intelligent than people who do not wear glasses.
14. Film stars are more interesting people than those in most other occupations.
15. My political opinions are more correct than most other people's.

THE NATURE OF PREJUDICE AND STEREOTYPICAL GENERALISATIONS

Research into prejudice owes much to the pioneering work of Gordon Allport, who published his groundbreaking book *The Nature of Prejudice* in 1954. Allport raised the notion that prejudice was the outcome of our tendency to generalise about others, and so to assign people to distinct social categories. By doing so we exaggerate the extent to which prototypical characteristics of that category are shared by all its members, and minimise individual characteristics which distinguish people from the general collective (Inman and Baron, 1996). This line of thought has been followed by subsequent investigators, who generally agree that prejudice involves holding negative attitudes towards others largely because of their perceived membership of some group (Worchel *et al.*, 1988). As Brown (1995, p. 8) sums it up, prejudice can be viewed as

'the holding of derogatory social attitudes or cognitive beliefs, the expression of negative affect, or the display of hostile or discriminatory behaviour towards members of a group on account of their membership of that group.'

Central to the process of bias formation is the observation that we make sense of a complex, contradictory and often unknowable social world by categorising and hence simplifying whatever is going on around us. Such categorisation enables us to perceive order in the world rather than random chaos. It is therefore necessary. We do not always have the time to observe each individuating trait of everyone we meet, particularly when the encounter is brief and occurs in the context of other events. Another, less fortunate, effect is that our communication with people is often mediated through the stereotypes we hold about their group. Such stereotypes assume that heterogeneous groups share more common behaviours, feelings and personality traits than they actually do (Leyens *et al.*, 1994). We are then inclined to view members of a group as interchangeable with other members of the designated category. Again, it can be seen that some of this is inevitable and often beneficial: nurses cannot know every single patient in detail, and must make a number of general evaluations based on diagnosis, age, prognosis and so on. This is despite the fact that no individual patient's overall illness profile ever accords to a notional statistical mean. Thus, the cost of any generalisation, however necessary, is that we fail to appreciate the full uniqueness of the whole person, ensuring that our stereotypes sometimes lead us into judgements which are both erroneous and biased.

Most of us are extraordinarily willing to categorise others on the basis of very limited information. This was well-shown by a newspaper report on the appointment of General Boonthin Wrongakmit as Assistant Police Director in Thailand some years ago. Speaking after his appointment he said, 'I shall be introducing an all-round shoot-to-kill policy towards our criminals. As police chief of North-East Thailand for 37 years I always used this policy.' Asked how he could be sure his men always shot the right people, the General replied: 'You could tell by the look of them' (cited in Hargie, 1992).

Moreover, we seem naturally predisposed to make the reduction of uncertainty a central aim during our interactions with others (Berger, 1987). Therefore, we resort to the perceptual short-cut of quickly identifying what this new person has in common with other people we have encountered in the past (Sutherland, 1992). Our initial and inescapably shallow categorisations are then often maintained because we tend to notice whatever supports our view-point while ignoring anything which goes against it (Dawes, 1994).

We also notice what people in a minority group do much more than we notice those in a majority group – precisely because of their minority status. For example, a black person in a predominantly white city will be more conspicuous than one where blacks pre-dominate. Given that anti-social behaviour is more noticeable than that which conforms to our norms or expectations this ensures that 'bad' behaviour by someone from a minority group is doubly likely to be noticed, commented upon and taken as evidence of a dominant behavioural trend among members of that minority group. We also have a tendency to see unusual events as somehow connected, even when there is no rational basis for assuming such a relationship (Hamilton, 1979). In terms of bias, a member of a minority group may behave badly, and because they do this becomes more noticeable. In turn, their membership of a minority group is more noticeable because it is more unusual. The suggestion is that we are likely to assume a connection between the two – what has been called an 'illusory correlation' (McArthur, 1980). It could reasonably be hypothesised, for example, that many readers will be inclined to assume a connection between forthcoming natural disasters, the occurrence of which is statistically inevitable, and the imminent arrival of a new millennium, even though there is no rational basis for such an inference. This explanation helps explain the persistent negative stereotypes which many people still hold of 'women drivers'. Despite the hostile folklore which abounds on this subject, actuarial evidence shows that they are safer drivers than men (Sutherland, 1992). Accordingly, many insurance companies (who know a thing or two about how to evaluate evidence) offer lower premiums to women. However, negative impressions were often formed in the days when a much lower proportion of women learned to drive than is now the case, and such impressions endure in spite of the evidence.

Stereotypes also become self-fulfilling. An employer may expect someone to fail, and so withhold the resources and support the person needs to succeed in their job. Their subsequent failure to perform well is then perceived by the employer as proof that their original perception was valid. Subsequently, other employees deemed to belong to the same category as this person will be more likely to be treated in the same discriminatory way. Additionally, relatively minor differences between people (such as their skin colour) are assumed to signify greater differences on other more important dimensions, such as leadership potential, sociability and intelligence (Leyens *et al.*, 1994). In this way, the process of stereotyping reinforces prejudice, reduces levels of contact between disparate groups and stimulates discriminatory practice.

In addition to minor differences being interpreted as a barometer of greater difference, it has been found that whites observing or hearing about a solitary black person's negative attitudes have their critical out-group perceptions strengthened (Henderson-King and Nisbitt, 1996). They were also more likely afterwards to avoid contact with black people or minimise the duration of interactions with black people when these proved unavoidable. Furthermore, a single negative event involving a black person was sufficient to lead participants into expressing in-group favouritism. It is interesting, in the light of this research, to speculate on the impact of OJ Simpson's trial on levels of intergroup communication between blacks and whites in the United States.

This has, among much else, major implications for multidisciplinary team working. A Fellini movie, *Orchestral Rehearsal*, features members of an orchestra talking in detail about what oboists, tympanists, violinists and bassoonists are like. As Brown (1986) points out, most professional groups categorise and define their subgroups. Within the medical field, doctors form stereotypes of psychiatrists, surgeons or proctologists – and nurses. In turn, the 'favour' is reciprocated by nurses, who also form and act upon stereotypes of other professional groups such as social workers, administrators, occupational therapists and so on. Bizarre misattributions of all kinds are then often maintained, precisely because they have been formed in a group context. For example, Venkatesan (1966) had subjects select the 'best' suit from three identical alternatives. When people chose individually they had an equal chance of picking any suit. However, when they were with others who had been primed to express a particular preference they all chose the suit singled out by the rest of the group. Furthermore, they stuck to their choice even when the others were no longer present, and insisted that the suit they had chosen was indeed different from the other two. This suggests that we interpret the agreement of others with our beliefs as a form of 'social proof' (Cialdini, 1993): in essence, we seize upon public support for our opinions as evidence of their correctness. Needless to say, everyone else performs the same operation on us. Thus, much of what we believe about different groups is little more than a shared hallucination inspired by conformity effects. As this discussion suggests, such perceptual distortions interfere with our ability to objectively appraise what another person is actually doing or saying, and so impedes clear communication.

THE IMPACT OF INTERPERSONAL EXPECTATIONS ON COMMUNICATION

A fruitful way to explore how stereotyping leads to biased communication practices is by considering how the beliefs we hold about other people and general social categories turn into *expectations*. Typically, we associate a range of traits (behavioural, personal, dispositional, motivational, emotional) with the people we assign to certain social categories (Jones, 1990). We develop a series of mental frameworks known as schemata to help us organise our impressions of others (Kagan *et al.*, 1986). Such impressions are often based on those descriptive terms most accessible to us, perhaps because they have been recently drawn to our attention (Zebrowitz, 1990). Thus, Langer and Abelson (1974) found that traditional therapists who were expecting to interview a 'patient' evaluated the person as more disturbed than therapists who were expecting to interview a 'job applicant.'

The results of this are very much in line with what is suggested by attribution theory: namely, that we interpret the actions of others in the light of what we assume their underlying dispositions to be rather than necessarily by what they do (Darley and Oleson, 1994). Thus if I expect you to be poor at games, clumsy in the kitchen or forgetful with messages it is likely that I will either not see disconfirmatory episodes or play down their significance, while I will also exaggerate the frequency of those occasions on which you conform to the attributional disposition I have formed of you. This has been called a 'perceptual confirmation effect' (Zebrowitz, 1990). While some of these expectations may be benign, such as the notion that nurses are nurturing, they are none the less dispositional expectancies which bias us towards interpreting a person's behaviour in a certain way. In short, they lead us to anticipate that a nurse will behave in a particular (predictable) fashion and, therefore, incline us to interpret his or her behaviour in such a way that it confirms our expectation. Of course, if we see enough of someone it is more likely that their individual personality will eventually take over and supersede category expectations of the kind under discussion. For example, it is not uncommon for white racists to feel hostile towards black people in general and treat black strangers badly, but nevertheless acknowledge that a particular black neighbour is a worthwhile person.

Furthermore, interpersonal behaviour evokes confirming behaviour from the target, and thus activates a self-fulfilling prophecy (Taylor, 1994). A fear of ageing (gerontophobia) may contribute to a morbid aversion towards elderly people, expressed in discriminatory or hostile practices during interviews (Thomas, 1988). In turn, such attitudes may encourage older people to act out the roles prescribed for them, thus creating a self-fulfilling prophecy (Phillipson, 1982). The 'confirmation' thus arrived at of our expectation reinforces it all the more.

As a further example of bias, a white person may assume that black people are unfriendly and either shun contact with them or transmit unfriendly signals themselves. This puts the black person off responding in a friendly manner. When the hostile expectation is responded to in like fashion the original prophecy has been confirmed, and the underlying feeling of bias reinforced. Not only do we see what our prejudice tells us we will see, but our own behaviour (founded on the prejudice) makes it more likely that what we are railing against will exist in the first place. In addition, research suggests that people tend to assume that whatever is repeated is true (Scheflin and Opton, 1978; Dawes, 1994). We also evaluate the correctness of our perceptions through ascertaining the extent to which they are shared by others, in a process of social testing. Thus, if we now find that our biased expectations are echoed back to us by others (or if we ourselves seek out opportunities to share them with other people) such conversations will form a pattern of repetition and become a further source of confirmation for our bias. In this manner, the unreal increasingly appears real.

Hostile expectations are capable of having a negative effect without reaching the stage of an interpersonal encounter (Darley and Fazio, 1980). For example, a senior nurse manager might be inclined not to interview members of a particular minority group for promotion. This becomes further evidence that they cannot do this sort of work: otherwise where are they? The consequence, moreover, is that the underlying bias is strengthened.

When a group is the subject of biased attitudes it is then discriminated against. It has been argued that we have a need to make sense of such marginalisation in a manner which reinforces our own self-image of superiority, while justifying or denying the existence of the discrimination to which such superior feelings give rise. Thus, Bobo and Kluegel (1991) investigated white stereotypes of African Americans, Hispanic Americans and Asian Americans. They found that whites needed to 'explain' the disadvantaged condition of the minority being observed: more precisely, to find explanations which justified it. Many alternative explanations for black disadvantage are available (for example, that the disadvantage is primarily the product of white prejudice and discrimination). However, to accept this would require self-criticism, and criticism might in turn be extended to social institutions with which many whites identify more closely than do members of minority groups. Thus, Bobo and Kluegel found that whites tended to assume a causal connection between the stereotypical traits ascribed to the minority groups and their social situation: that is, it was their own fault. In short, it was much more convenient to assume that their position of social disadvantage reflected their naturally inferior position than discrimination practised by the white society. This could be described as a perspective of 'illusory causality'. The tendency to blame those at the receiving end of bias for its effects is particularly pronounced among members of extreme hate groups. Thus, Ezekiel (1995, p. 75) cites Tom Metzger, a leader of White Aryan Resistance, as follows:

'I found so many Jews, and even when nobody was giving them any trouble they thought they were being persecuted, they're always looking for somebody to persecute them, and I think that many times they end up getting persecuted because of it.'

This tendency to seek confirmation and justification of our own attitudes, self-serving biases and consequent actions has been termed a reflex of self-justification (Tourish and Mulholland,

1997). We are basically motivated to see ourselves positively rather than negatively – although this mechanism breaks down if we are placed in an environment dominated by negative feedback (Seligman, 1975). However, the tendency to polish our own image predisposes us to seek supportive feedback on decisions made, behaviours adopted and the social groups to which we affiliate (Tajfel and Turner, 1986). Furthermore, the desire to affiliate is one of the most fundamental human attributes (Hargie and Tourish, 1997), since such affiliation provides us with a social identity, while it is easier to affiliate with groups which we see positively. The consequence is bias, discriminatory practice and a tendency to blame those at the receiving end of prejudice rather than ourselves for the socially disadvantaged position they occupy.

Nor are these difficulties simply the result of perceiving other people as belonging to groups (out-groups) – we also perceive ourselves largely in terms of the groups to which we belong (in-groups), and this in turn influences our perceptions of others (Brown, 1988). The tendency to stigmatise out-groups while rating in-groups favourably leads to an enhancement of contrast effect between groups (Campbell, 1956), in which the extent of differences becomes greatly exaggerated. For example, Hamilton and Bishop (1976) interviewed white residents in a Connecticut suburb into which new families had recently moved. They found that respondents were more likely to mention the arrival of a new family when it was black. A month later only 11 per cent of white respondents knew the last name of the black families, while 60 per cent of them knew the last names of the whites. Thus, blacks were seen as very alike (often without even the individuating marker of a last name), while the whites were accorded more individuality and became more memorable because of their perceived individual differences.

Such biases seem to reward us with a direct pay-off in terms of improved self-esteem (Zander *et al.*, 1960). Thus, Hunter *et al.*, (1996) found that when people experience evaluative intergroup bias, various facets of self-esteem (concerned with verbal ability, physical appearance, religion, honesty and academic ability) are enhanced. In short, when we denigrate members of another group it makes us feel superior, and we find such feelings of superiority rather agreeable. This process helps explain the observation that when we spot a flaw in the arguments of someone opposed to us (in politics, religion or in personal relationships) confidence in our own position grows, quite irrationally. This is akin to identifying a major design flaw in a neighbour's new home, and finding that our faith in the structural integrity of our own property rises as a result. In reality, every argument contains flaws. It is, therefore, an easy matter to spot contradictions in positions to which we do not subscribe. Since this strengthens our self-confidence it is a major explanation for the misplaced faith which many of us put in spurious arguments, outmoded political philosophies – and naked prejudices.

REDUCING BIAS

Given such a volume of perceptual constraints, can anything be done to eliminate bias? This has been a key concern of researchers for many years. So far, no simple solutions have been forthcoming, although many ideas have been proposed. Each of the major approaches suggested has grown out of a particular theoretical approach to prejudice and its various manifestations. It is worth exploring some of these in more detail.

The role of hardship

There is a certain intuitive validity to the notion that hardship causes frustration which, when it cannot be aimed directly at its cause, is then projected on to other groups – the 'frustration/ aggression hypothesis' (Dollard *et al.*, 1939). Such an analysis would suggest that fundamental social, economic and political transformation is required to eliminate bias. The hardship approach to prejudice formation and reduction has its origins in the research of Hovland and Sears (1940). They hypothesised that economic pressures explained high annual variations in the lynching of blacks in the USA: the greater the level of hardship in any one year the more likely it would be that the number of lynchings would increase. Likewise, some left-wing analysts have long argued that economic deprivation provides the fuel for sectarianism in Northern Ireland.

However, the experimental evidence on this issue is mixed. Some studies have indeed shown that manipulating levels of frustration creates or inflames hostile attitudes towards out-groups. For example, Miller and Bugelski (1948) arranged for the cancellation of an evening out which young men at an American camp had been looking forward to. They found that attitudes to Mexicans and Japanese, which they had prudently measured before the experiment began, deteriorated in the wake of the cancelled outing. Others have found no increase in prejudice among students after they failed certain academic tests (Stagner and Congdon, 1955). Furthermore, such an analysis does not explain why one group rather than another should become the focus of the aggression which has been displaced. An overemphasis on the role of hardship could also become a handy means of 'displacing' responsibility for ending prejudice on to government, rather than assuming it ourselves – a possible explanation for its intuitive validity. As we have already seen, much of what we find intuitively correct is actually wrong, or founded on self-serving biases.

A modified and more successful version of the frustration–aggression hypothesis has been 'relative deprivation theory' (Gurr, 1970). This proposes that the absolute level of deprivation does not cause prejudice – instead, the key factor is the relative nature of hardship which people experience (Stouffer *et al.*, 1949). For example, Vanneman and Pettigrew (1972) surveyed over 1000 white voters in four US cities. Respondents identified whether they felt they were doing better or worse economically than other whites. They also identified how they felt they were doing compared to blacks. Those who perceived themselves as doing worse than blacks were much more inclined to be prejudiced towards blacks, since, apparently, they had an out-group against which they could compare themselves. Rather than the absolute level of disadvantage producing prejudice, such feelings depended on a perception of disadvantage relative to another group viewed as doing particularly well. Those who only felt disadvantaged against fellow whites felt no such prejudice. Overall, this research suggests that uncertainty may indeed inflame prejudice (under certain conditions), largely as a result of the 'illusory correlation' effect discussed above. While this has implications for economic management, policy making and politicians, and certainly forms a worthwhile contribution to debate on the issue, it does not provide individuals with much guidance on how to manage their own communication episodes so that instances of prejudice are reduced. What can be done here to ease such problems?

Communicating to eliminate bias

The most influential theory of prejudice reduction has been the contact hypothesis, initially developed by Allport (1954). As its name suggests, this postulates that contact is the most important factor in reducing prejudice between different groups. However, as Allport and others quickly realised, there are many occasions when such contact exacerbates rather than reduces tension. Rival groups of football fans, crammed together in a football stadium, regularly show increased rather than reduced levels of conflict. However, the research literature broadly supports the notion that *close and sustained contact* reduces prejudice (Powers and Ellison, 1995), although it is important to understand more precisely the contexts in which such contact must take place if its benefits are to be realised. These have been summarised by Brown (1995) as follows.

1. Social and institutional support

This means that key individuals in the relevant society and in a number of its most vital institutions unambiguously endorse the notion of contact, and are overtly committed to its achievement. For example, integrated schooling in the USA has been more successful when teachers and the wider community come out in its support (Epstein, 1985). Such people and institutions are in a position to administer sanctions and rewards, are naturally looked up to by people for leadership and are therefore in a position to serve as role models for prejudice reduction. This could be conceived as a version of social learning theory (Bandura, 1977), which claims that we learn new behaviours and change old ones through a process of modelling, imitation and reinforcement.

In addition, cognitive dissonance theory proposes that if people change their behaviours in a particular direction it then becomes more likely that their attitudes will subsequently change, to come in line with the newly adopted behaviour (Festinger, 1957; Aronson, 1997). In this way feelings of dissonance, defined as an unpleasant awareness of the gap between behaviour and attitudes, is avoided. Thus, if people are compelled to behave in a less prejudiced manner their views will be more likely to change in line with their newly adopted and less biased behaviours. Accordingly, Thomson *et al.* (1995) argue in favour of strong institutional support for anti-racist practice, to involve granting the residents of any country full citizenship, regarding racist incidents as human rights violations and responding accordingly, and consciously rejecting any notions of a homogeneous, ethnically pure national identity. In addition, it is argued that laws against racism and discrimination are necessary and should be enforced. However, as they themselves note, notions of ethnic purity have grown within Europe (the euphemistic expression 'ethnic cleansing' is a recent excrescence on the language), in response to such unprecedented social phenomena as the collapse of the former Soviet Union.

2. Acquaintance potential

Contacts should be of sufficient frequency, duration and closeness to allow meaningful relationships to develop. Short-lasting contact may reinforce prejudice by activating stereotypical impressions, while its brevity does not afford those involved sufficient time to acquire detailed knowledge of each other and so go beyond the most obvious stereotypes. On the other hand, interpersonal contact is generally perceived as rewarding (Dickson *et al.*, 1993). If it lasts long enough such rewarding feelings challenge and displace stereotypes. Thus, a variety of studies suggest that integrated housing and schooling developments, over time, reduce prejudiced attitudes (Wilner *et al.*, 1952; Stephan and Rosenfeld, 1978).

3. Equal status

Contact needs to be between people of equal status, in order to have the maximum effect of reducing prejudice. For example, if prejudiced US whites interact with blacks mostly in the subordinate role as servants, impressions of their innate inferiority will be reinforced rather than eased (Brown, 1995). This increases the possibility that whites will treat new black acquaintances as if they occupy an inferior social position. The author of this chapter recalls meeting two well-off American women (one black and one white) who happened at the time to rent a house together in Los Angeles. However, the white woman was a well-known movie actress, which further gave her a high-status position and activated associated archetypes in the minds of acquaintances. Her friend reported that when people visited their house they often assumed that she was the maid, and treated her accordingly. (In reality, she had also been an actress and was now a published sci-fi writer.) On the other hand, cooperation between equals puts their essential human connection to the fore and reduces the group categorisation effect to negligible proportions.

4. Cooperation

If members of different groups, including those traditionally in opposition to each other, cooperate to achieve common goals, prejudice seems to be reduced. How this might work is illustrated by the work of Sherif *et al.* (1961), who conducted a highly influential series of studies into patterns of friendship formation among young boys in summer camps. Study participants were split into two groups. Care was taken to ensure that preexisting friends found themselves in different groups. These were then given separate activities and had minimal contact with each other for a few days. Furthermore, a number of competitions were organised between the groups (for example, tug-of-war contests). This led to hostility, with verbal abuse being directed against other groups and a number of physical attacks occurring. In-group bias was also rampant, while friendships formed with members of the new group rapidly replaced the old. The question then became one of how to reduce the tensions which had been generated. The solution hit upon by Sherif and his co-workers, after a number of failures, was to promote positive interdependence. For example, they arranged for a truck to break down miles from camp. This could not be started by one group on its own, but could be if two groups cooperated. After a series of such engineered incidents aggression and prejudice were reduced, while old intergroup friendships were reestablished.

A more recent example of how such insights can be adapted to particular situations comes from the work of Wolfe and Spencer (1996). They review what is known as 'the jigsaw method of classroom instruction'. Here, a lesson is divided into parts. Students are broken into multi-ethnic groups, while members of the group are given different parts of the lesson to learn. They are free during this stage to meet students from other groups who have been assigned the same part of the lesson. Students in each group must then learn the entire lesson by listening to individual students tell them about their section. This has obviously now been influenced by their interactions with people from other groups and from different ethnic backgrounds. The notion is that this approach helps people better appreciate what everyone else has to offer irrespective of their ethnic background, reduces rivalry for the teacher's attention (which can become a source of inter-ethnic conflict) and gives students of all aptitudes a chance to rehearse and to learn. Such an approach can be readily adapted to a variety of contexts, and could for example form the basis of training programmes involving people from a variety of professional back-grounds as a means of promoting interdisciplinary team working.

However, such collaborative approaches presume opportunities for interaction. An obvious problem with what is sometimes called 'multiculturalism' (that is, attempts to construct societies composed of people from different ethnic backgrounds) is that members of minority groups often have few opportunities to engage in cooperative activities with members of the dominant culture. Meanwhile, those interested in promoting division will maintain that different groups have competing goals and that the successes of one group disadvantage the other. For example, some would argue: 'Jobs are scarce. If members of your group gain employment it will be at the expense of my group. As a result, you and I are in hostile competition with each other.' Promoting intergroup contact, therefore, requires opportunities for cooperation around common goals, but this is often difficult to arrange, particularly if communities are segregated.

Assimilation or pluralism

A further dilemma facing those wishing to reduce bias is whether to ignore intergroup differences in the hope that assimilation will occur, or encourage people to openly discuss them. The evidence, in general, suggests that when intergroup differences are ignored prejudices either remain or become worse (Brown, 1995). The virus of prejudice does not self-destruct. Unchallenged, it replicates itself and mutates into hazardous new strains.

The challenges this poses are shown by a consideration of Education for Mutual Understanding' (EMU) programmes in Northern Ireland. These have been based on the assumption that 'relatively short term contact between small groups of individuals is an effective means of improving community relations generally' (Cornell, 1994, p. 33) – a notion which bears the imprint of the contact hypothesis, discussed above. However, such contact has often sought to deny or ignore dissimilarities between the Catholic and Protestant communities. When, despite such efforts, participants discover differences their expectations of the absence of difference are shockingly disconfirmed. This creates an even greater perception of differences than would have existed had they been openly articulated in the first place. Furthermore, as Cornell argues, when the participants return to their own community they may find that whatever new perceptions they have formed of 'the other side' are viewed as a violation of important community norms. In general, we dislike difference and exaggerate how much of it there is between in-groups and out-groups (Sutherland, 1992). As already noted, one of our primary human needs is to affiliate with others, while this is most easily achieved by conforming to in-group norms (Smith and Mackie, 1997). Accordingly, most people regard the social rejection involved in challenging in-group stereotypes as a price which is too high to pay. This means that newly acquired attitudes towards 'the other side' often atrophy on the person's return to their native social environment.

Furthermore, as Berry (1984) has pointed out, when prejudiced reactions are not acknowledged members of the minority group may be either discriminated against or pressurised to adopt the habits, language and culture of the dominant group. Ironically, this reinforces prejudice, since the minority group will resent such pressure and may respond by reemphasising the differences between itself and the dominant culture. Pressure to submerge one's cultural identity, therefore, tends to be counter-productive. The alternative is to acknowledge different value systems, cultures, linguistic traits, skin colours or other emblems of difference perceived to be important. These can then be utilised positively by all the people involved. Differences between groups can be recognised as a general cultural enrichment of society rather than a threat, and so become harnessed towards the achievement of common goals. Again, an obvious problem with this approach is that some people remain resistant to it, and seek to booby-trap the efforts which others make in this direction.

Such resistance may also be expressed as a fear of acknowledging difference, in case it inflames rather than reduces bias. Smyth and Campbell (1996) discuss this issue in connection to anti-racist and discriminatory practice (ARDP) within social work training in Northern Ireland. ARDP has involved raising the reality of sectarian divisions in the wider society for open discussion among social work students by trainers who come from both major traditions, and who openly draw their differing backgrounds to the attention of trainees. However, as Smyth and Campbell point out, some trainees have objected that discussing perceptions of difference could expose them to physical risks. This might well be a genuine fear, although, as the authors point out, it might also denote resistance to the difficult task of confronting sectarian attitudes on the part of some of the trainees themselves. It is, in general, easier, and certainly more satisfying, to recognise bias in others than in oneself. Addressing these challenges requires great care, sensitivity to feelings and strong diplomatic skills on the part of trainers, combined with a willingness to acknowledge their own biases. It also involves students learning how to listen respectfully to others, engaging in some self-disclosure and agreeing to preserve the confidentiality of whatever is discussed.

There are no data as to the overall impact of such approaches on prejudice or its applicability outside the context of social work. However, it could prove problematic in intergroup meetings where the people concerned lack the opportunity for interaction provided by an ongoing training programme. It also remains to be seen how such approaches would work among groups less favourably disposed to the values and norms of anti-discriminatory practice. The open acknowledgement of differences thus has much to commend it, but needs considerable skill on the part of facilitators and may require a receptive group(s) if it is to succeed.

PERSONAL COMMUNICATION STRATEGIES

Much of the discussion above dwells on societal initiatives to eliminate bias, and on initiatives (such as ARDP) which depend in the first instance on group-based interaction. A variety of important interpersonal communication strategies which we can utilise as individuals are also available to us. Fundamentally, communication practices aimed at reducing bias are concerned with improving the accuracy of our attributions (Gudykunst, 1994). It will be recalled that these are liable to fundamental distortion and, unless corrected, lead to stereotyping, the formation of prejudiced attitudes and discriminatory practice. As noted earlier, this creates wider social problems, but also inhibits the development of multi-disciplinary team working. Improving attributional accuracy stands to improve relationships with both patients and work colleagues from other professional backgrounds. Doing so involves perception checking and applying the principles of supportive communication.

Perception checking

Here, we describe what we think the other person's thoughts or feelings are, but do so without evaluating them. Assume for a moment that we are attributing the emotion of anger to another person. We could check our perception by saying 'I'm picking up a lot of anger. Are you angry?' This gives us ownership of own perceptions, helps us express them in a non-threatening manner and provides the other party with an opportunity to offer us corrective feedback. On the other hand, a comment such as 'Are you mad at me?' is not a perception check, since it avoids a direct statement of what we think the other person is feeling. The skill of reflecting is also useful in this context. Reflecting is concerned with 'presenting back to the other all or part of the message which has just been received' (Dickson, 1997, p. 160). Essentially, this involves restating in the listener's own words the affective and/or factual content of the utterance which has just been received. The central objective is to promote a common agenda and discourage misperceptions of key interaction goals.

Applying the principles of supportive communication

Various chapters in this book discuss, in one form or another, what has been termed 'supportive communication' (Albrecht *et al.*, 1994, Whetten and Cameron, 1991). This is concerned with the promotion of understanding, and so involves the replacement of categorisation effects with a greater awareness of traits specific to the people involved in a given interaction. The following guidelines indicate some of the main behaviours which represent such communication and which are, therefore, crucial to the elimination of bias:

1. *Focus your communication on specific behaviours rather than perceived personality characteristics of the other party* The rationale is that you can see and concretely describe what someone else does, but you can only reconstruct imaginatively what you think their motivation is. As this chapter has shown, many such attributions 'feel' right, but are nevertheless mistaken. Thus, it might be helpful to tell someone 'I felt intimidated when you slammed the door during our discussion. Do you think you could stop doing that when we next talk about X?' If the other party can imagine themselves slamming a door they are more likely to be receptive to the suggested behavioural change. However, if you tell them that they are 'aggressive', 'rude' and 'a bloody headache to work with', such general definitions will feel threatening, will probably appear erroneous and do not focus on specific behaviours which the other person can actually change. What does being 'a bloody headache to work with' look like, and how can the message recipient use such information to formulate a detailed behavioural response?
2. *Be congruent, not incongruent* This involves owning and admitting to one's own feelings, rather than denying what our non-verbals are probably telling the other person anyway.

Thus, it might be helpful sometimes to say 'Yes, I really was upset during that discussion' rather than 'I don't know what you're talking about. Everything is fine.' This facilitates open and honest communication about differences which, as we have seen, is often central to the elimination of prejudice, or to the dismantling of its harmful effects.

3. *Be descriptive towards others, not evaluative* The emphasis here is on objective description, leaving the other party free to draw their own conclusions about its moral content. A useful general rubric for such an approach is 'Here is what happened; this is what I did about it; this is what I suggest we do next that might ease the problem.' This is in preference to utterances such as 'Your behaviour was offensive', which again involves a generalised attack on someone's character rather than a helpful focus on specific behaviours which can be changed.

4. *Be conjunctive, not disjunctive* Communication should relate to the previous point made by the other party, rather than introduce a new issue, perhaps in the form of a counterproposal. You could therefore say 'You've just made the point X, and I think we should discuss it along with . . .' This is in preference to 'That is so interesting, but you've ignored the main issue completely, which I think is . . .' The latter approach raises issues when the other party is least receptive to what you have to say, and sets the stage for escalating conflict. It minimises the scope for mutual misunderstanding and the reduction of bias.

5. *Practice supportive and active listening* Many so-called conversations can be defined as 'two people taking turns at interrupting each other'. Supportive listening, on the other hand, involves paying attention to what other people say, summarising at regular intervals the main issues they have raised and then providing your response (Bostrom, 1990). It requires patience, and is the single most important ingredient of supportive communication.

6. *Accept responsibility for one's own prejudice* As suggested above, the open discussion of perceived differences is more productive than denying that they exist, and is in general a basic principle underlying conflict resolution (Donohue and Kolt, 1992). However, the manner in which this is done is crucial, since the projection of responsibility for relational breakdown on to others is one of the most popular but least fruitful of our international pastimes. It leads to degenerative communicative spirals, characterised by an escalation in fault-finding and overt

conflict (Willmot, 1995). In essence, we enjoy denouncing others (especially behind their back), but dislike accepting blame. One possibility, therefore, is that when groups discuss difficulties in their relationships the focus for each side should first be on identifying what they or their side has contributed to the breakdown, before engaging in the more pleasurable task of addressing what they think the responsibility of the other side is.

CONCLUSION

This chapter has argued that eliminating bias is achieved partly by adopting different behaviours, including different styles of communication, and partly through subjecting our own feelings to more critical scrutiny. Just because something 'feels' true doesn't mean that it is. Given the literature reviewed here on how stereotypes are formed and acquire a self-perpetuating character, it is certain that many of the things we most feel to be true of our social world are deeply mistaken. The key is to keep asking whether there is any scientific evidence to support our assumptions. Look again at the quotation which began this chapter, claiming that Aborigines have smaller brains than Australian whites. In fact, there is no evidence whatever to support such an assertion. Many more subtle expressions of bias must also be made explicit, compared to the evidence and, if needs be, discarded. Beyond this, we need to tolerate and welcome ambiguity, give up the idea that everyone can be pigeonholed, understand that diversity is not a threat and abandon the notion that uncertainty about other people can be eliminated. In the struggle to avoid the land-mines of prejudice our most precious asset is awareness.

Our own management of the communication process is also a vital factor in the elimination of prejudice. Among lessons to be drawn from the research is the uncomfortable finding that we tend to avoid contact with people belonging to stigmatised out-groups, misinterpret the communication they direct at us and engage in poor communicative episodes ourselves. This expands the distance between ourselves and those whom we perceive to be both different to us and possibly in some way inferior. There is, therefore, a twofold need to seek out interaction with those who are 'different', while avoiding the naive hope that such contact by itself will be sufficient to reduce bias. It is not. However, we can practise the principles of supportive communication, while guarding against the illusion that rapid change is possible. Bias, prejudice, stereotyping and social conflict have been features of human society since its inception. This does not mean that the problems to which they give rise are insurmountable. It does mean that struggling against them requires effort and an insight into the dynamics of prejudice formation. This chapter has outlined some of the communication strategies which should help all of us to approach other people first and foremost as people, and so learn to communicate beyond individual bias.

References

Albrecht, T., Burleson, B., and Goldsmith, D. (1994) Supportive communication. In M. Knapp and G. Miller (eds), *Handbook of Interpersonal Communication*, 2nd edn. London, Sage, pp. 419–49.

Allport, G. (1954) *The Nature of Prejudice*. Reading, Mass.: Addison-Wesley.

Aronson, E. (1997) The theory of cognitive dissonance. In C. McGarty and S. Haslam (eds), *The Message of Social Psychology*. Oxford: Blackwell, pp. 20–35.

Bandura, A. (1977) *Social Learning Theory,* Englewood Cliffs, NJ: Prentice-Hall.

Berger, C. (1987) Communicating under uncertainty. In M. Roloff and G. Millar (eds), *Interpersonal Processes: New Directions in Communications Research*. London: Sage, pp. 39–62.

Berry, J. (1984) Cultural relations in plural societies: alternatives to segregation and their sociopsychological implications, In N. Miller and M. Brewer (eds), *Groups in Contact: The Psychology of Desegregation*. New York: Academic Press.

Bobo, L. and Kluegel, J. (1991) *Modern American prejudice: stereotypes, social distance, and perceptions of discrimination towards blacks, Hispanics and Asians.* Paper presented at the American Sociological Association Meeting, Cincinnati, Ohio.

Bostrom, R. (1990) *Listening Behaviour*. New York: Guilford Press.

Brown, R. (1986) *Social Psychology*, 2nd edn, New York: Free Press.

Brown, R. (1988) *Group Processes*. London: Blackwell.

Brown, R. (1995) *Prejudice: Its Social Psychology,* Oxford: Blackwell.

Campbell, D. (1956) Enhancement of contrast as a composite habit. *Journal of Abnormal and Social Psychology*, 53, pp. 350–5.

Cialdini, R. (1993) *Influence: Science and Practice*, 3rd edn. New York: HarperCollins.

Cornell, J. (1994) Prejudice reduction through inter-group contact in Northern Ireland: a social–psychological critique, *Conflict Quarterly*, 14, pp. 30–46.

Darley, J. and Oleson, K. (1994) Introduction to research on interpersonal expectations. In P. Blanck (ed.), *Interpersonal Expectations: Theory, Research and Applications*. Cambridge: Cambridge University Press, pp. 45–63.

Darley, J. and Fazio, R. (1980) Expectancy confirmation processes arising in the social interaction sequence. *American Psychologist*, 35, pp. 867–81.

Dawes, R. (1994) *House of Cards: Psychology and Psychotherapy Built on Myth*. New York: Free Press.

Dickson, D. (1997) Reflecting. In O. Hargie (ed.), *The Handbook of Communication Skills*. London: Routledge, pp. 159–82.

Dickson, D., Saunders, C. and Stringer, M. (1993) *Rewarding People: The Skill of Responding Positively*. London: Routledge.

Dollard, J., Doob, L., Miller, N., Mowrer, O. and Sears, R. (1939) *Frustration and Aggression*. New Haven, Conn.: Yale University Press.

Donohue, W. and Kolt, R. (1992) *Managing Interpersonal Conflict*. London: Sage.

Epstein, J. (1985) After the bus arrives: resegregation in desegregated schools, *Journal of Social Issues*, 46, pp. 183–201.

Ezekiel, R. (1995) *The Racist Mind: Portraits of American Neo-Nazis and Klansmen*. London: Penguin.

Festinger, L. (1957) *A Theory of Cognitive Dissonance*. Evanston, Ill.: Row & Peterson.

Gudykunst, W. (1994) *Bridging Differences: Effective Intergroup Communication*. London: Sage.

Gurr, T. (1970) *Why Men Rebel*. Princeton, NJ: Princeton University Press.

Hamilton, D. (1979) A cognitive attributional analysis of stereotyping. In L. Berkowitz (ed.) *Advances in Experimental Social Psychology*, Vol. 12, New York: Academic Press.

Hamilton, D. and Bishop, G. (1976) Attitudinal and behavioral effects of initial integration of white suburban neighbourhoods. *Journal of Experimental Social Psychology*, 32, pp. 47–67.

Hargie, C. and Tourish, D. (1997) Relational communication. In O. Hargie (ed.), *The Handbook of Communication Skills*, 2nd edn, London: Routledge, pp. 358–84.

Hargie, O. (1992) *Communication: Beyond the Cross-roads*. Monograph, University of Ulster, Newtownabbey.

Henderson-King, E. and Nisbett, R. (1996) Anti-black prejudice as a function of exposure to the negative behaviour of single black persons. *Journal of Personality and Social Psychology*, 71, pp. 654–64.

Hovland, C. and Sears, R. (1940) Minor studies in aggression. VI: Correlation of lynchings with economic indices. *Journal of Psychology*, 9, pp. 301–10.

Hunter, J., Platow, M., Howard, M. and Stringer, M. (1996) Social identity and inter-group evaluative bias: realistic categories and domain specific self-esteem in a conflict setting. *European Journal of Social Psychology*, 26, pp. 631–47.

Inman, M. and Baron, R. (1996) Influence of prototypes on perceptions of prejudice. *Journal of Personality and Social Psychology*, 70, pp. 727–39.

Jones, E. (1990) *Interpersonal Perception*. New York: Freeman.

Kagan, C., Evans, J. and Kay, B. (1986) *A Manual of Interpersonal Skills for Nurses: An Experiential Approach*. London: Harper & Row.

Langer. E. and Abelson, R. (1974) A patient by any other name . . . : clinician group differences in labeling bias. *Journal of Consulting and Clinical Psychology*, 42, pp. 4–9.

Leyens, J., Yzerbt, V. and Schadron, G. (1994) *Stereotypes and Social Cognition*, London: Sage.

McArthur, L. (1980) Illusory causation and illusory correlation: two epistemological accounts. *Personality and Social Psychology Bulletin*, 6, pp. 507–19.

Miller, N. and Bugelski, R. (1948) Minor studies in aggression: the influence of frustrations imposed by the in-group on attitudes toward out-groups. *Journal of Psychology*, 25, pp. 437–42.

Pettigrew, T. and Meertens, R. (1995) Subtle and blatant prejudice in Western Europe. *European Journal of Social Psychology*, 25, pp. 57–75.

Phillipson, C. (1982) *Capitalism and the Construction of Old Age*. London: Macmillan.

Powers, D. and Ellison, C. (1995) Interracial contact and black racial attitudes: the contact hypothesis and selectivity bias. *Social Forces*, 74, pp. 205–26.

Scheflin, A. and Opton, E. (1978) *The Mind Manipulators.* New York, Paddington.

Seligman, M. (1975) *Helplessness.* San Francisco: W. H. Freeman.

Sherif, M., Harvey, O., White, B., Hood, W. and Sherif, C. (1961) *Intergroup Conflict and Co-operation: The Robber's Cave Experiment.* New York: Octagon.

Smith, E. and Mackie, D. (1997) Integrating the psychological and the social to understand human behaviour, In C. McGarty and S. Haslam (eds.), *The Message of Social Psychology,* Oxford: Blackwell, pp. 305–14.

Smyth, M. and Campbell, J. (1996) Social work, sectarianism and anti-sectarian practice in Northern Ireland. *British Journal of Social Work,* 26, pp. 77–92.

Stagner, R. and Congdon, C. (1955) Another failure to demonstrate displacement of aggression. *Journal of Abnormal and Social Psychology,* 51, pp. 695–6.

Stephan, W. and Rosenfeld, D. (1978) Effects of desegregation on racial attitudes. *Journal of Personality and Social Psychology,* 36, pp. 795–804.

Stouffer, S., Suckman, E., DeVinney, L., Star, S. and Williams, R. (1949) *The American Soldier: Adjustment During Army Life,* vol. 1. Princeton, NJ: Princeton University Press.

Sutherland, S. (1992) *Irrationality: The Enemy Within.* London: Constable.

Tajfel, H. and Turner, J. (1986) The social identity theory of inter-group behaviour. In S. Worchel and W. Austin (eds), *Psychology of Intergroup Relations.* Chicago, Ill.: Nelson, pp. 7–24.

Taylor, M. (1994) Expectancies and the perpetuation of racial inequity. In P. Blanck (ed.), *Interpersonal Expectations: Theory, Research and Applications.* Cambridge: Cambridge University Press, pp. 88–124.

Thomas, L. (1988) Images of Ageing. In S. Wright (ed.), *Nursing the Older Patient.* Cambridge: Harper & Row, pp. 9–23.

Thomson, J., Harris, M., Volkan, V. and Edwards, B. (1995) The psychology of Western European neo-racism, *International Journal on Group Rights,* 3, pp. 1–30.

Tourish, D. and Mulholland, J. (1997) Communication between nurses and nurse managers: a case study from an NHS Trust. *Journal of Nursing Management,* 5, pp. 25–36.

Vanneman, R. and Pettigrew, T. (1972) Race and relative deprivation in the urban United States. *Race,* 13, pp. 461–86.

Venkatesan, M. (1966) Experimental study of consumer behaviour, conformity and independence. *Journal of Marketing Research,* 3, pp. 384–7.

Whetten, D. and Cameron, K. (1991) *Developing Management Skills*, 2nd edn. New York: HarperCollins.

Willmot, W. (1995) *Relational Communication*. New York: McGraw-Hill.

Wilner, D., Walkley, R. and Cook, S. (1952) Residential proximity and inter-group relations in public housing projects. *Journal of Social Issues*, 8, pp. 45–69.

Wilson, T. (1996) Compliments will get you nowhere: benign stereotypes, prejudice and anti-semetism. *Sociological Quarterly,* 37, pp. 465–79.

Wolfe, C. and Spencer, S. (1996) Stereotypes and prejudice: their overt and subtle influence in the classroom. *American Behavioral Scientist*, 40, pp. 176–85.

Worchel, S., Cooper, J. and Goethals, G. (1988) *Understanding Social Psychology*, 4th edn. Chicago, Ill.: Dorsey.

Zander, A., Stotland, E. and Wolfe, D. (1960) Unity of group, identification with group, and self esteem of members. *Journal of Personality*, 28, pp. 463–78.

Zebrowitz, L. (1990) *Social Perception,* Milton Keynes: Open University Press.

Scoring system for 'Measuring interpersonal attitudes'

15–30

You understand the pitfalls of stereotyping other people, and attempt to approach most people you meet as unique human beings, with their own set of virtues and foibles. You categorise people and situations mostly to the extent that is necessary or unavoidable. You find bias extremely annoying, and are inclined to take a stand against it wherever possible.

31–45

You recognise that stereotyping others is a dangerous habit and try to do so only in so far as is necessary. However, you are inclined to do this rather more than you realise. You tend to draw too sweeping conclusions about the people you meet. On the other hand, you are aware of this and make some attempt to control your stereotyping urges. However, there is some room for improvement!

46–60

You are rather suspicious of anyone who is different to you, although you recognise that this sometimes leads you astray. You also draw conclusions too rapidly about people and groups of people based on particular incidents. You tend not to subject your view of others to much detailed inspection, and have a rather more confident view of the accuracy of your interpersonal perceptions than this survey would suggest is justified. Overall, you are more biased than you think and hold a number of assumptions which are clearly prejudiced.

61–75

You categorise other people with great enthusiasm. In your view people can be divided into positive and negative categories with relative ease, and you put most people in the negative category. You have a high but misplaced level of confidence in your own judgements. You believe that you can determine someone's character by the group to which you have assigned them, and you view such general considerations as an important factor determining how you relate to others. You have a great deal of work to do to reduce your existing level of prejudice.

CHAPTER EIGHT

Unconscious Communications

Raman Kapur

INTRODUCTION

Traditional models of communication within health care have relied mainly on learning theories whereby it is suggested that attention to overt and visible behaviours form the bedrock of therapeutic intervention (Hargie *et al.*, 1993). The incorporation of cognitive psychology within clinical interventions has facilitated movement away from the purely behavioural responses to attending to cognitive processes. These 'cognitive behavioural' interventions have recently been developed by Teasdale and Barnard (1993) where they take account of cognitive and affective processes. However, few models of communication have incorporated psychodynamic/ psychoanalytic perspectives into the everyday interactions that occur between community health care professionals and their clients. This chapter will outline some of the key concepts from psychoanalytic theory which will highlight interpersonal and intrapsychic processes that occur between nurse and patient. Unconscious processes such as transference, counter-transference and projection will be discussed and debated. An awareness of these hidden processes can offer community nurses a fuller picture of the patient's difficulties which can deepen their insight into how the patient is relating to him of herself and others. The chapter concludes with an example of a typical interaction between nurse and patient to illustrate the application of these concepts to practice.

TRANSFERENCE

A common experience for health professionals is to be experienced not as they are but either as someone else in the patient's past or a part of the patient's personality that has been projected on to them. This distortion of reality was called transference by Freud (1974) and proved to be one of his most significant discoveries in uncovering how experiences from the patient's past life can influence their current relationships with others. Many different definitions of transference exist in the psychoanalytic literature which are determined by each particular school of psychoanalysis. The classical Freudian definition places an emphasis on how significant others in the history of the patient may negatively and positively influence the patient's view of people they come into contact with. For example, individuals who have a history of aggressive and critical parents alongside similar experiences with teachers and others in authority will inevitably relate to newcomers in a similar way. This internalisation of negative experiences could then persuade the patient that all relationships are of a critical nature and thus to be avoided. This leads to the development of a 'harsh superego' whereby critical and negative judgements are both anticipated from others and also become part of the internal personality structure (Freud, 1919).

This traditional definition of transference differs from more contemporary formulations of this concept (Spillius, 1988) where there is a greater emphasis on 'internal object relations' in the activation of transference processes. This 'Kleinian' school of psychoanalysis places a greater importance on how reality is distorted by internal emotional processes within the patient. Theoretically, Melanie Klein (1935; 1963) suggested that the formation of personality occurs most crucially during infanthood rather than in childhood, as Freud had previously suggested. Kleinian theory emphasises the role of the mother in being able to 'contain' the infantile and aggressive impulses of the infant in the early months of like. The quality of this early containment would subsequently influence the development of harshness and aggression within the personality with a breakdown in this early maternal relationship giving way to the possibility of significant emotional disturbance in later life. The formulation of this damaged and disturbed personality would, in turn, lead to the development of relationships which are reminiscent of these early infantile unresolved, aggressive relationships. As such, according to Klein, the transference would be aetiologically earlier and much more aggressive than suggested by the Freudian formulation with the emphasis on how internal unresolved conflicts become reactivated in relation to interacting with others. These two definitions of transference have in common an emphasis on how unconscious processes become activated in present relationships which represent a significant distortion of reality. In Freudian terminology it may be that the nurse represents the mother or father in the patient's past and thus they will react as if the nurse were indeed that person. Alternatively, and I believe this to be the case when working with more disturbed patients, much earlier unresolved emotions will become located on to the mental health professional leading to the arousal of intense negative emotional states in patients whereby others, namely nurses, may be seen as persecutors. This 'negative transference' is often the hallmark of working with severely mentally ill patients (Kapur, 1991) whereby mental health professionals are seen as the enemy rather than the friend in the treatment process.

In sum, transference represents intense unconscious processes that exist in everyday human relations. These unconscious processes become more alive and intense in the relationship between mental health nurse and patient. The activation of early and often negative emotions places nurses in relationships where they are exposed to emotional states that are disproportionate and often unrelated to the reality of their current relationship with the patient. An aware-ness of these unconscious communications can help nurses under-stand more fully how the patient is experiencing and perceiving their relationship with them.

COUNTER-TRANSFERENCE

Within most mental and health care education and training, atten-tion to what we feel and think about relationships is virtually ignored and thus potentially vital data about patients and ourselves are difficult to locate or may be lost. Traditionally, emotional reactions to events in patients' lives have been peripherised for 'fear of getting too involved' and thus impairing clinical judgement. While there are, of course good reasons for this argument a consistently distant approach from our patients can lead to patients feeling ignored and isolated by those placed in a position to help them. Within psychoanalytic theory this reaction has been called counter-transference (Freud, 1974). Since the 1970's there has been a significant change in the definition of counter-transference where the response of the therapist/helping professional is no longer perceived as a problem to be analysed but rather provides important intuitive information about the state of mind of the patient, therapist and the relationship. A brief outline of the main theoretical and clinical debate over this term will be provided and then a definition which could be helpful for mental health professionals to use in their everyday practice illustrated.

The original recognition of emotional reactions from the therapist was seen by Freud (1919) and others as an impediment to therapeutic work. Thus, strong reactions indicated that further work had to be undertaken by the therapist to rid him or herself of potentially interfering processes with the patient. Thus, emotional reactions in the patient during the therapeutic encounter were recognised as legitimate and inevitable occurrences which required further work. This view of counter-transference was challenged by Kleinian psychoanalysis with the seminal paper by Heimann (1950) pointing to the usefulness of counter-transference as an instrument to understand the state of mind of the patient. Thus, reactions by the therapist such as joy, sadness, anger, despair and so on could be used not only to monitor the state of mind of the therapist but could give important clues about the patient. This involves a close and vigorous inspection of all felt emotional responses to differentiate their origins in either the therapist or the patient and so give a fuller picture of the therapis–patient relationship. For example, following a visit to a schizophrenic patient the community psychiatric nurse (CPN) felt that she had been humiliated and bullied; these feelings could have given important clues as to what the patient was doing to the CPN or what the CPN may have felt about working with a difficult patient. Within psychotherapy (Holmes, 1992) and psychoanalysis (Rosenfeld, 1987) many papers have been written on the counter-transference reactions of therapists to different types of patients (Searles, 1979). Inevitably the most extreme and disturbing experiences have been recorded with severely mentally ill patients who have stirred negative emotions up internally in others and consequently 'driven others mad' within mental hospitals. A well-known observation relates to the negative effects that this disturbed setting has on staff whereby, unconsciously, dysfunctional relationships with patients are repeated in staff teams. In taking our emotional reactions to patients more seriously we can understand both ourselves and our patients and allow ourselves to judge the impact of relationships more realistically, rather than allowing a potential accumulation of negative experience being built up in our psyche which may become manifest through our own dysfunctional psychological or psychosomatic reactions. In everyday life this is often described as the 'last straw' which leads to a 'breakdown'. Without insight, exploration and interpretation the impact of exposure to continued negative experiences could be ignored in the nurse, so leading to an emotional system that has become overloaded.

In mental health settings the exposure to negative human experiences is inevitable. We touch the lives of patients who have parents who have been lost or have reacted aggressively to them in their earlier lives. Through monitoring our own reactions to these events we can allow ourselves to be more open to these experiences and at the same time use this information to understand the patient. Importantly, we can also monitor how these experiences may be overloading our own personal and professional relationships. The story of the workaholic is common in organisational life. In mental health this can lead to burn-out if counter-transference reactions are totally ignored and thus remain unresolved.

A broad general definition of counter-transference is as follows: an awareness and legitimate recognition of our emotional reactions to events which can increase the repertoire of data we have to understand the reactions that are stirred up within us when we are interacting with others.

PROJECTIVE PROCESSES

Psychoanalytic and psychodynamic theories assign different levels of importance to the role of projective processes in the therapist–patient relationship. Simply stated this refers to the putting on to or into another person aspects of our personality. Typically, this would refer to accusations of dishonesty, bullying and superiority in others where, in reality, it is these characteristics in ourselves that cannot be accepted. Kleinian psychoanalysis places particular emphasis on projective processes as an unconscious way of the individual disowning parts/aspects of his or her own personality, especially those parts/aspects we do not like, and therefore projecting them on to others (Segal, 1973).

As early as 1895, Freud described the important mechanism of projection within the theory of drives. However, Freud did not develop this concept further into his theories of personality and psychopathology (Torras De Dea, 1989). Rather he continued his work through emphasising the etiological status of Oedipal conflicts within his overall framework of psychosexual development. In contrast, Melanie Klein (1963) gave this concept of projection central importance. In her theories, personality structure took place through projective and introjective processes between infant and mother. From the earliest moments, infants project their experiences of deprivation, rage and neediness on to the mother who may respond by either meeting these emotions positively through soothing the infant (positive introjection) or by putting back into the infant parts of their own personality such as deprivation, neediness and despair (counter-projection). In Kleinian theory positive mental health is determined by the final outcome of these projective/introjective experiences with the hope that good experiences will be greater than bad experiences, thus leading to the dissolution of negative projective processes over time.

Melanie Klein also went on to coin the phrase 'projective identification' (1946) which refers to processes whereby emotional states were put into others. This concept describes experiences in relationships whereby we have suddenly felt some strong emotional reaction within a relationship and cannot trace the origins of this in ourselves (for example, sadness, rage, despair, which may belong to the other person). Emotions have been placed internally into us and we find ourselves overwhelmed. Theoretically, Klein (1946) originally described negative aspects of projective identification whereby aggressive parts are placed in others. An example of this may be when a disturbed patient leaves us feeling hostile and critical after a heated exchange. However, more recently, other have recognised positive aspects of this style of unconscious communication (Spillius, 1988), whereby respect, warmth and affection can also be unconsciously communicated.

In being aware of projective processes, whether they be described as 'projection' or 'projective identification', the receiver of these communications requires sensitive counter-transference emotional apparatus to pick up the unconscious communications within projections. This analysis of these processes can lead to fuller and deeper understanding of the relationships between patients and others.

CLINICAL EXAMPLE

A 25-year-old male who has recently been diagnosed as suffering from schizophrenia is asked by his psychiatrist to see a female community psychiatric nurse in the health centre so that she can monitor medication and provide supportive counselling. This patient has struggled to accept how his diagnosis of schizophrenia can affect his life. He failed to keep the first appointment. Prior to the second visit the CPN had some difficulty in finding a quiet room in the health centre for the session.

The patient arrives ten minutes late for his second appointment saying he wasn't sure of the location. On walking to the interview room he apologises for missing his first appointment saying he wasn't given enough notice of the time. Immediately the patient arrives in the room he begins to ask personal questions about the CPN: 'Are you married?' 'Where do you live?' 'Have you got any children?' After his intense questioning he reports that he has stopped his medication and may be about to become homeless as his parents are about to throw him out. He comments on the perfume he smells on the CPN, saying it is soothing. He goes on to say that he has written a special story for this session about being a joyrider and then the IRA tell him to get out of Belfast. He goes to England where he initially feels safe but then becomes homeless. In the story he recalls a 'tramp' at London Victoria bus station who asks him for money: he can't give the 'tramp' any money. Towards the end of the interview he reports his sexual fantasies about black women and asks the CPN whether she can understand this sexual desire.

Commentary

One of the most important elements of any psychotherapeutic assessment is to pay attention to the initial moments of contact, whether this be by letter, phone or direct contact. While this is a hallmark of Kleinian psychoanalytic therapy (Hinshelwood, 1995), it is a technique which is useful across all therapeutic interventions. The first point of contact between the patient and the CPN was the comment by the psychiatrist that he should see someone else to 'help with his medication and offer some counselling'. At this early point the transference starts where the patient begins to form all sorts of fantasies (Segal, 1985) about the CPN. Examples of his fantasies are: Will the nurse force him to talk to comply? Will the nurse force him to talk against his wishes? Why is the psychiatrist asking for further help, is it because the psychiatrist is tired of him and is giving up? Is this the end of the psychotherapist–patient relationship?

It is at this early point that many paranoid anxieties can be stirred up in respect of the future contact with the CPN. We may enter a new therapeutic relationship with patients in the hope that they will view us as a benevolent helping authority figure, but this rarely occurs. Patients suffering from severe mental illness will often project their internal persecutory objects on to the new object (Stachey, 1934/1969) who will take on the emotional appearance of a strict, harsh and intensive figure.

To summarise, during this early stage of the professional contact, the patient will be searching his own mind to find reasons for the psychiatrist's referral to someone else. This new object (CPN) will become the recipient of his paranoid anxieties whereby he will project parts of himself on to the CPN. The initial transference will be distorted by the emotional state of the patient where he will most likely fear the potential annihilatory attacks from the CPN.

The second phase of the evolving therapeutic interaction is characterised by the patient missing the first appointment and arriving ten minutes late for his second appointment. This could indicate deeper anxieties within the patient relating to his fears about the new therapeutic relationship. At this point it would be useful for the CPN to pay attention to her counter-transference. How did she feel when the first appointment was missed – irritation, annoyance, impatience? Could these feelings represent the frustrations of the patient that were already being put into the CPN through the channel of projective identification and so give valuable clues as to the state of mind of the patient or could they represent unresolved issues within the CPN regarding unrealistic expectations? This reluctance of the patient to attend the appointment is further reinforced through his lateness for the second appointment and suggestion that the first appointment did not arrive on time. Here, the responsibility for attending the appointment has been put on to others; this disavowal or projection of responsibilities is a characteristic of a mentally ill state of mind (Kapur, 1991).

The next phase of the interview is characterised by the opening speech from the patient where he puts the CPN under pressure to disclose aspects of her life. Immediately, the focus to share information is on the CPN in this role-reversal. The patient, perhaps anxious at what this CPN may achieve through 'counselling' immediately 'turns the tables' wherby the CPN becomes the patient. This shift in focus not only allows the patient to feel that the pressure to talk is off him, but it also gains information about the personal availability of the CPN. In other words, is there an immediate sexualised/erotic transference whereby this 25-year-old male believes that this female CPN will 'take away' magically his mental, emotional and sexual deprivations? Again, this would be a feature of a mentally ill state of mind whereby intense and mercurial transference become established very early in the helping relationship (Bion, 1961). The comment on the perfume of the CPN and its soothing qualities may indicate the fantasy of the soothing breast (Klein, 1957) which the patient may hope will deal with his internal torment (Grotstein, 1979).

The patient then reports a story, which may have been a dream about being a joyrider and paramilitaries telling him he has to leave the country. This made a reference to how an internal mechanism could represent two dynamics. Either it may represent his own internal struggles when he finds some 'joy' in life that this new territory in his mind is attacked by an internal aggressive process where he is told that his more positive way of living is not acceptable in a mind inhabited by terrorists. In contrast, it may also represent a culmination of internal negative processes wherby any pleasure is taken in criminal acts, such as joyridimg, which can lead to further internal punishment for not dealing with his inner and outer life more constructively.

Next, the story of the homeless tramp could be a communication, in the transference, to the CPN of how he feels he has no emotional home. In Bowlby's (1988) terminology, he has no secure base (Holmes, 1992). The demand from the tramp for money may represent the paradox of his own situation where he finds those who are impoverished actually demanding resources from him. This inability to give the 'tramp' any money reflects his own deprived state;he may believe that relationships in life are about relating to people who have little resources and thus the possibility of his own deprivation being altered is doubtful.

Finally, at the end of the interview he hints at what might be the presence of an erotic/sexualised transference with the CPN. Here, it would be helpful for the CPN to be alert to these emotional reactions and keep in mind the possibility of a different relationship developing. A formal style of relating with the patient, minimising the use of first names along with little, if any, self-disclosure could help contain any difficult and intense sexual feelings that could otherwise spill into the professional relationship. The use of the CPN's own counter-transference responses could act as a valuable instrument to monitor the potential emotional disturbance within the relationship which could prevent intervention. For example, if the CPN recognises counter-transference reactions within herself wherby she believes the patient is becoming too intrusive and/or overfriendly, then there could be some firming of personal boundaries to ensure that the patient does not feel that other more sexualised ambitions could be fulfilled.

CONCLUSION

Human relationships contain a vast array of complexities that often occur at a hidden or unconscious level. These complexities are particularly apparent in the relationships that develop in working with patients who suffer from severe mental illnesses. Often, disturbing positive and negative emotions will be aroused which will have a significant influence on how the patient relates to others. The psychoanalytic concepts of transference, counter-transference and projection can help the nurse unravel some of the deeper meanings behind everyday communications and so facilitate opportunities for more effective interventions. Through paying attention to what the patient is doing to us (transference), how we react to the patient (counter-transference), what the patient may be putting into us (projection), we can formulate a fuller understanding of the state of mind of the patients. In the clinical example I have illustrated how paying attention to all of the events within the interaction can lead to several different hypotheses about what may be occurring. This careful attention to the emotional detail is a continuous process whereby observations are converted into formulations and retested in the alive relationship between patient and nurse. Through this process the patient may then feel that he or she is being truly listened to and thus understood.

References

Bion, W. R. (1961) Experiences in Groups. London: Tavistock.
Bowlby, J. (1988) *A Secure Base: Clinical Application of Attachment Theory*. London: Routledge.
Freud, S. (1974) *The Standard Edition of the Complete Psychological Works of Sigmund Freud*, vol. 5. London: Hogarth Press, pp. 1–24.
Grotstein, J. S. (1979) Demonical Possession, Splitting and torment of Joy: A Psychoanalytic Inquiry into the negative Therapeutic

Reaction, Unanalysability and Psychotic States. *Contemporary Psychoanalysis*, 15, (3) pp. 407–45.

Hargie, D., Saunders, C. and Dickson, D. (1993) *Social Skills in Interpersonal Communication*. Beckenham: Croom Helm.

Heimann, P. (1950) On Counter-Transference. *International Journal of Psychoanalysis*. 31, pp. 81–4.

Hinshelwood, R. D. (1995) Psychodynamic formulation in assessment for psychoanalytic psychotherapy. In C. Mace (ed.), *The Art and Science of Assessment in Psychotherapy*. London and New York: Routledge, pp. 155–66.

Holmes, J. (1992) *A Textbook of Psychotherapy in Psychiatry*. London: Churchill Livingstone.

Kapur, R. (1991) Projective processes in psychiatric settings. *Melanie Klein and Object Relations*, 9(1), pp. 16–25.

Klein, M. (1935) A contribution to the psychogenesis of manic-depressive states. *International Journal of Psychoanalysis*, 16, pp. 145–74.

Klein, M. (1946) Notes on some schizoid mechanisms, *International Journal of Psychoanalysis*, 27, pp. 99–1110.

Klein, M. (1957) *Envy and Gratitude*. London: Routledge.

Klein, M. (1963) *The Adult World and Other Essays*, New York: Heinemann.

Rosenfeld, H. (1987) *Impasse and Interpretation: Therapeutic and Anti-Therapeutic Factors in the Psychoanalytic Treatment of Psychotic, Borderline and Neurotic Patients*. London/New York: Routledge.

Searles, H. (1979) *Countertransference and Related Subjects. Selected Papers*. New York: International Universities Press.

Segal, H. (1973) *Introduction to the Work of Melanie Klein*. London: Hogarth Press.

Spillius, E. Bott (ed.) (1988) *Melanie Klein Today. Vol. 1 mainly Theory and Vol. 2 mainly Practice*. London: Routledge.

Stachey, J. (1934/69) The nature of the therapeutic action in psychoanalysis. *International Journal of Psychoanalysis*, 15, pp. 127–39. Reprinted in 1969 in *International Journal of Psychoanalysis*, 50, pp. 275–92.

Teasdale, J. D. and Barnard, P. J. (1993) *Affect, Cognition and Change*. Hove: Laurence Erbaum Associates.

Torras De Dea, E. (1989) Projective identification and differentiation. *International Journal of Psychoanalysis*, 70, pp. 265–74.

CHAPTER NINE

Health Promotion for Individuals, Families and Communities

Paul Fleming

INTRODUCTION

During the twentieth century the role of nurses in the community has expanded both in scope and in scale. The importance of the part played by community nurses in the delivery of primary health care has become increasingly recognised and established (NHSE, 1996).

One of the key roles for nursing in general is that of health promotion (UKCC, 1992a). Since the formalisation of the nature of health promotion by the World Health Organisation (WHO, 1984, 1956), there has been an ongoing debate on key questions such as 'what is health?', 'what is health promotion?' and 'how does health promotion differ, if at all, from health education?' Such questions indicate that there is still some confusion as to what is meant by the term 'health promotion'. This confusion is seen not only in nursing, but also in the wider world of the health promotion specialist (Delaney, 1994).

This chapter aims to: explore key questions regarding the nature of health and health promotion; demonstrate how current thinking regarding health promotion is applied to the various strands of community nursing, and highlight the importance of community nurses having the requisite skills to undertake advanced interactions related to health promotion. Such interactions are seen to take community nurses beyond the more traditional role of giver of health advice to one of facilitator of health gain through well-planned health promotion interventions.

It is also recognised that the involvement of community nurses in health promotion depends, to some extent, on how they are employed in the service (Gott and O'Brien, 1990). Thus nurses in the clinical area will participate in health promotion at a more face-to-face level of delivery while those in management will have greater involvement with strategic and planning issues.

HEALTH

During recent years many theorists have begun debating whether or not attempts to define health have been helpful (Ashton and Seymour, 1988; Kemm and Close, 1995). There is indeed a danger that spending inordinate amounts of time postulating on the issue could be a block to progress. However, it is helpful if professionals such as community nurses have a working conceptualisation of health to which they can relate so that when they adopt a health-promoting role they are aware of what it is they are promoting.

The starting point which is most often taken when discussing health is the World Health Organisation definition of health which was stated when the organisation began. The statement that 'health is a state of complete physical, social and mental wellbeing, and not merely the absence of disease or infirmity' (WHO, 1946) was appropriate to the time it was written. The world was emerging from the devastating effects of the Second World War. The establishing of a new organisation such as the United Nations, which gave the WHO its context, gave hope of human progress. There was a need, therefore, for the WHO to strike a note of optimism in relation to health. Thus, their definition of health, which was *aspirational* in character, described health as a perfect state to which the population of the world should aspire.

The problem of stating perfection is that it thus condemns the entire population of the world to a state of 'unhealthiness' as it is virtually impossible for anyone to ever claim to be in a *complete* state of well-being in all areas of their health (Seedhouse, 1986). On the other hand, the definition, in moving away from the its emphasis on absence of disease or infirmity, was shifting from a binary notion of well/sick, healthy/unhealthy to describing health as a more multifactorial entity. The seeds of holism in health were being planted.

Interestingly, by 1984 the tone of the WHO's thinking had changed. Health was now conceptualised as:

'the extent to which an individual or group is able, on the one hand, to realise aspirations and satisfy needs and on the other hand, to change or cope with the environment. Health is therefore seen as a resource for everyday life, not the objective of living: it is a positive concept emphasising social and personal resources as well as physical capabilities.'
(WHO, 1984, p. 23)

Here health is not an aspirational *end*, but a *means* to function in everyday life and to adapt to changing conditions.

Over the years numerous other definitions of health have been postulated which, when examined, fall into the two broad categories which are adapted from both of the previously cited WHO definitions. At one end of the configuration there are those which, like the 1948 WHO definition, are *aspirational* in that they aim for the perfect and therefore the unattainable. Within the other category there are those which, like the 1984 definition, are *functional*. These theorists describe the *health status* of the individual or group as a dynamic set of circumstances, states and expectations which combine to enable the individual to function and cope to his or her fullest potential (Dubos, 1960; Mansfield, 1977).

Functional definitions of health status are more useful to professionals such as community nurses in that they can identify the various factors which contribute to health status, and thus identify strengths and particularly needs in that status. Community nurses can then plan measures, within the scope of their role, which may provide health and social remediation or promotion. An examination of the literature demonstrates that health status may be represented as shown in Figure 9.1. This conceptualisation of health has been adapted from a synthesis of earlier work on defining health by scholars and researchers such as Aggleton and Homans (1987), Ewles and Simnett (1995) and Naidoo and Wills (1994). However, Figure 9.1 shows that the term *status* has been introduced. 'Status' has been used to indicate that health is a dynamic process. It constantly changes as the nature of its individual components and the consequent changes in the character of their interactions produce a cumulative status which changes throughout the lifespan.

In the model depicted in Figure 9.1, the inner circle represents the individual. Many theorists have chosen to describe the components of individual health in various ways. For example, Naidoo and Wills (1994) chose to express it as the interacting personal

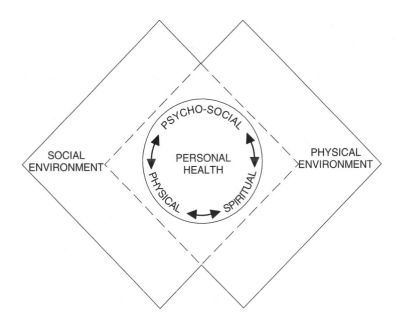

Figure 9.1   A holistic model of health status

components of physical, mental, psychological, spiritual and sexual health within the context of the physical and social environments. The personal components in Figure 9.1, however, are defined in three generic categories. This permits any topic area, such as sexual health, to be accommodated, as almost all health topics have physical, psychosocial and spiritual components.

Physical health status is aggregated by factors such as genetic inheritance, the functioning of the major body systems, the physical fitness to perform those functions which are necessary for each individual and the presence or absence of physically disabling factors. It should not be assumed that the presence of a disability necessarily lowers the health status – individuals can still achieve optimum physical health, for them, within the constraints of their disability.

In the past *Psychosocial health status* has been subdivided into mental, psychological and social health (Naidoo and Wills, 1994). However, it is evident that various factors impinge on both psychological and social functioning. Indeed, they are so inextricably linked that they are best categorised together. Psychosocial health is, therefore, composed of foundational factors such as levels of self-esteem, self-efficacy, body image, intellectual abilities and a sense of place in the various *people groups* in which individuals find themselves, such as family, workplace, community and wider society. All of these factors could be described as *states of being*. States of being are then expressed by the use of coping mechanisms which individuals use to deal with issues such as painful life events, stress, various levels of mental distress/disorder and the expression and control of emotions.

A further cadre of social coping mechanisms enable individuals to cope with the various relationships which are part of life: marriage and other sexual relationships, parent/child and other family relationships, peer group relationships, and relationships with authority such as work, the law and the church. All of these coping mechanisms may be used to try to give meaning and understanding to such life experiences and to enable people to deal with and resolve inner conflict. In so doing people become more able to empathise with others. It is perhaps also useful to note here that certain forms of learning disability may affect the way in which individuals relate to their social environment.

Spiritual health status (see Figure 9.1) relates to the personal belief system which produces the personal morality which gives meaning to the life of individuals. Often such a system will be closely linked to religio-cultural conditioning and will affect beliefs regarding gender, race, sexual orientation, respect for others and sexual mores as well as perceptions of issues such as the nature of society and family life. Perceptions of issues such as honesty, integrity and loyalty, to name but a few personal attributes, also contribute to spiritual health.

Moreover, each of these types of status is in itself inclusive of a wide range of factors. These broad, but inclusive categories of personal health status, therefore, begin to describe a holistic perspective on health.

It must also be recognised, however, that individuals do not exist in a vacuum. We live in environments which can largely be classified within two broad categories. In the model illustrated in Figure 9.1, both the social and physical environment are given equal prominence, thus recognising that both of these environments are, to a large extent, symbiotic. It also recognises that micro-environments such as the family and the workplace affect, and are affected by, the wider environments in which they exist.

The physical environment shapes, to some extent, the health status of individuals and communities by reason of features such as climate, altitude and other natural features, urban/rural location, and water and air quality. The same can be said of the social environment which is created from factors such as culture, political organisation and outlook, social class, gender and ethnicity. It is also affected by issues such as inequalities, communal violence and breakdown in law and order.

Further, the social environments which we create can have an effect on the physical environment. Thus a highly industrialised society gears its production to satisfy, for example, its consumer and defence needs. This can seriously affect both the quality of the physical environment and also the sustainability of its resources. Diminishing sustainability will ultimately have a detrimental effect on the health of individuals, families and communities. Such a situation has been recognised by both the Rio Summit with its emphasis on sustainability of resources (UN, 1992), and the United Kingdom's response to it in Local Agenda 21 (LGMB, 1994).

Another factor which must be taken into account by professionals such as community nurses when producing a working definition of health is that clients/patients also have their own views of health – the 'lay' concept. This may not necessarily concur with that of professionals. Williams (1983), for example, in a widely cited study of a group of older people in Aberdeen, found that the group studied regarded health as the ability to cope with and the strength to overcome the effects of disease. The loss of such an ability was seen as a weakness. Blaxter (1990) demonstrated differences in the manner in which women and men perceived health. While women perceived health as the ability to carry out daily tasks and as the absence of disease, men viewed it as being fit. Such perceptions must be taken into account when the community nurse is setting up projects which will address health needs. If people's perceptions are ignored, then the client/community may not recognise the interventions or accept them as relevant to their health.

Based on the holistic conceptualisation portrayed in Figure 9.1, and taking into account the lay perceptions of health, health status can now be defined as 'the cumulative effect of the dynamic interaction of the physical, psychosocial and spiritual aspects of the individual and the transactions that occur between these and the social and physical environments'. Such a holistic representation of health provides wide scope for promoting the health of individuals, families and communities.

HEALTH PROMOTION

The term *health promotion* first came into prominence in the 1970s and 1980s (Lalonde, 1974; WHO, 1984). However, it was the Ottawa Charter (WHO, 1986), conceived during the first International Conference on Health Promotion, which formalised the nature and scope of health promotion. The charter laid down five key areas of activity which were:

- building healthy public policy;
- creating supportive environments;
- strengthening community action;
- developing personal skills; and
- reorientating health services.

Subsequently health promotion was defined as: 'the process of enabling individuals to increase control over and improve their health' (WHO, 1984). This implied that health promotion was not a single activity but an approach that encompasses a number of activities which produce health gain but which are also derived from an overall aim to promote the health status of individuals and people groups. The increase of control implies the empowerment of individuals through a range of enabling measures which may have policy, education and service provision implications.

Thus, health promotion was seen as much more than a simple process of advice-giving which sought the outcome of changed health attitudes and behaviour. From this basis, there ensued a great deal of useful and informed debate which sought to clarify the theoretical basis of health promotion and to distinguish between health promotion and health education as discreet areas of endeavour. This quest for clarification led to a number of models and explanations of health promotion being postulated in the British literature (Catford and Nutbeam, 1984; Tannahill, 1985; French, 1990; Ewles and Simnnett, 1995; Tones and Tilford, 1994). The common strand which unites these models is that they all recognise that health promotion contains elements which focus on individuals, for example, lifestyle issues and structural (fiscal/ecological) elements (Macdonald and Bunton, cited in Bunton and Macdonald, 1992).

Further, Tannahill (1985) described health promotion as involving interactions between the overlapping spheres of health education, prevention and health protection. Health protection was achieved through policy development at various levels from legislation to voluntary agreements and codes. Later, French (1990) produced a typology of health promotion which included the four interlinked areas of disease management, disease prevention, health education and politics of health. One useful element of this typology was to show that health education was but one area of activity within health promotion which has been described as an umbrella term (Ewles and Simnett 1995; Downie *et al.*, 1997).

A further issue which arises in French's typology is the inclusion of disease management. It may be argued that if the cure or amelioration of disease raises and therefore promotes health status, then it should, by right, be included. Thus, when compared with Tannahill's model, the French (1990) typology, with its reference to disease management, goes beyond the three spheres of prevention, health education and health protection by including measures for the remediation of ill health.

Ewles and Simnett (1995) have also recognised the difficulty in interfacing health promotion with disease management and have attempted to address the issue to some extent by grouping those activities which lead to better health into categories. On the one hand there are illness and disability services, and on the other: 'positive health activities which are about personal, social and environmental changes to prevent ill-health and develop healthier conditions and ways of life' (pp. 22–3).

In parallel with the development of these models and typologies has been the development of various strategic approaches to health promotion. While a key focus of health promotion has always been the individual, the danger of victim-blaming (Tones and Tilford, 1994) has increasingly been recognised. Victim-blaming means that individuals can be made to feel that they, personally, are the authors of their own ill health. Linked to this have been several other developments in the wider debate regarding the organisation and nature of health promotion.

One such development has been the growth of a *settings* approach to health promotion which has been encouraged by the World Health Organisation (Tones, cited in Scriven and Orme, 1996). Here the *setting* is seen as any environment in which people spend significant parts of their lives such as workplaces, schools, hospitals, prisons, cities and communities. The settings approach aims to enhance health status through the development of a health-promoting environment. Such an environment is facilitated by interdisciplinary and intersectoral approaches. A number of key settings have been developed, for example, The Health Promoting Hospital (WHO, 1991, 1994), The Health Promoting School (WHO, 1993) and Healthy Cities (WHO, 1988).

Moreover, health strategies at national level such as *Health of the Nation* (DoH, 1992) are seen to encourage more innovative approaches to delivering health promotion. One notable strategy suggested in *Health of the Nation* was the encouragement of multisectoral approaches through the development of healthy alliances, such as intersectoral partnerships for health gain. Another innovative strategy is included in *Health and Wellbeing into the Millennium*, the Health and Personal Social Services Strategy for Northern Ireland (1997–2002) (DHSSNI, 1996). This involves the 'Targeting of Health and Social Need' and emphasises the importance of approaches such as community development. Such approaches are given much greater prominence than had previously been the case in the 1992–7 Northern Ireland Regional Strategy (DHSSNI, 1992). The theme of addressing inequalities in health has also been emphasised in the government White Paper on health (DoH, 1998).

The model depicted in Figure 9.2 attempts to reflect the recent shifts which have been evident in approaches to health promotion. The model is based on three premises:

1. The four core elements of health promotion (health policy, health education, health screening and monitoring and health empowerment) are interdependent and are likely to lead to integrated strategies where other core elements will be necessary constituents.
2. Health promotion strategies can be operationalised at either primary, secondary or tertiary levels of intervention.
3. Health promotion strategies can be developed not only for individuals, families and communities, but also for specific settings and for national initiatives.

Health policy

In the spirit of the Ottawa Charter (WHO, 1986) development of health-promoting policy is multilayered. Tones and Tilford (1994) would contend that health policy is at the core of health promotion and have described this as 'the primacy of policy' (p. 8). Health policy will include national legislation across a range of departments which have an input to health status, for example, Health, Education, Agriculture, Environment, Social Security and the

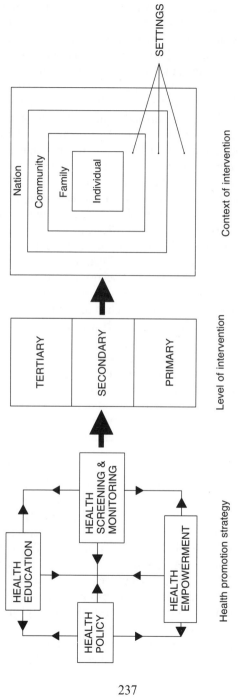

Figure 9.2 Model of health promotion

237

Treasury. Examples here are numerous but would include measures aimed at improving road safety, provision of safe food, health education in schools and measures for environmental protection.

In Great Britain, local authority regulation deals with policy areas such as housing, education, social services and environmental health. In the case of Northern Ireland only the latter remains within local authority control with all the others being organised, managed and delivered through quangos, this situation being known as the democratic deficit. Health authorities/boards and the commissioners of health care are recommended to develop commissioning policies which should be conducive to the promotion of the health of the communities which they serve. In proposals for the reform of commissioning for the beginning of the millennium, primary care-led commissioning teams comprising GPs and community nurses will be taking a lead in the provision of health care for their clients. The opportunity for community nurses to influence policy for the provision of health promotion is exciting.

Health care trusts (health and social services trusts in Northern Ireland), provide a range of health services which are responsive to the commissioners' requirements. They have the task of developing local health promotion policy which will inform the provision of health promotion services. Here again, community nurses have a key role to play in the shaping of policy.

Other areas of policy development are within individual organisations such as workplaces and schools, voluntary organisations, providers of a range of personal and community services and manufacturers. The latter are sometimes involved in producing and participating in voluntary codes and agreements such as the code on tobacco advertising.

It should be noted that the policy approach to health promotion leads directly to an ethical dilemma. One of the fundamental ethical principles of health promotion is that of *autonomy* (Beauchamp and Childress, 1995). Here the individual retains control of the decision whether or not to participate in a specific activity; it is also desirable that they participate in the planning process. The enhancing of autonomy is sometimes linked to the process of empowerment (Naidoo and Wills, 1994). Policy, such as legislation which leads to compulsion to participate, for example seat-belt wearing or compliance with no-smoking policies, necessarily introduces an element of *coercion* whereby autonomy is lost.

Admittedly, in terms of legislation, people in democratic societies could be said to have some control through the ballot box, but in other organisational settings, opportunities for participation in decision-making may be limited. This is an area of debate which health promoters must take into account when they decide how far legislation and regulation are in accord with an ethical approach to enhancement of health status.

Health education

Health education is a discipline which has been the source of much debate during the 1980s and 1990s. For the purposes of this chapter, health education is defined as any planned measure which aims to enhance health status/awareness through increasing empowerment of targeted individuals/groups by the facilitation of learning. Health education will include a number of activity areas which go well beyond the traditional notions of health information-giving and will take place at primary, secondary and tertiary levels.

Primary health education will facilitate learning in areas such as knowledge of primary risk factors of disease and related behaviour change measures. It also involves knowledge of services available and the development of life skills such as assertiveness, conflict resolution and lobbying. Primary health education is also concerned with initiating peer, family and community led approaches to the promotion of health and social wellbeing.

Secondary health education will facilitate learning in relation to screening and monitoring techniques and related services which are available. Tertiary health education could be better described as *patient* or *client education*. Here the target group is facilitated in learning which is related to established illnesses/conditions and the nature and outcomes of related remedial/rehabilitation measures.

One further area of health education which is slightly outside the scope of the approaches described above is that of *agenda-setting*. French (1990, p. 9) describes this as 'putting health on the agenda of policy makers'. It is also about helping people to develop their own health agendas. This is somewhat different in emphasis from the view of Tones and Tilford (1994) who see agenda-setting as the process whereby governments test the public's acceptance of certain proposed health-related legislation.

Health screening and monitoring

At their most basic, health screening and monitoring attempt to introduce prevention at the earliest possible opportunity. They usually involve secondary-level health interventions which include the provision of screening at the personal level and seek to identify diseases, conditions and health-denoting factors at an early stage. Examples are screening for female cancers through pap smears and mammography, coronary risk factors through well-person (MOT) clinics and child developmental surveillance. The majority of these screening procedures are carried out within the remit of general practice and primary health care. This is a key role for community nurses in that they are often involved in the organisation, delivery and evaluation of such services.

Comparable monitoring processes exist at the wider environmental level. Key agencies monitor factors such as air and water quality, hygiene standards in areas where food is prepared and home safety assessments. This type of monitoring is carried out by a number of agencies such as environmental health departments and health and safety agencies. The National Rivers Authority and various other regulatory bodies perform similar duties at a societal level through monitoring related health and social issues.

Health empowerment

Health empowerment, unlike the other elements described in this model, does not rely primarily on professionals providing the impetus for its operation. It describes health and social issues which individuals and communities identify and undertake on their own behalf and within their own control to enhance their health status. People develop health-promoting measures through empowerment within their personal lives and/or within the life of a community. Subsequently, they take steps to work towards health gain. Empowerment can emerge as the result of becoming skilled in a wide range of communication processes which enables people to take individual or collective action. Thus, professionals such as community nurses can assist people to become empowered through a range of measures which increase their own sense of control and ownership of their health status. This may often involve the facilitation of health and social knowledge and communication skills development.

It should be noted, however, that it is debatable whether or not professionals can empower clients or patients *per se*. A more apt description might be that professionals facilitate clients to become more empowered. It is evident, however, that when the mode of health promotion is client-led, this gives the opportunity for individuals or groups to seek to further their own empowerment. Examples of how they may achieve change are: choosing to lobby for the provision of new services or changes to services; forming self-help groups; negotiating for changes in environments and communities at local and national levels; influencing policies affecting health at local and government levels; or undertaking and advancing learning which will enhance self-growth as well as group (community) development.

The model of health promotion illustrated in Figure 9.2 is appropriate, in whole or in parts, for use by all community nurses and midwives. The question must be asked, however, how community nurses can enhance their health-promoting role through a systematic approach to health promotion organisation. Before developing a *model* of health promotion delivery, community nurses need to ensure that they are aware of both the context for their health promotion planning and also the skills which are necessary for advanced interactions.

HEALTH PROMOTION PLANNING CONTEXT

It seems obvious that the context within which community nurses deliver health promotion is the community where they provide a service to individuals and families. These terms in themselves bear further scrutiny before the health promotion planning pathway (see Figure 9.3) can be applied. On first impressions, the concepts of the individual, family and community may seem self-evident. It may be prudent, however, to examine each of the three concepts in more detail before attempting to ask what people's needs are and how these will be met.

Individuals are not simply lone entities who can be viewed in isolation. The model of health (Figure 9.1) suggests that any client or patient is a member of many social networks. These networks exist in physical environments and cannot thus be seen in isolation. Their current health knowledge, beliefs and behaviour will have been formed by many influences such as family, peers, education, the media, culture and socioeconomic status. It would be naive, therefore, for professionals to believe that they can devise a health promotion input which does not take all of these influences into account.

Similarly, those who seek to deliver health-promoting inputs to families must question what they mean by the term 'family'. The concept of family is now a matter for debate as common usage may be based on assumptions which never really existed (Weir, cited in Gough *et al.*, 1994). Attempts at definition inevitably lead to such as that found in Beckmann Murray and Proctor Zentner (1989, p. 46) where a number of configurations is possible:

'The family is a social system and primary reference group made up of two or more persons living together who are related by blood, marriage or adoption or who are living together by agreement over a period of time.'

This type of definition brings into question traditional views where 'family' has meant a nuclear family which consisted of a male and female parent who were usually married prior to procreating a number of offspring. This basic assumption has been increasingly challenged by a number of factors. First, there has been the gradual breakdown in the traditional configuration of the family and increasing recognition of other family structures. Lone parenting has become more common, divorce rates have increased, and parenthood outside marriage has become more acceptable. Second, changing work patterns have meant that significant numbers of children spend larger proportions of their time with 'second families' which may consist of those who provide their child-minding facility, such as child-minders and grandparents. Third, an increasingly multicultural society has introduced other definitions of family life. Extended families and dislocated families necessitated by the needs of migrant workers are but two in this category. Thus, those who promote health with families must ascertain what their client group mean by the term 'family'.

With regard to promoting health with communities, again, like 'family', the term 'community' must be defined. The most common way in which community is defined is in terms of geographical, cultural or social stratification (Naidoo and Wills, 1994). Thus any geographical location from an isolated rural backwater or various sizes of municipality through to nations can form a geographical community. It must, however, be pointed out that *community* can also be used to describe a group of people who share a common characteristic. Such a characteristic may be gender, ethnicity, sexual orientation, a shared disease entity, disability or disorder. The permutations of such communities provide a constant challenge for community nurses.

Having established the context of health promotion, it is now necessary for community nurses to identify the skill mix which will be necessary to enable them to undertake advanced interactions in health promotion. Only when such a repertoire of skills is identified and adopted can community nurses move to consider issues related to health promotion planning.

COMMUNICATION SKILLS FOR ADVANCED INTERACTIONS IN HEALTH PROMOTION

Advocate and mediator

The role of advocate has been a clearly identified health promotion role since the Ottawa Charter (WHO, 1986). The role of the nurse as advocate has also been formally recognised by their professional body (UKCC, 1992b). Advocates, it has been argued, actively seek to represent the interest of relatively underprivileged and marginalised groups. Their role is to redress, at least in part, the imbalances in power that occur in society (Tones and Tilford, 1994).

Based on this working definition, community nurses may regard advocacy as representing the needs of clients/patients to nursing management structures as well as to other providers of health and social services and all interested others. The difficulty for community nurses in this role, which is recognised to be both complex and controversial (Sines, 1996), is that fulfilling the role of advocate may bring them into conflict with their own employers. This is particularly so if the role is seen by employers to be outside the scope of their professional function. Therefore, a community nurse may find that while the employing authority's priorities for health promotion may be related to the lifestyle issues of clients, such as smoking and nutrition, the priorities of the clients may centre on issues such as financial benefits or the promotion of road safety for their children. In such a situation community nurses may feel caught between the employer's epidemiologically proven need to promote changes in lifestyle and the autonomous rights of clients to pursue other agendas and, indeed, to reject the lifestyle initiatives.

To reconcile these two seemingly conflicting roles, nurses may adopt the role of *mediator*. This role, adapted from that described in the Ottawa Charter (WHO, 1986), involves utilising the ethical principle of justice which can be conceptualised as the resolution and reconciliation of competing claims. Here, community nurses will endeavour, through using negotiation skills, to mediate and reconcile the conflicting expectations of both groups (not to mention others who may also have a view on the matter) and produce an agreed solution.

Negotiation skills that bring about solutions to two opposing points of view require: that, the community nurse be open-minded enough to accept both views without preconceived judgements; working towards preventing either party ending up feeling hurt or left out; agreeing ground rules for negotiation; identifying existing areas of agreement; and subsequently seeking compromise on areas of disagreement.

Educator

The role of health educator is one which is well-established for community nurses. However, it appears that the roles of educator and advice-giver have often been confused. There has been a long-held tradition that advice-giving was, in itself, sufficient. This has been exemplified in the oft-heard phrase, 'we give them the information and it's up to them what they do with it'.

Perhaps the confusion surrounding the efficacy of advice-giving has emanated from the use of the KAB (knowledge–attitude–behaviour) model of health behaviour change (Kemm and Close, 1995). Many people who have tried to lose weight or to stop smoking can attest to the fact that they may *know* the advantages of such a behaviour change and their attitudes are such that the change is highly desirable. However, the problem is that sound knowledge and favourable attitudes do not necessarily turn into desirable behaviour change. Thus, the simple act of information-giving may lead to attitude change, but this will not necessarily lead to behaviour change. However, as Kemm and Close (1995) rightly point out, empowered choice can only become reality when people have the relevant information.

The role of educator must go beyond advice-giving. One way in which this can be achieved is through brief motivational interventions (Rollnick *et al.*, 1992). Such interventions, which draw on the work of Prochaska and DiClementi (1986), recognise that clients will learn when they are in a state of readiness to do so. A brief synopsis of this model shows three key aims: (1) during a series of brief interventions lasting approximately ten minutes each, clients may be facilitated to identify the necessity to make a choice in relation to a specific health behaviour change; (2) the model continues by helping clients to recognise their state of readiness to change the behaviour; and (3) clients are presented with a choice of behaviour-change strategies and subsequently choose the one which they feel most comfortable to participate in.

In the wider arena of facilitating health behaviour change, communication skills development such as assertiveness skills, behaviour modification techniques and education on the judicious use of services may be necessary.

Much has been written elsewhere regarding the more detailed elements of the planning process (Naidoo and Wills, 1994; Ewles and Simnett, 1995; Kemm and Close, 1995; Tones and Tilford, 1994). The purpose of the remainder of this chapter is, therefore, to focus on the key communication skills which underpin advanced interactions in health promotion with particular reference to community nurses. Having established the context and the repertoire of skills necessary for advanced interactions in health promotion, it is now possible to proceed to describing the multi-phase health promotion planning pathway.

THE MULTI-PHASE HEALTH PROMOTION PLANNING PATHWAY

Phase one: needs assessment phase

An examination of Figure 9.3 shows that assessment of need is a key task which all community nurses undertake during their initial professional education. Completion of community profiles, general practice population profiles and neighbourhood studies are commonplace methods of assessment of need. Community nurses need the ability, time and resources to create and maintain appropriate databases on which assessment of need can be compiled. However, this type of data is not, in itself, sufficient. Questions must be asked about what types of need are being assessed and whose needs are being considered. In answering these questions a helpful method of conceptualising need was advanced by Bradshaw (1972).

1. *Normative needs* are those where the need of a defined individual, family, or community is identified by a key decision-maker such as a professional or public representative. In this type of need the mechanisms used for identification maybe quite different. Professionals from statutory/voluntary organisations

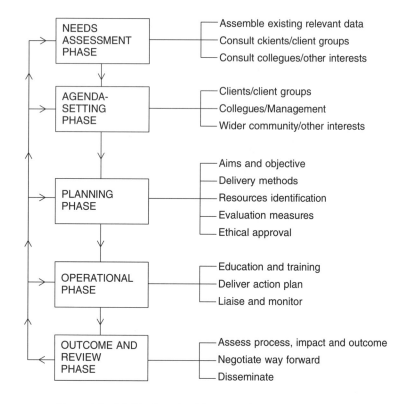

Figure 9.3   Multi-phase health promotion planning pathway

with time and skill will, most often, base their assessment of normative need on the comparisons between epidemiological and demographic evidence compiled, for example, in a community profiling exercise and observed clinical/social factors for individuals. The professionals involved will then identify norms against which need is assessed. If clients fall short of the defined norms, they can then be said to be in normative need.

2. *Expressed needs*, on the other hand, are the felt needs of individuals and communities which have been articulated and noted by professionals. They are ascertained by consulting individuals and communities about their perception of need, usually through good quantitative and qualitative survey work. Such needs have the unfortunate habit of not always matching the normative needs as defined by professionals. Often, those who are not used to articulating need are not even sure what

their needs are. A not uncommon experience for those involved in ascertaining expressed need is the ambiguity involved when asking individuals and communities what they perceive their needs to be; to be given the reply, 'What have you got to offer?'

The added complication of expressed needs is that they raise inconvenient issues for officialdom. Thus, for example, while a health authority may consider smoking a priority health issue for individuals and their communities, the community may be more concerned with the lack of child-care facilities. Similarly, the authority may consider immunisation a top priority while parents may be more concerned by the hazardous traffic conditions where they live. In both cases, the expressed needs will have direct resource implications for the statutory services and this may not always be welcome. Community nurses have the task, therefore, of attempting to reconcile the normative and expressed health and social needs of individuals, families or communities. They may have to balance the dual role of agents of their employers and advocates for their clients/patients.

3. *Comparative need* involves the identification and comparison of models of good practice in relation to health promotion. Clients or communities who are not in receipt of equally good interventions may be said to be in comparative need to those who are. This type of need will often be a good bargaining chip for community nurses. They can, in the first instance, inform their own practice by reference to other research identifying evidence of good practice. Subsequently they can use this evidence-based practice to encourage their own and other organisations to consider providing health promotion inputs for the 'in-need' clients and communities.

Phase two: agenda-setting

Once the appropriate needs have been identified nurses must proceed to develop a strategy to ensure that the needs are met (see phase two of the model depicted in Figure 9.3). The task at this stage is to facilitate *agenda-setting* (French, 1990; Tones and Tilford, 1994). Here, community nurses will attempt to place the relevant health promotion issue on the agenda of the individual or community being worked with. The aim here is to produce informed decision-makers. Community nurses will do this through their ability to motivate, educate and listen to their clients.

Agenda setting also requires the community nursing team – both face-to-face practitioners and managers – to use *negotiation* and *advocacy skills* with colleagues from a range of other disciplines. By forming healthy alliances (DoH, 1992) to place the needs of the individual/community on common agendas, community nurses can help to facilitate colleagues and others to learn about and act on behalf of relevant client groups. Such an approach is in line with the call for partnerships which has characterised World Health Organisation and Local Agenda 21 thinking (WHO, 1978, 1986, 1997; LGMB, 1994). The aim here is to produce informed professionals who can meet the challenges presented by clients or carer groups. Also, by participating as members of healthy alliances, community nurses can present the panoply of assessed needs of the community to key decision-makers. Attempts can thus be made to win optimal resources from within community nurses' own employing authority and/or other parties which may prove to be sources of support.

At the same time, community nurses may need to negotiate with the community to help them come to a realistic assessment of what is possible within the resource restraints which are often present. They may also facilitate the meeting of need by pointing the community towards other sources of assistance, encouraging the judicious use of existing resources and services and, when possible, the funding and provision of new ones. It may also be possible to put the community in touch with pressure groups which may be able to provide lobbying assistance that is outside the scope of the remit of the community nursing team. Thus by employing the communication skills of negotiation and facilitation, community nurses aim to produce *informed individuals, families and communities* who may be receptive to health promotion interventions/ initiatives.

Phase three: planning phase

Once the health and social needs have been established, the community nurse has achieved agreement on the health issue which is to be addressed and appropriate agenda-setting work has been done, then the role of planner comes into play. For some relatively simple inputs, such as an information-giving session, the nurse will be able to plan alone and unaided. For more complex initiatives, community nurses will often be involved in planning teams. The community nurse may, as with the needs assessment phase, need to employ motivation, negotiation, advocacy, mediation and facilitation skills such as information-providing, networking facilitating and conflict resolution, to name but a few.

On entry to the planning phase of the pathway (see Figure 9.3), community nurses must be able to pursue a coherent plan of action. Regardless of the type of strategy being adopted, five discreet steps will have to be negotiated in the planning phase of the pathway.

1. Identification of an appropriate strategy

This may involve helping individuals and communities to take action for health gain. If community nurses are to be the main health promoters in the programme, then they must also ensure that they have the requisite knowledge and skills to perform effectively. In addition to the generic skills which have been outlined for the pathway, what other types of skills may be involved?

When working with individuals and families, community nurses may be involved in helping clients to identify specific health problems and to work towards appropriate solutions through the use of counselling skills which may be supplemented, as appropriate, with health education. Clients' levels of empowerment will therefore be increased to assist them in addressing their own health issues and needs.

If, on the other hand, the health promotion work is designed to work in partnership with the community, then community nurses may find themselves facilitating, or at least participating in, strategies such as community involvement/participation or community development. With reference to community participation, the community is involved in the planning process to varying degrees. Involvement of the residents of the community in a health promotion programme can vary from simply assuring they all receive the appropriate information regarding the proposed programme through to increasingly complex levels of consultation, involvement, implementation and evaluation. At the more complex levels, joint planning and delegation of authority to the community to make decisions regarding the programme may be possible. Beyond this, the community makes all the key decisions and is facilitated to accomplish its own goals (Ewles and Simnett, 1995). At all levels of community involvement, community nurses may thus find themselves liaising with and facilitating the members of the community in its involvement with all stages of the programme.

Community development, unlike community involvement, relates to the community being empowered to identify its own health and social needs and to decide on key ways in which those needs should be met (CHIR/LCHR, 1987). At each stage of the process the residents of the community retain control of the process. This differs from community participation in that professionals will not primarily lead the process. The role of community nurses would, therefore, be to facilitate the process of defining need and to act as facilitators/supporters of the community as it seeks to have its needs met. Needs are usually met through policy change and service/resource provision.

2. Setting mutually agreed and realistic aims and objectives

Setting out a mutually agreed aim or goal is skilled in so far as it must be realistic and appropriate for the client group. It is better to move incrementally and set relatively easily attained goals which produce a sense of achievement in the clients than to aim for the grandiose or unattainable which may lead to demoralisation for all concerned. The main aim is the outcome that should be achieved from the overall programme.

Similarly, the objectives, which are the steps by which an overall aim is achieved, must be realistic, achievable and relevant (Ewles and Simnett, 1995). The setting of objectives should, if possible, be in discussion with the client group and relate to the achievement of specific *outcomes*. When planning outcomes, the health promotion planner should beware of the assumption that the main outcome of health promotion is always behaviour change. This may not be necessarily so. Many situations may call for the facilitation of *empowerment* of clients or communities through: improved knowledge of services available; negotiating changes in service provision; providing child care to support the activities of the programme; ensuring that transport is provided to services; and by providing low-cost food or clothing. Educational objectives may focus on facilitating learning in the cognitive (knowledge), affective (attitudinal/feeling) or conative (behavioural) domains.

Development of communication skills such as assertiveness, conflict resolution, getting the most from meetings and/or from other professional bodies and voluntary organisations may also be required. All of these advanced interaction skills go beyond the more conventional talks, leaflets and posters which have been the mainstay of so-called health promotion in the community. Where community nurses are not directly involved in such health promotion measures, they may act as referral agents for the community to the appropriate providers.

3. Identifying resources

Identification of resources will, to some degree, determine what objectives can be achieved. It will also require community nurses to make a realistic assessment of what they may need to negotiate for. Resource provision could fall into three main categories: financial, human and physical.

Financial resources will often be the determining factor which will decide whether or not a programme will be feasible and also what other resources will need to be sought. Community nurses may be involved in helping individuals or client groups to identify sources of funding and also be involved in the often time-consuming process of making applications for funding.

Human resources involve a wide range of people. Within the context of this chapter the key resources are the community nurses themselves. Colleagues in community nursing and primary health care teams may also provide valuable support. The client group may act as a resource by contributing to the strategy by, for example, forming self-help groups for mutual support and engaging in the lobbying of statutory providers of services as well as all local public representatives. Others may be able to negotiate the use of facilities in the community or arrange for the collection of funds if necessary. Local personalities may also be helpful in reinforcing specific messages or providing publicity to advertise the issue/topic area. Help may also be obtained from specialist voluntary organisations of other statutory bodies.

Physical resources, again, cover a wide range which may include: arranging suitable facilities in which to meet; ensuring appropriate equipment to provide crèche or fitness facilities; and providing catering equipment and accessible transport for clients. Audio-visual and print materials which are necessary to support health education initiatives require community nurses to have the ability to draw up criteria for choosing appropriate resources. With the explosion of the information superhighway the need for clients to have access to on-line information and to be able to network through the Internet will become more apparent.

4. Evaluation

It must also be remembered that the process of evaluation must be built into the strategy during the planning stage. Three aspects of evaluation must be taken into consideration – *process, impact* and *outcome* (Hawe *et al.*, 1990). The indicators (criteria) which will be used for evaluation must be chosen when the aims and objectives are stated.

Process evaluation will measure the acceptability of the programme to the clients and the quality of the constituent parts of the programme. Impact evaluation will measure the immediate outcomes of individual objectives and outcome evaluation will assess whether or not the overall aims of the programme have been achieved. The indicators which can be used to monitor evaluation can include epidemiological factors, to measure changes in disease rates such as incidence, prevalence and standardised mortality ratios.

Evaluation of the learning outcomes that have occurred in knowledge, skills, and attitudes/beliefs may be assessed using the following factors:

- Assessment of health-related learning is designed to evaluate knowledge gain that has occurred in areas such as coronary risk factors and cancer-screening services.
- Behaviour change may be measured by identifying, for example, the percentage of clients who have stopped smoking, changed their diet or developed a specific skill such as a successful tooth-brushing technique.
- Attitude and belief change may come about as the result of facilitating clients to make decisions about integrating disabled and marginalised people into the community, thus helping to reduce stigma through the process of normalisation and facilitating measures which may lead to increased levels of self-efficacy.
- Monitoring of service use may be evaluated by auditing the number of people attending drop-in centres or screening clinics; what they achieved from the staff in terms of health information and health gain; how the services could be improved; and, for example, the number of leaflets distributed on certain topics.

5. Ethical approval

Once a plan has been formulated it may be necessary to obtain ethical approval, particularly if community nurses are going to offer some form of intervention which may involve risk, no matter how minimal. Some examples of current controversial areas are offering lifestyle checks such as blood pressure monitoring; bereavement counselling; peer education regarding sexuality and sexual orientation; and contraception for people with learning disabilities. Ethical considerations are embodied within the UKCC's (1992b) injunction to always act in a client's best interests. Moreover, ethical health promotion will always attempt to ensure that a client's autonomy is respected, that the intervention will do good, and will, at the very least, do the client no harm. Issues such as confidentiality and anonymity would also be taken into account.

Phase four: operational phase

Once the planning phase has been finalised, an action plan should be drawn up. This will give a sequential outline of the programme and will, if possible, have a time-scale built in. It will also outline milestones by which certain elements of the programme will be completed to ensure that the planning team can monitor the project and validate that it is on target for successful completion. If possible, one key person should be identified to manage the project. This person should be responsible for the conduct of the project and for reporting on the achievement of specific milestones and objectives and ultimately for the overall success (or failure) of the project aim.

Community nurses may find themselves involved in pre-implementation negotiation with clients, communities and colleagues to ensure that everyone is in agreement with the programme to be implemented. This process will also be necessary during the implementation phase as liaison and monitoring will be necessary on an ongoing basis. This is the point where community nurses may particularly find themselves acting in the role of diplomat. It would be hoped that conflicting or varying expectations would have been reconciled in the earlier parts of the pathway (see Figure 9.3), but when the difficulties of real life impinge on an ideal plan and ensuing conflicts arise, it may be necessary for the community nurse to act as a mediator and address and resolve operational problems.

The provision of education and training may also be necessary prior to the running of the programme. For example, education and training in groupwork skills may be required. Here community nurses must decide whether or not they have the necessary knowledge, skills and resources within their own profession to provide training or whether 'experts' from the specific area should be employed. Decisions regarding the actual planning and delivery of the training may involve bringing together a small task team to ensure that relevant views are represented and to share the workload. Each of these elements will become, in itself, a small-scale programme which should be based on the same planning process. Education and training may vary in extent from a simple awareness-raising exercise prior to implementation to more complex skills development.

The other issue which must be considered at this point is to ensure that the evaluation measures which were agreed at the planning phase are being implemented. This will be important to demonstrate accountability and achievement and to inform any subsequent health promotion programmes. Practically this may involve the community nurse in facilitating, or indeed creating, the design, administration and analysis of evaluation tools. This may involve purchasing expertise from researchers and/or statisticians to support each element of the evaluation process.

It may well be that modifications to the programme will be necessary during implementation as a result of monitoring process issues. Negotiations for such modifications will again call for a prudent application of communication and networking skills. Negotiating the final element of this phase of the pathway should find the community nurse with the process completed (successfully or otherwise) and the evaluation data should be available for dissemination.

Phase five: outcome and review phase

This is the phase which is most often neglected or delayed in its completion. Often, in the relief of having achieved a reasonably successful operational phase, there is a temptation to neglect the writing-up of a final report and/or an article for publication. By choosing not to follow this phase to completion, much valuable experience and learning may be lost. Failing to disseminate knowledge to others can result in health promoters making unnecessary mistakes and wasting scarce resources. It is, therefore, important that those involved in the programme are given the opportunity, in light of formal and informal evaluation data, to affirm and celebrate those elements of the programme which went well and to identify and learn from those elements which were less successful.

Once this process has been undertaken it is then possible to negotiate a way forward. In some cases, a discreet programme will have ended, but in many instances the professionals involved will wish to negotiate where and how they will proceed with their health promotion work.

In such cases it would be helpful to revisit earlier stages of the pathway and use it as a checklist to decide where changes should be made. Joint proposals could then be made to relevant decision-makers in relation to approval for a more province-wide provision of the new strategy as well as for funding and staffing.

The final element of this phase is the dissemination of the programme outcomes. It is important that community nurses share both their successes and their failures. Too often, only the successful outcome is written about, thus losing a valuable learning opportunity. Lack of success is part of professional experience and professionals should not be afraid to acknowledge this and to learn from it. Community nurses should recognise that there are a range of forums where they can share their experience.

Writing academic papers is important as this should ensure rigour at all stages of the process. However, it should also be noted that the current pressures on academics to publish make it somewhat more difficult to achieve an early publication in high-profile academic journals which are heavily over subscribed. It must also be noted, however, that a well-written journal article for the more popular elements of the professional press may well reach a wider readership and encourage further work in the author's field of study. Finally, it is important that a cogent final report is assembled which will reflect well on the programme by highlighting relevant issues related to methodology, funding and other resources, the outcomes of the programme and plans for future development.

CONCLUSION

This chapter has sought to highlight the key role of community nurses in promoting the health and social well-being of individuals, families and communities. It emphasised the importance of having a clear understanding of the key communication skills that are required for advanced interactions in the area of health promotion. The chapter continued by outlining an holistic approach to health and this definition was used to describe an innovative model of health promotion. This model of health promotion was designed to embrace a number of key activities which community nurses may utilise to facilitate health gains for individuals, families and communities.

Further, the multi-phase pathway for health promotion planning described a number of steps which, when followed logically, may facilitate community nurses to carry out the important task of providing their clients with high quality health promotion opportunities. As the new millennium approaches, the provision of such health-promoting opportunities targeted at individuals, families and communities provides community nurses with exciting challenges as they continue to search for new and creative ways to promote and improve health status. Moreover, client expectations in the future will, no doubt, match the mood of a new century.

References

Aggleton, P. and Homans, H. (1987) *Educating about AIDS*. London: NHS Training Authority.

Ashton, J. and Seymour, H. (1988) *The New Public Health*. Oxford: Oxford University Press..

Beauchamp, T. L. and Childress, J. F. (1995) *Principles of Biomedical Ethics*. Oxford: Oxford University Press.

Beckmann Murray, R. and Proctor Zentner, J. (adapted by C. Howells (1989) *Nursing Concepts for Health Promotion*. London: Prentice-Hall International (UK).

Blaxter, M. (1990) *Health and Lifestyles*. London: Routledge.

Bradshaw, J. (1972) The concept of social need. *New Society*, 19(30), pp. 640–3.

Bunton, R. and Macdonald, G. (1992) *Health Promotion Disciplines and Diversity*. London: Routledge.

Catford, J. and Nutbeam, D. (1984) Towards a definition of health education and health promotion. *Health Education Journal*, 43(2, 3), p. 38.

Community Health Initiatives Resource/London Community Health Resource (1987) *Guide to Community Health Projects*. London: NCVO.

Delaney, F. (1994) Nursing and health promotion: conceptual concerns. *Journal of Advanced Nursing*, 20, pp. 828–35.

Department of Health (1992) *Health of the Nation: A Strategy for Health in England*. London: HMSO.

Department of Health (1998) *Our Healthier Nation – A Contract for Health*. London: HMSO.

Department of Health and Social Services for Northern Ireland (1992) *Regional Strategy for the Health and Personal Social Services 1992–1997*. Belfast: DHSSNI.

Department of Health and Social Services for Northern Ireland (1996) *Health and Wellbeing into the Millennium*. Belfast: DHSSNI.

Downie, R. S., Tannahill, C. and Tannahill, A. (1997) *Health Promotion Models and Values*, 2nd edn. Oxford: Oxford University Press.

Dubos, R. (1960) *Mirage of Health*. London: Allen & Unwin.

Ewles, L. and Simnett, I. (1995) *Promoting Health: A Practical Guide*, 3rd edn. London: Scutari Press.

French, J. (1990) Boundaries and horizons, the role of health education within health promotion. *Health Education Journal*, 49 (1), pp. 7–10.

Gott, M. and O'Brien, M. (1990) The role of the nurse in health promotion. *Health Promotion International* 5 (2), pp. 137–43.

Gough, P., Maslin-Prothero, S. and Masterson, A. (1994) *Nursing and Social Policy – Care in Context*. Oxford: Butterworth-Heinemann.

Hawe, P., Degeling, D. and Hall, J. (1990) *Evaluating Health Promotion*. Sydney: MacLellan & Petty.

Kemm, J. and Close, A. (1995) *Health Promotion Theory and Practice*. London: Macmillan.

Lalonde, M. (1974) *A New Perspective on the Health of Canadians*. Ottawa: Government of Canada.

Local Government Management Board (1994) *Local Agenda 21 Principles and Process – A Step by Step Guide*. Luton: LGMB.

Mansfield, K. (1977) *Letters and Journals*. London: Pelican Books.

Naidoo, J. and Wills, J. (1994) *Health Promotion, Foundations for Practice*. London: Bailliere & Tindall.

NHS Executive (1996) *Primary Care: The Future*. Leeds: NHS Executive.

Prochaska, J. and DiClementi, C. (1986) Towards a comprehensive model of change. In W. R. Miller, and N. Heather (eds), *Treating Addictive Behaviours: Processes of Change*. New York: Plenum.

Rollnick, S., Heather, N. and Bell, A. (1992) Negotiating behaviour change in medical settings: the development of brief motivational interviewing. *Journal of Mental Health*, 1, pp. 25–37.

Scriven, A. and Orme, J. (eds) (1996) *Health Promotion – Professional Perspectives* (1996) London: Macmillan/Open University Press.

Seedhouse, D. (1986) *Health: The Foundations of Achievement.* Chichester: John Wiley & Sons.

Sines, D. T. (1996) Advocacy. In S. Twinn, B. Roberts and S. Andrews (eds), *Community Health Care Nursing – Principles for Practice.* Oxford: Butterworth-Heinemann.

Tannahill, A. (1985) What is health promotion? *Health Education Journal,* 44 (4), pp. 167–8.

Tones, K. (1996) The anatomy and ideology of health promotion: empowerment in context. In Scriven and Orme (1996).

Tones, K. and Tilford, S. (1994) *Health Education – Effectiveness, Efficiency and Equity,* 2nd edn. London: Chapman & Hall.

United Kingdom Central Council for Nursing, Midwifery and Health Visiting, (UKCC) (1992a) *The Scope of Professional Practice.* London: UKCC.

United Kingdom Central Council for Nursing, Midwifery and Health Visiting, (UKCC) (1992b) *Code of Professional Conduct for Nurses, Midwives and Health Visitors.* London: UKCC.

United Nations (1992) *Report of the United Nations Conference on Environment and Development,* Annex 1 – The Rio Declaration on Environment and Development. A/CONF. 151/26 (Vol. 1) New York: United Nations.

Weir, H. (1994) The family and social policy. In Gough *et al.,* (1994).

Williams, R. G. A. (1983) Concepts of health: analysis of lay logic. *Sociology,* (17)2, pp. 185–204.

World Health Organisation (1946) *Constitution.* Geneva: WHO.

World Health Organisation (1978) Alma Ata Declaration. Geneva: WHO.

World Health Organisation (1984) *Health Promotion: A Discussion Document on the Concepts and Principles.* Copenhagen: WHO Regional Office for Europe.

World Health Organisation (1985) *Targets for Health for All.* Copenhagen: WHO Regional Office for Europe.

World Health Organisation (1986) *Ottawa Charter on Health Promotion, An International Conference on Health Promotion.* Copenhagen: WHO Regional Office for Europe.

World Health Organisation (1988) Healthy Cities Papers 1, 2 and 3. Copenhagen: WHO Regional Office for Europe.

World Health Organisation (1991) *Budapest Declaration on Health Promoting Hospitals.* Copenhagen: WHO Regional Office for Europe.

World Health Organisation (1993) *The Health Promoting School.* Copenhagen: WHO Regional Office for Europe.

World Health Organisation (1994) *Health Promoting Hospitals – Aims and Concepts, Strategies and Possibilities for Participation in the Network.* Copenhagen: WHO Regional Office for Europe.

World Health Organisation (1997) *Jarkarta Declaration.* Geneva: WHO.

CHAPTER TEN

Communicating with Challenging Clients

Pauline Irving and Diane Hazlett

INTRODUCTION

The issue of working with challenging people is one which will be familiar to all community nurses. It is a truism that some clients are more difficult to help than others, due to diagnosis, personal characteristics or poor interpersonal skills, but it is surprising that there is very little in the literature that directly addresses this issue. The guidance that does exist tends to be rather anecdotal in nature and focuses on two areas: first, types of difficulties are delineated and, second, the communication skills thought most appropriate are identified and discussed. This approach is typified, in the business context, by Markham (1993, p. 9) who states:

> 'There is no way you can make difficult people change and suddenly become sweet and amenable. Such change can only take place when the individuals concerned desire it and work towards it. So, if you can't change *them*, the only thing you can do is change your own *reaction to them*.'

Markham (1993) goes on to identify thirteen different types of difficult people and presents strategies for dealing with them. Such an approach is problematic for several reasons. In the first place it locates the problem firmly with the client. The term 'difficult people' is a pejorative one that does not take account of the complexities of the communication process or interpersonal relationships. Use of the term 'challenging people' is much less value-laden and more positive. Windahl, Signitzer and Olsen (1992) point out that modern definitions of communication have moved away from the mechanistic message–channel–receiver models towards conceptualisations which emphasise 'mutuality and shared perceptions' (p. 6). The success of communication is the responsibility of both participants in any interaction. Approaches to problem situations which identify one participant as 'difficult' ignore the complexities of the communication process and can encourage stereotyping and stigmatisation of clients. They also encourage manipulative types of behaviour on the part of the professionals who could see themselves as dealing with a problem rather than working with an individual. Any analysis of communication with challenging people must take account of both participants and the communication process itself.

Communication is at the heart of community nursing practice. In a review of patient attitude surveys Ley (1988) pointed to a high level of dissatisfaction with the interpersonal aspect of health care. Fletcher (1997) asserts that nurses see themselves as uniquely placed 'to blend physical and emotional support into care' (p. 43). However, he questions the ability of the profession to deliver this in practice, citing studies which found that nurses were perceived as not being helpful in their response to emotional need. For example, a study of HIV/AIDS care indicated that nurses were not seen as the main source of emotional support by patients. Irving and Long (1993) discuss the role of counselling in health promotion and present case studies to illustrate the central importance of the emotional aspects of care. Dickson (1989) supports a holistic view of health care encompassing both physical and psychosocial aspects and argues for increased attention to be paid to the interpersonal component during education and training. Working with challenging people puts strain on the nurse's interpersonal skills and weaknesses in this area are more evident in such situations.

In examining the issue of challenging people a number of factors need to be considered. It has already been argued that communication success or failure is the responsibility of both participants. It therefore follows that any model attempting to explain challenging communication scenarios needs to examine the role of both the client and the nurse in addition to aspects of the communication process itself. This chapter presents such a model. A model for working with challenging people that takes account of the helper, the client and the process will be outlined. The focus will be on the two participants in interactions and less attention will be paid to the communication process itself since this has been discussed in detail elsewhere in this book. Common reasons for difficulties will be examined and constructive strategies suggested. At the end of the chapter two specific examples of challenging groups will be considered: working with people with communication disorders; and working with anger or aggression. A more detailed discussion of strategies will be presented in order to illustrate general points.

A MODEL OF CHALLENGING COMMUNICATION

An examination of work with challenging people needs to address the problem on at least three levels:

1. the client;
2. the nurse;
3. the communication process.

Clients can present problems for a variety of reasons. Some of these can relate to physical or psychiatric conditions which interfere with the communication process. For example, stroke patients, by virtue of their condition, often have difficulty expressing themselves. Many psychiatric conditions like schizophrenia and depression can interrupt the smooth progress of communication. Later in this chapter strategies geared towards overcoming such difficulties are presented in detail. Client problems can also arise from personal characteristics separate from any medical condition. Markham's (1993) discussion presents a number of such 'personality types' and although rather stereotyped can have some validity in forming the basis for the formulation of communication approaches. More generalised personal characteristics like shyness, aggression or a reluctance to talk about personal material can also pose problems, as can communication skill deficits and styles. Again these will be discussed later in the chapter. The handling of personal material can create problems in itself. Hill *et al.* (1993) investigated covert processes in counselling and psychotherapy and identified taboo areas such as sexuality that tend not to be spoken of easily in therapeutic situations. They also looked at the impact of misunderstanding on the part of the helper.

The second participant, the nurse, can also bring problems to the helping situation, in terms of attitudes, beliefs, personal characteristics and life experience. Fletcher (1997), in a review of studies, questions whether or not nurses always bring to the care situation the positive attitudes that characterise the ideal world. Similarly Burnard and Morrison (1991), in an investigation of client-centred attitudes in nursing, found that empathy, genuineness and acceptance were not always evident. Lindlow (1992), in a discussion of self-advocacy, highlights the importance of 'mentalism' (Chamberlin, 1988) as a barrier to communication. This attitude is rooted in the training of mental health professionals whose focus on seeking symptoms of mental illness can interfere with the client's expression of feelings, as such expression can be seen as a symptom. Read and Wallcraft (1992) speak as 'survivors of the mental health system' (p. 4) and, in guidelines for mental health workers, (p. 15), say:

'Don't dismiss our complaints and worries as symptoms of our "mental illness". Too often people's physical illnesses have been disregarded, women sexually molested in hospitals and hostels have not been believed, and genuine grievances have not been taken seriously.'

Setting aside personal issues, workloads and time constraints can inhibit communication. Salvage and Buxton (1997, p. 56) present a view of the community nurse as being overworked and under pressure:

'She complains of being overworked and feeling demoralised, and perhaps developing a persecution complex. She says she doesn't feel valued or listened to, and constantly feels she must prove herself.'

Under such circumstances it is hardly surprising that personal issues have the potential to be brought into the professional arena.

Training also plays an important role. Dickson (1989) makes the case for a 'systematic and structured framework' (p. 345) for teaching communication skills. Although this is now more fully addressed in nurse education programmes its importance cannot be overemphasised. In any interaction the nurse is both a professional and a person. Self-awareness is an important prerequisite of effective communication.

The third element in the equation is the communication process itself. One frequently voiced concern is high caseloads and lack of time. If communication is rushed it is less likely to achieve its objectives. By definition community nurses work with clients in situations that are not always conducive to easy communication. A health visitor working with a new mother in her home may have the simple difficulty of not being able to speak to the client alone and obviously interruptions have a negative effect on the interaction. Social conventions can lead to situations where the client tries to be sociable, pleasant and welcoming to a visitor and baulks at disrupting a rewarding social relationship by introducing anything negative. It is not uncommon for new mothers to want to impress the professional with how well she is coping and consequently anxieties and worries are not easily brought out into the open.

Communication difficulties can be seen as arising from the client, the nurse or the situation and are often the result of the interaction between all three elements. If the difficulty is seen as centred on the client the solution will also be seen as residing there. This is important because how the problem is conceived is a vital element in developing solutions. Self-awareness and openness on the part of the helper are a vital part of effective helping and it is challenging and professional to examine the problem from different angles.

REASONS WHY CLIENTS MAY BE RESISTANT

Egan (1990) suggests that resistance and reluctance are a normal part of the helping process. He believes that clients tend to become resistant if they feel they are being coerced in some way but there are many other reasons why this may occur. Some clients do not understand why help is necessary in the first place and may be defensive about the value of the intervention. Counselling and helping are often misunderstood and can be perceived in a negative way. Seeking or being referred to a counsellor can be seen as evidence of weakness. It should also be remembered that the counselling encounter can be an unfamiliar situation to many people and clients can be unsure of how to participate effectively. This obviously points to the importance of how encounters are handled at the beginning. It is vital that clients understand the reason and the structure for any session if they are to participate fully. Hargie, Saunders and Dickson (1994) point to the importance of set induction which should have social, motivational and cognitive components. This needs to be coupled with effective closure which allows clients to ask questions, summarises key points and actions and makes links with future encounters. The busy community nurse described by Salvage and Buxton (1997) often feels that he or she is pressed for time and it is these very important elements at the beginning and end that are often rushed or overlooked. This is linked to problems associated with assumptions. Just because a professional understands the professional role does not mean that clients are equally familiar and may have different agendas. A study by Irving and Dunne (1994) into the information needs of health centre users found that a large number were unaware of even basic information on services available.

Some clients may, through past experience, have developed negative attitudes towards the helping process or the organisation the helper represents. Issues of trust and confidentiality are particularly important. In addition the helper may be perceived as too dissimilar in terms of such factors as attitude, sex, race, religion and social class. This can be linked to the client's own defensiveness if he or she perceives the helping process as implying that they are in some way inadequate or weak. By resisting the process, it is possible to maintain their own self-esteem. Similarly, the client's own need for personal power may be fulfilled by resisting what they perceive as being a powerful figure or process. Furthermore, some clients may feel the need to test out the nurse's level of support and competence by displaying negative attitudes or behaviours. Other difficulties can arise from the client's ambiguity towards change when the price of change can be seen as too high with too few pay-offs. The client's conception of the type and degree of change required may differ from the helper's.

The interview situation and the type of helping model used may also pose problems for the client. Many people feel ill at ease in one-to-one interactions with professionals. Some find it difficult to cope with the verbal medium which dominates such interactions. Some find difficulty in talking about personal issues (Hill *et al.*, 1993) which can be governed by a sense of strong taboos in certain areas of work like sexuality. On a simpler level many individuals have difficulty talking the language of emotions as this is not a usual or acceptable interactional style. The question 'How do you feel?' is often very hard to answer. The helping model itself can be problematic with clients feeling potentially confused, threatened or irritated by perceived lack of structure or an overly didactic or evaluative approach. Research into client perceptions of counselling suggests that clients value practitioners' interactions characterised by the client-centred attitudes of genuineness, acceptance and empathy but which are also perceived as structured and forward-moving (Oldfield, 1983; Elliot, 1985; Heppner and Rosenberg, 1992).

The above issues are only some of the factors which may inhibit the client's cooperation in the helping setting. It is also important to remember that clients can feel overwhelmed by the number and magnitude of their problems and perceive the task as too difficult. They can be discouraged by feelings of impotence or even panic. Such feelings need to be out in the open and dealt with if progress is to be made. Helpers need to be evaluating the process, constantly seeking to identify resistance and trying to understand its roots. Egan (1990) points out that such difficulties are a normal part of the helping process and should be worked with on that basis. Before looking at helpful responses to such resistance, and in line with the model presented in this chapter, it is important to look at possible sources of difficulty and resistance emanating from the helper.

REASONS WHY HELPERS MAY BE RESISTANT

As previously stated, problems in a communication situation may be construed as coming from the helper. It is often easier for helpers to attribute blame to the client than examine their own role in the process. However, such attributions may be premature and could represent defensiveness. The nurse's self-awareness, reflection and openness are important components in causal attribution. It is challenging to be open to the possibility that the nurse could be a contributory factor. A simple example of this can be seen in the helper's response to client resistance. Egan (1990, p. 173) observes:

'Helpers, especially beginning helpers who are unaware of the pervasiveness of reluctance and resistance, are often disconcerted by them. They may find themselves facing unexpected feelings and emotions in themselves when they encounter these behaviours in clients: they may feel confused, panicked, irritated, hostile, guilty, hurt, rejected, meek, or depressed. Distracted by these unexpected feelings, they may react in any of several unhelpful ways.'

Such a picture should be easily recognisable to most community nurses. If honest attempts at helping the client are rejected it is easy to get disheartened and begin to label and blame the client. Helpful responses to client resistance will be discussed later but it is useful to look at possible unhelpful responses at this stage. These could include:

1. accepting guilt and trying to placate the client;
2. becoming impatient or hostile;
3. doing nothing and hoping the problem will disappear;
4. lowering expectations of either client or helper;
5. trying to win the client over with 'love';
6. blaming the client;
7. engaging in a power struggle;
8. playing the role of scapegoat;
9. handing direction to the client;
10. giving up;
11. referring the client;
12. colluding with evasion;
13. directing the interaction; and
14. labelling the client. (Egan, 1990)

It is important for reflective practitioners to monitor their own performance in order to identify unhelpful responses. Supervision is an important safeguard here, in that defensive reactions are usually more evident to outsiders rather than participants in any interaction.

In any nurse–patient interaction participants are relating on a professional and a personal level. In Chapter 7 of this book Dennis Tourish examines individual bias in interpersonal interaction. He argues that most of us are subject to such biases, which have the potential to disrupt the communication process. Stereotyping and labelling are particularly harmful in that they result in the deindividualisation of clients into social groups rather than human beings. This is the process underlying the concerns expressed by Read and Wallcraft (1992) in their guidelines for mental health professionals. They argue that the diagnostic labels used can lead to a dehumanising relationship where behaviours are seen as symptoms rather than genuine reactions to difficult situations. The same is potentially true of labels relating to physical illness. The label can be used to define the interaction in overly rigid ways. Professional knowledge and training are important here. Wheeler and Turner (1997) investigated the attitudes and experiences of counsellors working with people with alcohol problems. In general, generic counsellors did not feel comfortable working with this group and feelings of competence increased with greater experience. However, it can be argued that the more knowledge and experience a counsellor has the greater the danger of stereotyping. Specialist knowledge can be a double-edged sword. At the personal level counsellors whose own alcohol intake was more than eight units a week were less likely to take on this type of client.

It is important to remember that each of us as professionals is the constant in all our helping interactions. In developing effective interactions the central role of self-awareness cannot be overemphasised. O'Farrell (1988, p. 83) points out:

'Seeking to understand how we are likely to react in given situations and to different people, and learning what triggers our emotional responses gives us the opportunity to see what is preventing us from achieving our ideal selves.'

It is essential that helpers are aware of what client behaviours trigger certain responses in themselves. For example, what kinds of feelings does a client's anger provoke in us? Many different types of response are possible including embarrassment, fear or anger. How do these feelings relate to behaviour? Do we try to diffuse the situation or become confrontational? The understanding of our own reactions is vital before we can cope with those of another person. Strategies for dealing with anger and aggression are discussed in more detail later in the chapter.

Rogers (1957) presents the core condition for therapeutic change, which make great demands on the helper as a person. Empathy is central to understanding another's pain and involves us as helpers in a deep awareness of the client's situation as if we were that person. Helpers also need to be what Rogers describes as congruent; this is often referred to as genuineness, but Rogers's conception involves a strong element of self-awareness. Congruence not only involves being genuine with another person but also with ourselves. The final condition of unconditional positive regard relates to our acceptance of another person. Rogers places great emphasis on the unconditionality of that acceptance. Being non-judgemental is seen as basic to counselling encounters; however, it can be a difficult task for helpers to suspend their own beliefs and values. Value clarification is an important aspect of self-awareness. There can be an apparent dilemma between being our true selves in the encounter and not letting our own values direct the process. Obviously, the first step is to examine our own values carefully and systematically. O'Farrell (1988) suggests that although we cannot suspend our own beliefs during an encounter we can suspend expression of them by accepting the client's right to choose the way forward and the standards to be applied to any decision-making.

One way of conceptualising the issue of self-awareness is presented in the Johari Window, which incorporates internal and external factors. Figure 10.1 shows four aspects of self at various levels of accessibility. Figure 10.1 illustrates that we can share the area known to us but not to others, the 'hidden area', by self-disclosure; feedback from others can reduce the 'blind area', which is known by others and not ourselves. The reduction of the 'blind' and 'hidden' areas can in turn lead to the reduction of the 'unknown area'. Thus the combination of insight and external information can lead to an overall increase in awareness. Self-disclosure can be seen as an important catalyst in promoting more meaningful feedback from others, remembering that self-disclosure needs also to be of the right type. Knox *et al.* (1997) investigated client perceptions of the effects of helpful and unhelpful counsellor self-disclosure in long-term therapy. They found that helpful self-disclosures were characterised by the following: first, they occurred when clients were discussing important personal issues; second, they were perceived as intending to normalise or reassure the client; and finally, they consisted of personal non-immediate information about the counsellor. However, Knox *et al.* (1997) did find differences between clients in their desire for counsellor self-disclosure. At one end of

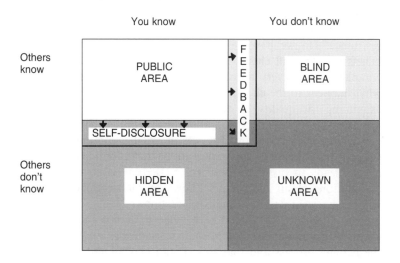

Source: Luft and Ingham (1955).

Figure 10.1   Johari Window

269

the spectrum some clients seem to have a virtually insatiable interest in the counsellor as a person, 'even arranging to meet with another client of the same therapist to share information about the therapist' (p. 282). Other clients preferred to keep a distance and worried about blurring the boundary between the professional and the personal. There is always a real danger that self-disclosure can shift the focus away from the client or if handled insensitively belittle the problem or demean the client in some way. As with all interpersonal skills judgement is required about usage.

This section has looked at the nurse as a possible source of difficulties within a professional encounter. As previously stated it is potentially threatening but ultimately valuable to consider our own role in any communication problems. Self-awareness is an important precursor of effective communication. The next section suggests helpful responses to communication difficulties.

HELPFUL RESPONSES WITH CHALLENGING CLIENTS

As discussed above, the type of response made if clients appear to be reluctant, resistant or apathetic is influenced by the helper's initial causal attributions regarding the difficulty. Such attributions will in turn influence the choice of intervention, of which a number of possibilities exist. First it is important to explore our own resistance. Do we have self-defeating beliefs? Examples of such beliefs are: that all clients must like us, that we have to succeed completely with every client or that we are solely responsible for what happens to the client. Coupled with this is the importance of examining the quality of our own interventions. Have we been insensitive or misunderstood the client's needs? Symon (1997) considered the role of explanation in good communication and suggests that 'failing to give explanations for procedures and events always leads to dissatisfaction' (p. 594). It is vital not to make assumptions about the client's knowledge of treatments or even what is expected within a single interaction.

Egan (1990) asserts that it is of value to accept and work with clients' resistance and to accept some resistance as a normal part of the helping process and that this should be explored and worked with in a positive way. He suggests the need to invite participation, at each step of the therapeutic process, to maximise shared expectations. As examined earlier perceived coercion can be a basis for resistance. Egan (1990) suggests that helpers need to establish a 'just society' with clients based on a mutual understanding and respect. It is also important to attempt to create a 'taboo free' climate within the interaction. Other suggestions from Egan (1990) include searching for incentives, involving significant others as resources and trying to get resistant clients into situations where they are responsible for helping others. Obviously the involvement of others can be a delicate issue particularly if that person is perceived as part of a coercive process to get help for the client.

It is of value to prize the client's self-responsibility in the helping situation. This can more naturally lead to the client feeling in control of what is happening. On the other hand some clients can shy away from what they perceive as unwanted responsibility (Elliot, 1985). For example, it is often difficult for clients to make decisions about treatment as they may feel that they lack information or expertise. As in many other instances the helper needs to walk a very fine line here. However, an open collaborative relationship, in which the client is involved at each stage of the healing process, is the best basis for progress. Hill *et al.* (1993) point out that when helpers misunderstand what the client is trying to say or focus on the wrong issues, clients very rarely correct them. It is important to keep evaluating that the client understands and is in agreement with what is going on.

Sometimes simple measures can help, for example, changing the situation, structure or setting of a session. Not all clients work best in their own homes, other people may be present, or 'social graces' may interfere with the professional role. It is important to provide the client with the time and space to explore their difficulties and an appropriate pace is a vital ingredient. This needs to be tailored to client perceptions. There is little point in the helper charging towards the finishing line, if the client is not ready. Changing the medium employed can help overcome barriers. Some clients are more comfortable writing down their concerns. Fantasy exercises and visualisations can also be of assistance. It is important to be creative here and keep trying different approaches. Client needs and experience should always remain the focus and the essential role of empathy cannot be overemphasised. Some clients feel overwhelmed by their problems. It is useful to begin with setting small mutual goals, thus reducing the problem to manageable targets which can be tackled individually. This approach can allow for early success and consequently boost confidence. Judicious use of reinforcement is a useful technique. Behaviour can be shaped by reinforcing

271

successive change of the kind wanted. For example, rewarding quiet clients for talking can increase involvement.

A number of interpersonal skills can be used to encourage participation. Initially it is important to attend to all of the client's communications, particularly non-verbal messages. In this way problems can be identified earlier in the relationship. Listening skills are also vital in developing communicative understanding. With clients who are not responding adequately it is always tempting to become more directive and begin to dominate the interaction. The use of silence, positive reinforcement and open probing questions is much more likely to be effective. Helpers should adopt a reflective style focusing on the resistance itself; this is an aspect of immediacy. It is important to remember the degree of threat which may be created by attention to aspects of clients' lives and the perceived risks inherent in the disclosure of sensitive material to a relative stranger. Helpers should be prepared to back off if necessary and return to issues when the client is more prepared.

Effective responses to difficult communication situations are often rooted in respect and understanding of the client's perspective. It is easy to blame another person, and stigmatise them as difficult, simply because they do not fit in with our preconceived notions of how they should respond in a given situation. Explanation and clarification of the helping process, role expectations and what is involved in learning should be constant themes within and helping relationship. Trust can only be created if we are trustworthy and perceived as being such. A final thought involves the overly cooperative client; if clients show no resistance whatsoever this may be cause for concern and it is worth exploring if agreement is only superficial and not translated into action. For example, many people promise to make lifestyle changes like losing weight or giving up smoking, but this is difficult for many. In these cases it is relatively easy to assess if only lip-service is being paid, but in others it can be much more difficult. The skills of challenging within the helping relationship might be what clients need to move to constructive action. For example, helping to 'normalise' feelings of anxiety in relation to a problem may encourage clients to do what is necessary to manage their problems more effectively. Egan (1994) outlines the communications skills that support the process of challenging. They are:

1. Information-sharing – giving or helping clients access needed information.

2. Advanced empathy – sharing views with clients about their experiences, behaviours and feeling to help them develop new perspectives.
3. Helper self-disclosure – sharing appropriate experience with clients as a way of modelling non-defensive self-disclosure.
4. Immediacy – discussing aspects of your helping relationship to improve the working alliance.
5. Summarising – helping to put together pieces of the clients' stories in order to see the bigger picture and move on in the helping process.

By establishing the framework for the relationship, the nurse can often relate to the clients with more flexibility, helping them at each stage to challenge themselves and move forward.

ILLUSTRATIVE EXAMPLES OF CHALLENGING COMMUNICATION

As a conclusion to this chapter, two examples of challenging communication are presented: working with individuals with communication disorders; and working with aggression and anger. In this section more detailed strategies are developed in order to illustrate general principles discussed earlier.

Working with clients with communication difficulties

We have discussed the constraints of communication with clients who, in spite of difficulties, have the capacity to respond appropriately and participate within the helping relationship. However, a nurse in the community will increasingly have contact with people who have specific communication disorders. This may be with someone who is suffering a gradual loss of ability to communicate through illnesses like Parkinson's disease, motor neurone disease or multiple sclerosis. In this case, the person's anxiety about the future for themselves and others they are responsible for may be reflected in periods of depression and despair. Dalton (1994) describes the emotional consequences of such conditions, which can include feelings of humiliation from their slurred, dysarthric speech. Many reflect on how they feel others see them, such as being less intelligent. One client explained that she refused to talk to anyone she did not know after having being accused of being drunk.

The communication, physical emotional effects of brain damage due to strokes, tumours or cerebral infections can have even more devastating effects, as the onset is usually sudden and unexpected. The loss of speech and language can lead to confusion as the client struggles to understand a conversation or explanations as to what has happened. As a helper in this context, the community nurse may find it difficult to communicate at an appropriate level without an understanding of how the speech or language pattern has been affected. Counselling in these situations tends to focus on reassurance, advice or giving information to the clients or care givers. Continuity, however, is crucial to developing the helping relationship with the client and carers in this situation. Brumfitt and Clarke (1983) see not only 'the loss of life-roles as threatening the sense of self but the loss of speech and language abilities and limb function as contributing to the confusion as to who they are' (pp. 97–8).

Language function is not affected where cancer of the larynx leads to laryngectomy. However depression and anger are often experienced in the realisation of the diagnosis itself and the experience of total voice loss. Dalton (1994) reminds us that our voice is so much part of our identity that without it, we feel diminished, 'unwhole'. This condition is manageable with tracheo-oesophageal valving, allowing many laryngectomees to 'vocalise' with fluent, effective communication. In instances where it is not possible to achieve pseudovoice, laryngectomees may reject artificial voice aids, choosing instead to whisper or write what they want to communicate. This may be sufficient for the client to communicate his or her needs, but often this affects interactive ease.

Communication problems in children can severely affect their social and emotional development. Gordon (1991) confirms that 'reduced ability to comprehend and use language will hinder cognitive and social development and there is known to be a high incidence of emotional and behavioural problems among such children' (pp. 86–9). The stigma attached to a delay in speech and language development may affect the development of the child's self-concepts, resulting in disruptive behaviour, fear of failure, avoidance of social situations or poor self-esteem (Rinaldi, 1991).

Extreme anxiety from the anticipation of speech failure may lead to withdrawal and low expectations of their communication or social competence. Hall (1991) showed that children with only mild articulatory errors were viewed more negatively by their classmates in judging their ability to communicate, their status as peers and how they would develop as teenagers. Communication with children and adolescents may be more challenging, as they may be unable to assert themselves verbally, or have been subject to teasing and bullying. All professionals involved with communicatively impaired children need to be sensitive to their psychological, educational and social needs.

Client expectations of the helping relationship in this situation need to be clarified. The community nurse may be one of many health care professionals in contact with the client or carer at any stage in their treatment. If expectations about their condition are unrealistic or the extent to which treatment can improve their ability to lead a normal life again, the interaction between the client, carer and nurse will be adversely affected.

Situations where clients find it difficult to come to terms with their communication problems demand skilful interaction and management. Communication within the health care team should be clear, consistent and continuous to ensure that there is no conflict in strategies, style or approach. In reality, the community nurse may be in more regular contact with the client than other members of the clinical team. It is useful to access information from the speech and language therapist on how to tailor communication, specifically the level of interaction for the client's individual needs. This can greatly enhance the communication process, allowing the community nurse to focus on what he is saying rather than how he is saying it.

Andrews (1995) outlines the effects on the family which result from serious loss of communication: 'disruption of the family system, changes in family roles, family guilt, overprotectiveness and the depletion of carers' energy' (p. 337). Often their reaction to the crisis have a direct bearing on the client's ability to cope and maintain a sense of dignity. This requires effective interaction to explore the meaning of the psychosocial changes in the person and their family. By allowing their feelings to be brought to an awareness level and accepted in a non-judgemental way, the community nurse can support and facilitate more effective coping strategies.

The clarity of the nurse's communication is particularly important for some client groups. Howell and Bonnett (1997) examine the influence of speaking clarity on communication with the hearing-impaired. Speakers employed in this study all had a minimum of five years communicating with the hearing-impaired listeners who had a bilateral hearing loss which had occurred in adulthood. 'Unclear' speech was obtained by instructing speakers to speak as they would in normal conversation. 'Clear speech was obtained by instructing them to speak as clearly as possible, as if they were communicating in a noisy environment, or with a hearing-impaired listener. In addition, they were asked to enunciate consonants carefully, to avoid slurring words together and place stress on the content words.

The clarity of the speech was then assessed by intelligibility tests with the hearing-impaired subjects and from self-ratings about the speaker's ability to communicate with such listeners. Speakers who considered themselves to be good communicators had a high number of their target words identified than poorer communicators. Howell and Bonnett (1997) conclude that it is difficult to specify elements which differentiate clear from unclear speech in this context. They suggest that the prosody of the speaker, involving stress patterns, pauses and pitch movements as well as rate variation and nasalisation of stretches of speech, can effect clarity and intelligibility of communication. Results also suggest, however, that a confident communicator has great awareness of the client's interactive needs.

As stated earlier, the nurse and client are partners in the therapeutic process. Andrews and Schmidt (1995) suggest that it is 'the quality of the collaboration, rather than the skill of the clinician alone, that predisposes a successful outcome' (p. 263). Pettigrew (1977), in investigating therapeutic communicator style, found that the therapeutic communicator was more precise, friendly, attentive, relaxed, dominant and impression-leaving than the general communicator. Similarly, Norton (1978) believed that an attentive friendly and relaxed style indicated willingness to provide feedback, empathy and encouragement, stating that relaxed clinicians are calm and collected and are perceived as being con-fident and in control. Clearly personality characteristics can max-imise the effectiveness of interaction with the communicatively impaired client and their carers. Parkinson and Rae (1996, p. 150) conclude that it is necessary

'to be aware of the four dimensions of relating to clients with communication disorder (ongoing attention to oneself, the client, the therapeutic space outside influences). These can only be successfully developed experientially, with close supervision and personal growth work on the part of the practitioner over time.'

Working with aggression and anger

Angry or aggressive clients can pose great problems for the helper. By definition this type of client tends to be uncooperative and there is often an inadequate or damaged helping relationship. As with all communication situations it is important to understand where both parties are coming from. Helpers need to try to understand the basis for anger and need to understand their own reactions to it. Thomas (1997, p. 83) advocates the importance for each of us of talking through our anger, suggesting:

'Nurses encounter angry clients in all types of clinical settings. Pathogenic coronary-prone or cancer-prone patterns are often observed. However angry behaviour is learned and can therefore be changed. Nurses should assess their clients' style of anger management and encourage verbalization of feelings with a supportive listener. By discussing anger-producing incidents, self-understanding, assimilation and acceptance are facilitated.'

It is certainly true that nurses have a responsibility to help clients understand and manage their own anger but many are unsure of the strategies available to cope with aggressive encounters. Knowledge and training are of importance here. Haber et al., (1997) showed that there was a difference in the way that registered nurses and nursing assistants responded to aggressive behaviour, with registered nurses selecting fewer behaviours that required physical intervention. Coid (1991) points out that helpers do not simply need skills to cope with aggressive clients but also need to understand why they are behaving in this way, pointing out that 'Aggressive clients are usually complex with a multitude of problems besides those of threatening behaviour and poor anger control' (p. 97).

It is important for helpers to recognise that preconceived attitudes towards aggressive clients may make the situation worse. Aggression can stem from feelings of helplessness or low self-esteem. It is all too easy to set up a vicious circle in which the helper's approach can exacerbate the situation. There is no single right way to deal with an aggressive client but some practical guidelines can assist inexperienced helpers. Initially, it is useful to consider the physical environment of the interview. Both parties need to be able to feel relaxed. Heavy objects which could be used as missiles should be removed in advance of the interview. Chairs should be positioned at a non-confrontational orientation, preferably at 45 degrees (Hargie *et al.*, 1994). If possible position chairs so that both the helper and the client have a way out if necessary, for example, sideways to the nearest door. It may also be useful to have furniture between yourself and the client. It is unadvisable to conduct the interview with the client standing; always encourage the client to sit down. Such measures help give confidence to the interviewer which is an important factor in facilitating a successful outcome (Coid, 1991).

Aggressive or violent outbursts disrupt the normal 'rules' of interaction. It is essential that the helper maintains a sense of purpose and is not diverted from this. Non-verbal behaviours, such as gaze, degree of proximity or posture, are very important in managing difficult encounters. Too much eye contact (prolonged staring) can be interpreted as a lack of genuineness. Hermonssen *et al.* (1988) have considered the importance of postural lean in communicating the core conditions of counselling (see Chapter 5 in this volume). Forward postural lean is associated with high levels of the conditions, whilst a more backward-leaning posture can convey disinterest. In situations where the helper is afraid, backward lean may indicate a desire to protect oneself. However, it is the client's perception which is important and if he or she feels the counsellor is indifferent this may lead to a heightening of tension.

Simple techniques for diffusing a threatening situation include: using the client's first name as frequently as possible; keeping interjections simple, including clear statements of what you want the client to do, which can be usefully repeated; and, above all, avoiding getting involved in arguments. If clients are projecting anger against a designated group, do all you can to let them see you as a person, not as a role representative. Some basic self-disclosure can help here. In addition it can be helpful to let the client know the effect their behaviour is having on you as a person. Personalising the situation in this way can have a calming effect.

Coid (1991) suggests a three-stage model for dealing with aggressive clients:

- Stage one: assessment and calming the client
- Stage two: history-taking and counselling
- Stage three: formulation and termination

This framework forms a useful structure for practice. Each stage will now be considered in more detail in order to highlight helpful strategies and techniques.

Stage one

Before the session it may be useful to collect as much information as possible, from as many sources as possible, about the client. This forms a pre-interview assessment. Helpers should also take into account potential influences on the client's attitude or mood immediately prior to the session. For example, what are the waiting facilities like, who will greet the client and how will the client be greeted, will the session start promptly? Preplanning can play an important part in managing potentially difficult encounters. Personal introductions should be polite and formal and the client should be told clearly who you are and what your role in seeing them is. It can be helpful to try and ascertain the client's feelings about coming to the session at this point; misperceptions may be identified which, if clarified at an early stage, may affect the course of the interaction. At an early stage it is important to try and identify the sources of any anger and to whom it is directed. It may be helpful here to remember Thomas's (1997) assertion that helping clients express their anger verbally and more constructively can have therapeutic effects beyond a single encounter.

Stage two

It is at this point that the helper begins to try to manage the client's aggression. It is important to attempt to understand the nature of the client's feelings and their origin. The general objective is to gradually reduce the level of anger and arousal by getting the client to express his or her feelings in a controlled manner. This process can be both time-consuming and stressful. The community nurse's assertiveness skills play an important role at this point. Aggressive clients try to change the rules of the professional relationship and dominate the space around them as well as anybody within it. The helper must maintain the boundaries between what is acceptable and what is not. Hopson and Scally (1981, p. 117) define assertiveness as involving:

'directly telling someone what you want or prefer in such a way as to appear neither threatening or punishing, nor in putting down the other person. It is not aimed simply at getting what you want if getting what you want means trampling over the needs of others. It is about standing up for your rights but not at the cost of violating the rights of others. It is about being open about one's feelings – both negative and positive. It also involves being able to express what you want without experiencing undue anxiety while doing so. It involves being totally honest about one's feelings.'

This definition is clearly in line with the characteristics of the self-aware helper discussed earlier. Hargie *et al.* (1994) present the verbal and non-verbal components of assertive behaviour. Verbally the importance of factors like clarity in statements, explanation, acknowledgement of the other person's point of view, praise and attempts at discovering a mutually acceptable compromise are noted. Non-verbally assertive behaviour involves: 'medium levels of eye contact; avoidance of inappropriate facial expressions; smooth use of gestures while speaking, yet inconspicuous while listening; upright posture; direct body orientation; appropriate paralinguistics' (pp. 281–2).

Assertiveness is important in maintaining boundaries with aggressive clients and minimising their attempts at domination. It should not be forgotten that the helper also has rights in the situation. It can be helpful for helpers to be able to identify warning signs. These can include: progressive anxiety and fearfulness in the interviewer and awareness of loss of control; dehumanisation; failure to follow clients' train of thought which could indicate losing touch with reality; and behaviour like sexual innuendo or increased proximity which may indicate the point of no return (Coid, 1991).

Stage three

This stage involves formulating the client's main problem and offering possible solutions. This may not be easy if the client had a preconceived notion of how problems should be tackled. It is often best to have simple goals in the short term. Egan (1990) presents guidelines for action planning which may be useful here. He advocates a three-step process involving: developing strategies; choosing a 'best-fit' strategy; and formulating action plans. Clients should be encouraged to develop subgoals. If complex goals are broken down in this way, sequenced and related to the strategies needed to accomplish them, they are more likely to be achieved.

Many aggressive clients are afraid and confused by their feelings and may fear they are 'going mad' or 'cracking up'. Coid (1991, p. 111) suggests:

'Patients who behave aggressively are often profoundly distressed and later grateful for the opportunity to have shared their problems with a caring professional who is able to make sense of the chaos of their emotions and experiences.'

It is important that helpers assist clients to make sense of their experience and offer ways forward which have positive benefits.

In conclusion, Newell (1994, pp. 102–3) offers a list of basic survival tactics with aggressive clients:

1. minimise likelihood of aggression by adopting a client-centred approach and in particular offering the client respect;
2. be aware of the effects of aggressive behaviour on our own emotions, and avoid compounding the problem;
3. adopt submissive postures in response to aggression;
4. share with the client the effect their behaviour is having on you;
5. encourage the client to explore the source of their anger using open questions;
6. try not to engage in self-justification;
7. reinforce periods of non-aggression with attending behaviours;
8. if aggression is expected plan for it in seating arrangements and the availability of support;
9. avoid over-reacting to histories of aggression by being overly defensive;
10. if you feel unsafe or unable to concentrate terminate the interview.

There should be a limit to the helper's expectations of what can be achieved and interview objectives may need to be scaled down as a result of the client's behaviour.

CONCLUSION

This chapter had considered the issue of communicating with challenging clients. At the outset it was stated that this is a difficult area to summarise. Although it is acknowledged that some situations are more challenging for the professional than others, there is very little literature on the subject. The main contention in this account is that challenging communication should not be equated with difficult clients. Automatically, attributing blame to the client can lead to problems in the helping relationship. In such circumstances it is possible for the client to become labelled and stigmatised and the helper to become manipulative. Any analysis of communication difficulty must take account of both participants in the interaction and the communication process itself. The importance of the nurse working on self-knowledge and self-awareness has been emphasised throughout the discussion. It is important that, we as professionals, are aware of our own strengths, weaknesses and blind spots, if we are able to be of positive assistance to clients. Rogers's (1957) core relationship conditions should always be borne in mind as the ideals of ant helping relationship. Difficult situations tend to be those in which we find problems in being genuine, empathic and accepting. Characterising the client as difficult will have a negative effect on acceptance. This chapter has examined sources of difficulty in both the helper and the client and suggested approaches to working with these effectively. The inclusion of two specific examples of challenging situations helps to illustrate how general guidelines can be translated into practice. The communication principles proposed tend to be those which will have a positive effect on any interaction. However the skills of the helper are most severely tested in challenging situations.

References

Andrews M. L. (1995) *Manual of Voice Treatment*. San Diego: Singular Publishing Group.

Andrews, M. L. and Schmidt, C. P. (1995) Congruence in personality between clinician and client: relationship to ratings of voice treatment. *Journal of Voice*, 9(3), pp. 261–9.

Brumfitt, S. and Clarke, P. (1983) An application of psychotherapeutic techniques in the management of aphasia. In C. Code and D. Muller (eds), *Aphasia Therapy*. London: Edward Arnold.

Burnard, P. and Morrison, P. (1991) Client-centred counselling: a study of nurses' attitudes. *Nurse Education Today*, 11, pp. 104–9.

Chamberlin, J. (1988) *On Your Own*. London: MIND.

Coid, J. (1991) Interviewing the aggressive patient. In R. Corney (ed.), *Developing Communication and Counselling Skills in Medicine*. London: Routledge.

Dalton, P. (1994) *Counselling People with Communication Problems*, Counselling in Practice, 3. London: Sage, pp. 6–8.

Dickson, D. (1989) Interpersonal communication in the health professions: a focus on training. *Counselling Psychology Quarterly*, 2(3), pp. 345–66.

Egan, G. (1990) *The Skilled Helper: A Systematic Approach to Effective Helping*, 4th edn. Pacific Grove, Calif.: Brooks/Cole Publishing.

Egan, G. (1994) *The Skilled Helper: A Problem-Management Approach to Helping*. Pacific Grove, Calif.: Brooks/Cole Publishing.

Elliot, R. (1985) Helpful and non-helpful events in brief counseling interviews: an empirical taxonomy. *Journal of Counseling Psychology*, 32(3), pp. 307–22.

Fletcher, J. (1997) Do nurses really care? Some unwelcome findings from recent research and inquiry. *Journal of Nursing Management*, 5, pp. 43–50.

Gordon, N. (1991) The relationship between language and behaviour. *Developmental Medicine and Child Neurology*, 33, pp. 86–9.

Haber, L., Fagan-Pryor, E. and Allen, M. (1997) Comparison of registered nurses' and nursing assistants' choices of intervention for aggressive behaviour. *Issues in Mental Health Nursing*, 18, pp. 113–20.

Hall, B. (1991) Attitudes of fourth and sixth graders towards peers with mild articulation disorders. *Language, Speech and Hearing Services in Schools*, 22(1), pp. 334–40.

Hargie, O., Saunders, C. and Dickson, D. (1994) *Social Skills in Interpersonal Communication*, 3rd edn. London: Routledge.

Heppner, P. and Rosenberg, J. (1992) Three methods of measuring the therapeutic process: clients' and counselors' constructions of the therapeutic process versus actual therapeutic events. *Journal of Counseling Psychology*, 39(1), pp. 20–31.

Hermonsson, G., Webster, A. and McFarland, K. (1988) Counselor deliberate postural lean and communication of the facilitative conditions. *Journal of Counseling Psychology*, 35(2), pp. 149–53.

Hill, C., Thompson, B., Cogar, M. and Denman, D. (1993) Beneath the surface of long-term therapy: therapist and client reports of their own covert processes. *Journal of Counseling Psychology*, 40(3), pp. 278–87.

Hopson, B. and Scally, M.(1981) *Lifeskills Teaching Programmes: No. 1.* Leeds: Lifeskills Associates.

Howell, P. and Bonnett, C. (1997) Speaking clearly for the hearing impaired: intelligibility differences between clear and less clear speakers. *European Journal of Disorders of Communication*, 32, pp. 89–97.

Irving, P. and Dunne, A. (1994) An empirical basis for the formulation of strategic communication objectives at a local level. *Health Services Management Research.* 7(1), pp. 56–65.

Irving, P. and Long, A. (1993) Counselling in health promotion: a nursing perspective. *Journal of the Institute of Health Education*, 31(4), pp. 126–32.

Knox, S., Hess, S., Peterson, D. A. and Hill, C. (1997) A qualitative analysis of client perceptions of the effects of therapist self-disclosure in long-term therapy. *Journal of Counseling Psychology*, 44(3), pp. 274–83.

Ley, P. (1988) *Communicating with Patients.* London: Chapman & Hall.

Lindlow, V. (1992) Just lip-service? *Nursing Times*, 88 (December 2), pp. 49–63.

Luft, J. and Ingham, H. (1955) *The Johari Window: A Graphic Model of Interpersonal Relations.* Los Angeles, Calif.: University of Los Angeles Press.

Markham, U. (1993) *How to Deal with Difficult People.* London: Thorson.

Newell, R. (1978) *Interviewing Skills for Nurses and Other Health Care Professionals.* London: Routledge.

Norton, R. (1978) *Communicator Style.* Beverly Hills, Calif.: Sage.

O'Farrell, U. (1988) *First Steps in Counselling.* Dublin: Veritas.

Oldfield, S. (1983) *The Counselling Relationship: A Study of Clients' Experience.* London: Routledge & Kegan Paul.

Parkinson, K. and Rae, J. P. (1996) The understanding and use of counselling by speech and language therapists at different levels of experience. *European Journal of Disorders of Communication*, 31, pp. 140–52.

Pettigrew, L. S. (1977) An investigation of therapeutic communicator style. In R. Ruben (ed.), *Communication Yearbook 1*, New Brunswick, NJ: Transaction Books, pp. 593–604.

Read, J. and Wallcraft, J. (1992) *Guidelines for Empowering Users of Mental Health Services*, London: MIND.

Rinaldi, W. (1991) The meaning of moderate learning difficulties at secondary school age. *CSLT Bulletin*, ISSN 0953-6086.

Rogers, C. R. (1957) The necessary and sufficient conditions for therapeutic personality change. *Journal of Counselling Psychology*, 21, pp. 95–103.

Salvage, J. and Buxton, V. (1997) Assessing the health of community nursing, *Health Visitor*, 70(2), pp. 56–7.

Symon, A. (1997) Improving communication: apologies and explanations. *British Journal of Midwifery*, 5(10), pp. 594–6.

Thomas, S. (1997) Angry: let's talk about it! *Applied Nursing Research*, 10(2), pp. 80–5.

Wheeler, S. and Turner, L. (1997) Counselling problem drinkers: the realm of specialists, Alcoholics Anonymous or generic counsellors. *British Journal of Guidance and Counselling*, 5(3), pp. 313–26.

Windahl, S., Signitzer, B. and Olsen, J. T. (1992) *Using Communication Theory*. London: Sage.

CHAPTER ELEVEN

Clarifying Communication for Advanced Interaction

Ann Long

INTRODUCTION

Community health care nursing is not a single concept. Rather, it comes about as the result of a combination of various interrelated and overlapping concepts that amalgamate to form the unique profession of community health care nursing. The title 'community nursing' suggests that individuals 'nurse' communities and they do. It is widely accepted that embraced within this term is the concept that community nurses also 'nurse' all individuals and families who reside in those specific communities which nurses are allocated to.

However, although some of the residents within the community may not require nursing interventions, community nurses have a duty to promote the overall health and social well-being of the total population of the community they serve. They do this mainly through the provision of health promotional activities which encompass the needs of individuals and families within their relational, cultural, religious and social circumstances including the ecological and environmental health of the planet.

The title 'community nursing' also suggests that those who carry out this work are active interventionists and that their activities are founded on scholarship and research. Community nurses are also autonomous, independent, interdependent and dependent on other human beings for their daily living. Thus, initiating, maintaining and closing relationships are part and parcel of being human (see

Chapters 2 and 3) and nurses are equal with other people in this respect.

Furthermore, as human beings we are all capable of being influenced by communication events in the existential 'here and now'. This suggests that we spend all of our lives relating with 'self', other human beings, our global environment and, for some of us, a Supreme Being of our own understanding. In order to fulfil these meaningful relationships we need to communicate. Hence, communicating is an inherent component of being human and, therefore, it is the most fundamental characterisation of nursing. Indeed, it could be said that sensitive and compassionate communication is the *sine qua non* of true nursing care. To be sure nursing and communicating are joined together. They are symbiotic. It would be very demanding for nurses to demonstrate that they effectively 'care' for another human being without communicating. Equally, it would be very difficult to communicate effectively and compassionately without 'caring'. If we believe this to be true, then the manner in which community nurses communicate with people does have either a positive or negative impact on the quality of their nursing care and consequently on the success or failure of the healing process.

This introductory argument concludes by suggesting that sensitive, compassionate and effective communication is the foundation on which nursing stands. Communication exists at the heart and soul of nursing and caring and it is a very powerful energy that drives nursing care forward. Indeed, without communication, nursing could not really be called nursing.

NURSES BRINGING ENLIGHTENMENT TO THE PROCESS OF NURSING

Where does communication in nursing begin? It seems obvious that in order to carry out the activity of nursing all nurses must develop a knowledge and acceptance of 'self', as all nurses bring their 'self' with them when they choose to enter nursing as a career. This means that they bring their life histories of success, pain and discontent as well as everything they have learned from those experiences. Consequently, they also bring their own powerful internal healing resources in terms of their unique human characteristics, creativities and gifts.

287

The term 'self' is a particularly difficult concept to define since much of the interpretation we attach to it derives from essentially private experiences of a kind that are difficult to communicate about or agree upon. Interpretation of experiences is a form of internal communication that is both secret and safeguarded. Private communication also appears to be an important tool of intellectual adaptation whereby people regulate their mental activities to solve problems and make new discoveries (Vygotsky, 1962, 1978). How we communicate with (our) 'self' internally determines how well we will communicate with others. If we cannot convey that we care for (our) 'self', would it be possible to affirm that we care for others? If we have difficulty loving or respecting our 'self', is it possible for us to love others? The way in which we communicate that we care for and physically, emotionally and spiritually nurture self is the starting point. From it all other forms of communication will follow. Egan (1994, p. 11) used this concept admirably when describing counsellors:

'Ideally, they are first of all committed to their own physical, intellectual, social, emotional and spiritual health . . . for they realise that helping often involves modelling the behaviour they hope others will achieve.'

LOCATING SELF

For the purpose of this chapter the term 'self' refers to our inner-most being, our essence (Wilber, 1981). The 'self' is what an individual is when considered separately from others. It is 'me' in my individuality, in my inwardness, in my uniqueness (Ferruci, 1983). It is my closeness with my own self in times of solitude (Long, 1997a). However:

'we entertain a notion of the integrity and completeness of our own experience in that we believe all parts of it to be relatable because we are, in some vital sense, the experience itself.'
(Bannister, 1984, p. 60)

An examination of this citation shows that we extend the notion of 'me' into the notion of my world. We regard experiences and events as more or less related to us. We delineate boundaries which separate the events and situations that concern us and those that are irrelevant to us. This differentiation of experiences and events and the interrelationship that exists between those parts that concern us help us to build our personal world. It becomes a world that is either comfortable or uncomfortable to live in, or a world that fluctuates between comfort and discomfort depending on our acceptance of 'self' coupled with the challenges, obstacles and growth blocks that are scattered in front of us as we live our lives and write our personal histories through our personal life experiences.

ENLIVENING NURSING

Life, therefore, is a journey; it is a time span. We accept that we are essentially the same person now as we were ten minutes ago, or even ten years ago. We know that our circumstances may have changed in many respects but we have a feeling of continuity, of having a 'life'. This includes being aware that we are living a life that is like billions of other lives, and yet it is also unique (Brown, 1981). Furthermore, we can view our history in a variety of ways, but how we see it, the way in which we interpret it, is a central part of our 'being'. Similarly, it is also possible for us to imagine our future lives.

> 'you are led through your lifetime by the inner learning creature, the playful spiritual being that is your true self. Don't turn away from possible futures before you are certain you don't have anything to learn from them. You are always free to change your mind and choose a different future.'
> (Bach, 1982, cited in Dakman, 1992)

Likewise, as well as believing we have a life we also think of ourselves as making 'choices' and of being identified by our choices. For example, we made a decision to become 'a nurse', it was our intention. So we took certain deliberate steps which enabled us to achieve this decision, and we are prepared to accept responsibility, when challenged, for the choice we made.

Unfolding with the 'self' is the concept of 'becoming a person and self realization' (Rogers, 1993). Becoming a person:

'is "me" considered in relationship with other human beings, in my social context, in my solidarity, "in-touchness" or communion with others in moments of sharing, in times of listening.' (Long, 1997a, p. 499)

In other words we can only define 'self' by distinguishing it from and comparing it with other human beings. Indeed, the 'self' has been defined by Kelly (1955, 1969) as a bipolar construct of self versus others. Distinguishing 'self' from others implies that others can be viewed in the same way: as 'persons' or as 'selves'. Bradshaw (1996, p. 26) had this to say:

'our reality is shaped from the beginning by relationships. We are "we" before we are "I" . . . our individuality comes from the social context of our lives.'

Comparing ourselves with other human beings infers that others have experiences that are comparable to, although not the same as, our own. It seems reasonable to deduce, therefore, that all other human beings experience themselves as a 'self' too.

Fundamental to the notion of attempting to define the concept of 'self' is the view that we, as human beings, have the quintessential ability to reflect on the idea of 'self', which involves standing back and viewing it. The paradox intricately woven into this contemplation of self means that we have the ability to do two things simultaneously: (1) we experience and (2) we reflect upon our experience, summarise it, comment on it and analyse it. Therefore, the capacity to reflect is both the source of our commentary on self and a central part of self-awareness and the experience of being a 'self' (Bannister, 1984). As far back as 1925, Mead had meaningfully defined this paradox in terms of the 'I' and 'me', referring to the 'I' who acts and the 'me' who reflects upon the action and goes on to reflect upon the 'me' reflecting on the action.

BRINGING YOUR INNER REALITY TO NURSING

Relating this argument to nursing, those community nurses who have a sense of 'self' have an inner reality, something fundamentally as precious as life itself because it distinctly affects the way in which they experience their 'self' and the way they relate with others. Marie Louise von Franz (1975, p. 114) said the experience of 'self'

'brings a feeling of standing on solid ground inside oneself, on a patch of eternity, which even physical death cannot touch.'

The statement 'standing on solid ground inside oneself' is profound. At the heart of the debate this means that those community nurses who embrace that solid ground inside themselves will probably trust themselves, possibly respect themselves and undeniably have the internal capacity to reach out and trust other human beings (clients/patients/colleagues), thus enhancing and advancing their relationships with self and others.

Standing on solid ground, however, does not mean that those nurses will be dull and static or egocentric. Community nurses who possess a sense of inner reality will still find themselves acting and reacting in ways that are spontaneous, childlike and sometimes incomprehensible (Berne, 1972). Rogers (1993) suggests that the mentally healthy person is one who can experience and express the whole range of emotions and thus has the ability to be open to and accepting of one's own experiences. For Rogers (1993) this means that they do not have to walk around all of the time with smiles on their faces. Being mentally healthy involves individuals not trying to control their emotional reactions but being able to accept and embrace their feelings as they are (George, 1990). Being human means we will be affected by the way other people judge us or react to us. But those individuals with a sense of inner reality are not *dependent* on the power of others to offer or withdraw 'status', 'acceptance', 'love' or 'meaning'.

Kelly (1955) argued that we derive our picture of ourselves through the mirrored reflection we have of other people's picture of us. He was arguing here that the central evidence we use in understanding ourselves is other people's reaction to us, both what they say of us and the implications of their behaviour towards us. He did not say, however, that we take other people's views of us without challenge. That would be impossible because people have very changing and often very dissimilar reactions to us.

Kelly (1955) continued this argument by reasoning that we 'filter' others' views and opinions of us through using our 'construing goggles' (p. 8) to determine our perceptions of them thus enhancing our 'experience corollary' (p. 8). To be sure, community nurses do not come to find that inner reality, that solid ground inside, solely by self-contemplating or even through analysing their own histories. They build up a continuous and changing picture of themselves out of their interactions with other people. Moreover, those nurses who experience a sense of inner reality:

'• need not shrink from contact with others, nor are the compelled to be with someone else in order to know that they are alive;
• can choose to be alone without feeling condemned to loneliness;
• know they are someone and that they do have a place on this Earth;
• are free to take themselves largely for granted; and,
• they are who most of us would choose to be like (and can become).'
(Dowrick, 1993, p. 9).

And so it follows that when community nurses become self-aware and develop an understanding and acceptance of 'self' they change. Knowledge of 'self' brings with it insight into the motives and attitudes that govern their behaviour and this insight has the power to alter that behaviour. It seems fair to assume that self-aware community nurses are the dynamic multiplication of their understanding of their world (of nursing) and of themselves. Changes in what they know about themselves as well as in the way in which they come to know it are changes in the kind of people (nurses) they are.

Taking this line of argument a step further, it seems reasonable to postulate that if nurses believe this to be true about themselves, it is also true about other people (clients/patients). Therefore, if clients/patients are facilitated to come to know themselves, the closer they will come to solving (at least in part) their health and personal problems. This self-changing element of self-knowledge may also be the very basis of living a worthwhile and self-fulfilling life.

KNOWLEDGE, SKILLS AND A UNIQUE INDIVIDUALITY

It is reasonable to assume, therefore, that nursing goes far beyond the provision of clinical skills and therapeutic interventions that are based on the knowledge that underpins those activities. Each chapter in this book has highlighted evidence that nurses are more than 'the knowledgeable doer' that the UKCC (1988) asserted the 'ideal' nurse of the future should be. This declaration suggests that nurses are practical people but that their practice needs to be based more on knowledge than it presently is. This seems to be a reasonable enough idea but by placing an emphasis on *knowing* and *doing*, a third and, to me, the most vital mode of function, namely being, has been overlooked (Long, 1995).

Using an example from medicine, back in 1957, Balint (p. 1) had this to say about general practitioners: 'by far the most frequently used drug in general practice was the doctor himself'. This is as true today as it was then about nursing (Long *et al.*, 1998). Nurses are their own, or perhaps the patients', most important 'utensil' and they employ this as a catalyst for change mainly through: (1) being there for the individual; (2) employing the communication skill of attentive listening which is encased within (3), the therapeutic use of 'self'. Each of these concepts will now be examined.

The experience of being

The experience of 'being' is central to understanding the concept of 'self'. Assagoli (1978) claimed that 'being' is and always has been a touchstone for healing and human development. The nurse's ability to 'be' with and for the patient is the most important way he or she needs them to be psychotherapeutic. The concept of 'being' within the therapeutic relationship has been eloquently explored in Chapters 2 and 3 of this book. It suffices to state here what 'being' with and for communicates to me. It suggests that rather than being practical people, that is 'knowledgeable doers', nurses require to have a degree of passivity, and embraced within this, a high proportion of listening skills on their part, if patients/clients are to benefit from 'being' nurses who have developed an inner reality and who utilise the therapeutic use of 'self'.

Attentive listening

The art of attentive listening is interesting in itself on two counts: first, the nurse becomes less of a 'doer' and attends primarily to 'being with' the patient in their time of need, and second, the patient becomes empowered through the process of self-awareness and insight as patients have all the healing resources they require inside themselves. It is very interesting that most patients go to the doctor hoping he or she will prescribe a 'cure' when in actual fact they bring their cure with them in the first place. Attentive listening and the interactional skills that accompany it facilitate individuals to work through their own needs and problems in participation with nurses. As the result of this therapeutic time spent together sharing their stories, people are facilitated to make and take their own health decisions (see Chapter 5). Further, listening attentively suggests that nurses also use non-verbal communication as a powerful agent of change and healing.

The therapeutic use of self

The therapeutic use of self has been defined as:

> the unique attributes of the nurse, coupled with the salience of what he or she says, feels, thinks and believes, when accepted and introjected, can lead to the client internalising positive experiences of self . . . and to the nurse appreciating the nature and use of self as a therapeutic catalyst (Long, 1995, p. 257).

Hence, in all aspects of community nursing, nurses individualise their interventions and use their own special and unique attributes and characteristics to an advantage when working knowledgeably with patients/clients (Beck 1991). Corey (1997, p. 5) has summarised this superbly, saying:

> 'the kind of person a therapist is or the way of being he or she models is the most critical factor affecting the client and promoting change.'

So far it has been argued that communication is inherent in the notion of being human and, therefore, it is intrinsic to effective nursing care. It has been further contended that the idea of the nurse using his or her self as a catalyst for healing and growth is the most fundamental ingredient a nurse can bring to a therapeutic relationship. Indeed, Rogers (1993, p. 62) maintained: 'Most of all I want him [the client] to encounter me as a real person.' (See Chapters 2, 3 and 5.)

CHOICE AND THE COMMUNICATION CONTINUUM

In addition, making choices and being responsible for the consequences of those choices was viewed as a crucial element contained within the notion of concept of 'self'. It follows that we also have to make choices with regard to reading, understanding and responding to communication messages that are related to us. It is evident that ways of responding may be calibrated on a positive–negative communication continuum and that there are as many configurations within this continuum as there are messages conveyed. In truth, some messages that are communicated to us may mean the exact opposite of what we have read, interpreted and subsequently responded to.

Transmitting contradictory messages

Research has shown, for example, that sometimes proximity (or physical closeness) indicates intimacy or emotional closeness (Marsh, 1994). At other times proximity can indicate exactly the opposite: invasion of personal privacy and physical threat. When a stranger stands close to us we can experience fear or even a rise in blood pressure (Clore, 1977). Nurses in the hospital situation often invade a patient's private space: a room that is their 'home' for the period of time they are in hospital and which is personified by the screens which surround their beds.

However, as nurses, we rarely reflect on this as it is 'our' ward and we feel we have a 'right' to be there. Working in the community is completely different. Nurses do need to reflect on how they enter, maintain, respect and close all encounters which are held within the individual's territory (Marsh, 1994). Of equal importance, this invasion of privacy includes the use of touch. It also encompasses the ability to show concern rather than nosiness when asking questions which nurses may use as a rite of access into another person's world of thoughts, feelings, perceptions and life experiences (Long, 1995).

Contrary meanings may also be read into the use of eye movements and gaze. Gazing at an individual's eyes can often indicate an intense liking. Argyle and Cook (1976) and Marsh (1994) have shown that the more often we look at another person's eyes the more interested and accepting of them we are. However, staring and gazing can also be threatening. This is particularly noticeable in persons who are vulnerable, anxious or mentally ill. An intense stare can be used as a threatening cue both in animals and in humans. The stare may be enough to produce an oversecretion of adrenalin, hence causing the person who is stared at to be frightened or to take flight. There are at least two pieces of research to support the 'fear or flight' notion. First, it has been shown that those who are stared at when they stop at traffic lights are known to move faster from the crossing when the lights turn green (Ellesworth *et al.*, 1972). Second, it has been demonstrated that as interviewers progress into more deep and personal questions interviewees reduce eye contact when giving answers (Carr and Dabbs, 1974). Thus, on the positive–negative communication continuum, eye contact can indicate either threat or power, as well as liking. Do you know when you use eye contact to threaten people or as a powerful 'tool' and when you use it to show you like them? Are you sure you can interpret the correct meaning when others are using these 'tools'? What are the differences between the two bipolar communication experiences? Now, have a go at answering the questions in Box 11.1.

How did you make your decisions? The answer may be that not only is the verbal–non-verbal system one that helps us to understand the meaning of people's messages but that the non-verbal communication system is a system within a system. The parts work together to help us clarify the meanings intended in particular situations. For example, a cue, such as a raised tone of voice or crying, never happens in isolation. A complex interrelationship exists between the raised tone of voice and non-verbal cues such as facial expression and between crying and non-verbal cues such as posture and facial expression. The way in which we can try to understand the full relational messages is to attend to a pattern of cues, both verbal and non-verbal, and not focus on just one.

VIEWING THE WORLD OF COMMUNICATION THROUGH NURSING LENSES

Seeing the richness of communication through nursing lenses may be described as analogous to looking at a hologram. If individuals look at only one part of a hologram then they will fail to see the complete picture (Bandler and Grinder, 1979). However, if they change their focus and choose to look at several different aspects, then they may be able to 'read', interpret, understand and respond with compassion to the holistic message inscribed on the hologram.

Consider, for example, your reading and understanding of a person sitting with hunched shoulders, head between knees and crying and another person throwing confetti, waving a white handkerchief and crying. Both are shedding tears but without observing and reading the complementary signals it would be difficult to attach meaning to the complete scenario.

Put simply but meaningfully, words are like music and we all know that as an orchestra plays, the sound of music is more than the total sum of the individual players (Perls, 1970). So too, with communication. The reading and understanding of the message is much more than merely listening to the spoken words. We must read 'between the lines' and listen to the 'music' that accompanies the words. Therein lies the difficult part.

Box 11.1   Interpreting bipolar meanings

- When and how may a touch be described as intimate and when is it physically and emotionally painful?
- When does a 'friendly' smile become a flirtatious 'come on'?
- When does a comforting hug take on a sexual meaning?
- How do you decide if a voice is raised to protect you from having an accident or to shout at you and put you down?
- How might you know if someone is laughing *with* you or *at* you?
- When does a very low tone of voice signify anger and when does it signify calmness?
- When does a blush signify embarrassment and when does it denote a lie or deception?
- When does a laugh signify that the person is using a defence mechanism to hide their emotional pain and when does it signify a sense of humour and a fun time?
- When a person says 'It doesn't matter' how do you know that it really does matter?
- How do you interpret the difference between tears of joy, sadness, grief and despair?
- How do you distinguish between complimentary and sarcastic statements?

SEEING THE WORLD THROUGH PATIENTS' LENSES

Real nursing care involves striving to perceive the non-verbal world of feeling and thinking through the 'lenses' of the people in need of our care. This involves working in a proactive way in order to ensure respect for their dignity as human beings and promote healing as well as to prevent further hurt and pain. It is exceptionally difficult to enter the person's world of 'quiet desperation' (Thoreau, 1944) and see and feel events as they experience them.

Chapter 1 of this book has shown that most of the complaints that are forwarded to the Complaints Department of the NHS are related to problems with communication. It is evident that we, as nurses, sometime tend to interpret the communication behaviours of others incorrectly. Inaccurate interpretation of the meanings of communication messages leads to incorrect responses and a mixture of messages which may leave patients and carers more confused and bewildered than ever.

As professionals it is incumbent on us to take responsibility and endeavour to read the patients' cues and try to understand the patients' point of view as they are the vulnerable ones. The fact that they need our care helps us realise they are going through some of the most critical experiences in their lives. This, however, does not mean that patients and carers cannot read and understand our communication. Indeed, because of their vulnerabilities, they may be even more hypersensitive to 'feeling' our manner of (non-verbal) communication. In truth, therefore, non-verbal communication is particularly relevant in all nursing relationships. Indeed, it has been estimated that non-verbal cues exert 4.3 times more effect than does verbal behaviour on the impressions formed of a speaker (Argyle, 1983; Walker and Trimboli, 1989). Even when such results have been challenged on the grounds that the methodology used in the studies was poor, the potency of non-verbal communication is still accepted.

EXPLORING THE VITALITY OF NON-VERBAL COMMUNICATION

More up-to-date research has shown, for example, that shy and lonely people have poor non-verbal communication skills (Patterson, 1988; Muncer and Gillen, 1997; Rokach and Brock, 1998; Black and Bruce, 1998). Shy people were found to be nervous, embarrassed or socially incompetent, their non-verbal communication indicating that they criticized both themselves and their humiliating feelings in encounters. Spitzberg and Canary (1985) found that lonely people have poorly adapted eye movement, smiles, gestures, nods and so on. The authors concluded that this was partly because they had essentially disengaged from the social world and, therefore, had stopped trying. Similarly, it was found that shy and lonely people become passive in encounters and have a poor view of themselves and of their encounters with others (Vitkus and Horowitz, 1987).

There is a high probability that there are many shy and lonely people in nursing and the reverse is also true: community nurses must come into contact with a number of shy and lonely people during their careers. Similarly, there is also a high probability that there is a number of arrogant and egotistical people in nursing who display many challenging behaviours towards colleagues, patients and carers and the converse is also true: community nurses may have to cope with the challenging behaviours of clients as part of their everyday work. These ideas have been eloquently explored and examined in Chapter 10.

INTERNAL INTERACTIONAL SYNCHRONY AND RECEPTIVENESS

Poor quality of non-verbal communication skills can basically take two forms: (1) inadequate or faulty internal synchronisation of the thoughts we think and the emotions we feel; and (2) inferior or inaccurate reading, assimilation and interpretation of the internal communication. The former, internal interactional synchrony, refers to our ability to integrate our feelings with practice basically to do what we mean. Take two examples: to act sad if we feel sad or to act hurt if we feel hurt. This is self-awareness which is a process of the conscious mind coming into synchrony with the unconscious (Peck, 1987, p. 28). Alternatively, the latter, receptiveness, alludes to the ability to work out what other people mean, by observing their non-verbal communication, accurately reading and interpreting their intention, and authentically responding.

We are all somewhat naive at utilising both of these faculties. For example, I may see my male colleague coming out of a 'special' clinic and refrain from acknowledging him in case I embarrass him.

Why might this be? Perhaps my colleague was actually slinking out of the clinic instead of walking (poor internal interactional synchrony) or perhaps his posture was tensed up and closed rather than open (again poor internal interactional synchrony). Alternatively, perhaps I *just thought* my colleague was slinking or *just thought* he looked 'closed' because of his posture (poor receptiveness). More unsuspecting still, perhaps the fact that I had just consumed a few alcoholic drinks caused my social psychological judgement to be faulty.

In summary, an analysis of the complexity involved in correctly interpreting this scenario means that it is important to pay attention to the context in which the totality of interaction cues are shown, which in turn helps other people to understand the meaning of the non-verbal behaviour itself.

We have acknowledged that internal interactional synchrony (conveying what you feel and think) and receptiveness (working out what the other person feels and thinks) are important aspects of the communication process. Now let us attempt to look at these aspects within the context of the nurse–patient relationship.

An examination of the concept of internal interactional synchrony in the nurse–patient relationship shows that patients are aware of very few central rules in this setting. Two that are taught from childhood are: make sure you are clean; and speak the truth (Argyle and Henderson, 1984). Having such rules already suggests there is a power differential. This implies that as well as being ill and in need of nursing care, patients also feel a sense of powerlessness and concurring anxiety. This may mean that they will not be able to say how they feel and think (convey internal interactional synchrony) perhaps because they may feel inferior to the professional. It seems reasonable to assume, however, that they will expect emotional and psychological support from nurses (see Chapter 5).

Furthermore, as far back as 1956, Szasz and Hollander identified a form of doctor–patient relationship which they termed 'mutual participation'. An analysis of their writings when transposed to nursing shows that a more therapeutic relationship takes place where the nurse and the patient are mutually interdependent and where 'power' is more evenly distributed. This suggests that patients need another element in the nurse–patient relationship; they need to feel equal in status to the nurse. It is clear, therefore, that not only their 'symptoms' and 'clinical features' concern patients but the social, psychological and communicative elements, including how they are dealt with, matter a great deal too.

Nurses do offer some psychological support by giving patients information about the meaning of their illness and they provide health promotional knowledge which is known to prevent further deterioration. If these aspects are not dealt with in a sensitive and convincing manner this could lead to further misunderstanding and alienation on the part of patients, hence leaving them more anxious and confused than ever. Furthermore, even when this is all the psychological support nurses offer, there are at least four areas of potential misunderstanding: (1) The patient may require information but may not be aware which aspect of information is the most important for him or her to know; (2) the patient requires different information according to the stage of the healing process; (3) the nurse may explain the information in a way that the patient finds difficult to comprehend; and (4) the patient may be in a state of shock and numbness. Therefore, he or she may unconsciously utilise the defence mechanism of denial in order to cope with painful information. This means he or she may not *hear* any information given at that time. These four areas will now be dealt with in greater depth.

Patient information requirements

With respect to patient information requirements, it has been shown that patients expect more general issues to be covered than simply those that relate directly to the illness. Martha Rogers was aware of this in 1970 when she used the example of a woman's need for information following a mastectomy. The nurse in this instance focused on the woman's wound and physical well-being whilst the woman wanted information on how long she would have to stay in her daughter's home, annoying her and disturbing 'her own little family'.

In order to be truly receptive, therefore, humanistic nursing care must begin with listening to patients' 'stories', their life histories of pain and distress, and opportunities must be provided to allow them to explore their thoughts and feelings with nurses at their own pace and in their own way, using their personal code of language. It has been cited that 'Hearing the patient's true message is the *sine qua non* of a great physician' (Pickering, 1978, p. 554). This is as true today as it was then about the caring nurse. In terms of receptiveness, people need to be accepted as human beings first before their medical or nursing histories as well as their clinical features are dwelt upon. Being respected for who and what I am as a person in a

301

receptive manner can make me feel worthwhile and hence this alone may make me want to recover. In an altruistic way offering this form of care to patients/clients can also make nurses feel more skilful in their jobs and more valuable as people. Caring for people as individuals also means that nurses must be prepared to provide holistic care for their non-medical, non-nursing needs and to anticipate their needs and attend to them in a proactive way.

Information appropriate to stage of healing process

With regard to providing information appropriate to the stage of the healing process, after reading Rogers's (1970) example, it becomes patently obvious that patients need different information depending on and relating to their stage of the healing process as well as their cultural, social, familial, economic and spiritual circumstances.

Information symbolised as compassionate nursing care

Lack of information germane to skilled nursing care demonstrates how many nurses use the jargon of the medical profession which has a myriad of complex terms, thus giving the information an air of formality. Many contemporary nurses may even use the jargon of the marketeer which helps distance them from the human/compassionate elements of nursing care (Long, 1997b). In reality, it has been shown that patients would rather have communication that is psychologically supportive (caring) than communication that is neutrally informative or indeed humorous (Linn and Di Matteo, 1983).

The previous chapters in this book have very clearly shown that patients/clients and their carers respond not only to evidence-based clinical treatment but also to the way they are personally cared for as human beings. The community nurse's personal qualities, attributes and characteristics coupled with the way in which he or she uses them through the channel of communication within the therapeutic relationship can influence the outcome of nursing care (Orth et al., 1987). It follows, therefore, that the more we are cared for in a personal and non-punitive manner, the less embarrassed, humiliated and defensive we will be.

This may be especially so in intimate nurse–patient relationships where people may have to undress and struggle to fit into a hospital gown which is open at the back and perhaps three sizes too small for them. Intimacy, for some people, may also mean that nurses may touch their bodies in places where they have never been touched before or certainly may not have been touched for years. Moreover, it must also be remembered that intimacy refers to much more than making physical contact with others. When people share their life experiences with nurses, uncovering their innermost thoughts and feelings, this, too, is an intimate relationship.

The use of defence mechanisms

Patients (and indeed nurses) may utilise unconscious defence mechanisms such as denial or rationalisation to protect themselves from the overwhelming impact of 'bad news'. (For further information see Chapter 6.) When nurses are conveying this type of information they should always be aware that there may be a 'numbed' reaction and that consequently only a small part of the information may be heard. In order to deal with this effectively nurses should give patients time to be 'receptive' and to allow the information to 'soak in', and inform patients they will return to them (say twenty minutes later) to give them the opportunity to ask questions and to explore their thoughts and feelings in depth. Too much information too soon can be devastating. The psychological blow (the bad news) that causes shock may require people to pull down the receptive 'shutters' on their minds and consequently they may become numb and emotionally 'close down'.

A rich communication thread that is skilfully embroidered within every chapter of this book is the reality that scholars, practitioners and researchers have begun to understand more fully the extent to which the nurse–patient relationship can contribute to the promotion of health and well-being and the facilitation of healing and recovery. Cast your mind back over the writings in this book and answer the questions in Box 11.2.

VIEWING THE LEARNING OF COMMUNICATION THROUGH A COGNITIVE LENS

It has been well-documented throughout the book that communication skills can be taught. However, can the problems we face with regard to how we interpret, understand and subsequently respond to the meaning and significance of therapeutic interactions

---

Box 11.2   Communication in the nurse–patient relationship

- What do you consider to be the most important skill in nursing?
- What is the most meaningful quality a nurse brings to nursing care?
- Why is the nurse–patient relationship a significant aspect of the healing process?
- How might we improve our communication skills in community nursing?
- How would you convey to patients that you respect and accept them as worthwhile human beings?
- How might you communicate to each patient that the 'here and now' encounter is special, is a happening that can never occur again, and is a time span that is part of both of your life histories?
- What skills and attributes would you use to convey to patients that they have added to your personal growth and development as much as you have added to theirs?
- If you were asked to plan a programme on 'communication skills for community nurses', what ten recommendations would you make and why?

---

be similarly taught? After completing the answers to the questions in Box 11.2, it seems obvious that sometimes we know we do not know all of the answers; frequently we think we do but we are wrong and occasionally we have an idea that is partly right. This is one of the reasons why communicating is so complex, mysterious and dynamic.

Of particular relevance to the teaching and learning of the deeper and more meaningful processes involved in advancing communication in nursing is Vygotsky's (1962, 1978) sociocultural theory of cognitive development. Vygotsky's theory has recently attracted much attention among Western developmentalists, providing a valuable service by reminding us that cognitive growth, like all other aspects of development, including communication, is best understood when studied in the cultural and social contexts in which it occurs. All communication, therefore, is affected by the beliefs, values and tools of intellectual adaptation passed to individuals by their culture. His theory offers a new lens through which to view the learning and advancement of communication in nursing.

Communication with self in terms of internal speech and with others using specific social processes helps nurses to plan strategies and regulate their behaviour so that they are more likely to accomplish their goals. Examined through Vygotsky's theoretical lens, communication may thus play a critical role in cognitive development by making nurses more organised and efficient problem solvers. Further, according to Vygotsky (1962) people's (nurses') minds develop as they take part in cooperative dialogue with 'skilled partners' on communication skills that are specific to nursing, and incorporate what 'skilled tutors' say to them about communication into what they say privately to themselves. As social communication is translated into internal private communication, the culture's preferred method of thinking and problem-solving, that is, the tools of intellectual adaptation, work their way from the communication of competent tutors and practitioners into the nurse's own repertoire of thinking, feeling and communicating.

Vygotsky (1978) refers to three main stages of development when applied to communication in nursing. The first stage is the vague syncretic stage during which the nurse depends primarily on actions or on spoken words. Responses, therefore, would be on a trial and error basis until nurses found the 'right' responses to feel comfortable with themselves. The second stage is the complex stage during which nurses have the ability to use responses of varying complexity but still are not proficient at identifying the 'right' response at the right moment. The potential concept is the third stage which occurs when nurses are able to cope with the individual relevant nuances of the communication encounter but cannot handle all of the verbal and non-verbal cues at the same time. Using the terminology Vygotsky (1978) used in his theory and skilfully integrating it with nursing shows that when nurses have the competence to communicate in a sensitive and compassionate manner they will have reached communication maturity in nursing.

According to Vygotsky many of the important 'discoveries' people make occur within the context of cooperative or collaborative dialogue between a skilful tutor, who may model the activity and who transmits verbal scholarship and research, and a novice student who first seeks to understand the theoretical concepts and eventually internalises the relevant theory and research and uses it to regulate his or her own communication performance. Vygotsky

(1978) further suggests that advancement of communication skills occurs when nurses have the ability to mentally manipulate several different concepts at the same time while simultaneously reflecting on the relationship that exists between them.

The importance of socially skilled communication in nursing cannot be underestimated. It seems obvious and imperative, therefore, that nurse education and training should begin with and continue to advance the art of communication during all modules of study. Moreover, nurses should never become complacent about their abilities to compassionately communicate, nor should they ever conclude that because they have previously studied communication they do not need to learn any more about it. Effective and therapeutic communication must be monitored, maintained and enhanced as we change and grow and cope with our own personal and professional experiences. The art of communication is, after all, integral to the art and science of nursing.

References

Argyle, M. (1983) *The Psychology of Interpersonal Behaviour*, 4th edn. Harmondsworth: Penguin.

Argyle, M. and Cook, M. (1976) *Gaze and Mutual Gaze*. Cambridge: Cambridge University Press.

Argyle, M. and Henderson, M. (1984) The rules of friendship. *Journal of Social and Personal Relationships* 1, pp. 211–37.

Assagoli, R. (1978) *Psychosynthesis: A Collection of Basic Writings*. New York: Penguin.

Bach, R. (1982). Cited in A. J. Dakman (ed.) (1992) *The Observing Self*. Boston, Mass.: Beacon Press.

Balint, N. (1957) *Anatomy of an Illness*. New York: Norton.

Bandler, R. and Grinder, J. (1979) *Frogs into Princes*, Moab, Utah: Real People Press.

Bannister, D. (1984) *Psychology for Teachers,* London: BPS and Macmillan.

Beck, A. T. (1991) Cognitive therapy: a 30-year retrospective. *American Psychologist*, 46, pp. 368–75.

Berne, E. (1972) *What Do You Say After You Say Hello?* London: Corgi Books.

Black, B. and Bruce, M. E. (1998) Treating tuberculosis: the essential role of social work. *Social Work in Health Care*, 26(3), pp. 51–68.

Bradshaw, J. (1996) *Creating Love*. Deerfield Beach, Fla.: Health Communications.

Brown, M. J. (1981) Discovering the self. *Psychosynthesis Digest*, 1(1), pp. 20–38.

Carr, S. E. and Dabbs, J. M. Jr (1974) The effects of lighting, distance and intimacy of topic on verbal and visual behaviour. *Sociometry* (37) pp. 592–600.

Clore, G. L. (1977) Reinforcement and affect in attraction. In S. W. Duck (ed.), *Theory and Practice in Interpersonal Attraction*. London: Academic Press.

Corey, G. (1997) *Theory and Practice of Counselling and Psychotherapy*. 6th edn. Pacific Grove, Calif.: Brookes Cole.

Dowrick, S. (1993) *Intimacy and Solitude: Balancing Closeness and Independence*. London: The Women's Press.

Egan, G. (1994) *The Skilled Helper, a problem-management approach to helping*. Pacific Grove, Calif.: Brooks Cole.

Ellesworth, P. C., Carlsmith, J. M. and Hensen, A. (1972) The stare as a stimulus to flight in human subjects: a series of field experiments. *Journal of Personality and Social Psychology*, 21, pp. 302–11.

Ferruci, P. (1983) *What We May Be*. Wellingborough: Turnstone.

Franz, M. L. von (1975) *Carl Gustav Jung: His Myth in Our Times*, New York: Putman.

George, R. L. (1990) *Counselling the Chemically Dependent: Theory and Practice*. Boston, Mass.: Allyn & Bacon.

Kelly G. A. (1955) *The Psychology of Personal Constructs*, Vols I and II. New York: Norton.

Kelly, G. A. (1969) *Clinical Psychology and Personality: The Selected Papers of George Kelly*, ed. B. A. Maher. New York: Wiley.

Linn, L. S. and DiMatteo, M. R. (1983) Humor and other communication: preference in physician–patient encounters. *Medical Care*, 21, pp. 1223–31.

Long, A. (1995) Community mental health nursing. Cited in D. Sines (ed.), *Community Health Care Nursing*, Oxford: Blackwell Science.

Long, A. (1997a) Nursing: a spiritual perspective. *Nursing Ethics*, 4(6), pp. 496–510.

Long, A. (1997b) Avoiding abuse amongst vulnerable groups in the community: people with a mental illness. Cited in C. Mason (ed.), *Achieving Quality in Community Health Care Nursing*, London: Macmillan Press.

Long, A., Long, A. and Smyth, A.(1998) Suicide: a statement of suffering. *International Journal of Nursing Ethics*, (5)1, pp. 3–15.

Marsh, D. (1994) *Eye to Eye: How People Interact*. London: Guild Publishing.

Mead, G. H. (1925) The genesis of the self and social control. *International Journal of Ethics*, 35, pp. 251–73.

Muncer, S. J. and Gillen, K. (1997) Network analysis and lay interpretation: some issues of consensus and representation. *British Journal of Social Psychology*, 36(4), pp. 537–51.

Orth, J. E., Stiles, W. B., Scherwitz, L., Hennrikus, D. and Vallbona, C. (1987) Patient exposition and provider explanation in routine interviews and hypertensive patients' blood pressure control. *Health Psychology*, 6, pp. 29–42.

Patterson, M. L. (1988) Function of non-verbal behaviour in close relationships. In: S. W. Duck, D. F. Hay, S. E. Hobfoll, W. Ickes and B. Montgomery (eds), *Handbook of Personal Relationships*, Chichester: Wiley.

Peck, S. (1987) *The Road Less Travelled*, London: Simon & Schuster.

Perls, F. S. (1970) Dream seminars. In J. Fagan and I. L. Shepherd (eds), *Gestalt Therapy Now: Theory, Techniques and Applications*, Palo Alto, Calif.: Science and Behavior Books.

Pickering, G. (1978) Medicine on the brink: the dilemma of a learned profession. *Perspectives in Biology and Medicine*, Summer, 79, pp. 73–91.

Rogers, C. R. (1993) *On Becoming a Person*. London: Constable.

Rogers, M. E. (1970) *An Introduction to the Theoretical Basis of Nursing*. Philadelphia, Pa.: F. A. Davis.

Rokach, A. U. and Brock, H. (1998) Coping with loneliness. *Journal of Psychology*, 132(1), pp. 107–127.

Spitzberg, B. H. and Canary, D. (1985) Loneliness and relationally compentent communication. *Journal of Social and Personal Relationships*, 2, pp. 387–402.

Szasz, T. S. and Hollander, M. H. (1956) A contribution to the philosophy of medicine: the basic models of the doctor–patient relationships. *Archives of International Medicine*, 97, pp. 585–92.

Thoreau, T. (1944) cited in *Alcoholics Anonymous* (1984) 3rd edn. Aylesbury: Hazell Watson & Viney.

United Kingdom Central Council for Nursing, Midwifery and Health Visiting (UKCC) (1988) *P2,000: A New Profession for Practice*. London: UKCC.

Vitkus, J. and Horowitz, L. M. (1987) Poor social performance of lonely people: lacking skills or adopting a role? *Journal of Personality and Social Psychology*, 52, pp. 1266–73.

Vygotsky, L. S. (1962) *Thoughts and Language*. Cambridge, Mass.: MIT Press.

Vygotsky L. S. (1978) *Mind in Society: the development of higher mental processes*. Cambridge, Mass.: Harvard University Press.

Walker, M. B. and Trimboli, A. (1989) Communication affect: the role of verbal and non-verbal content. *Journal of Language and Social Psychology*, 8, pp. 229–48.

Wilber, K. (1981) *Up from Eden*. New York: Doubleday.

Index

Note: page numbers in **bold** type refer to illustrative figures or tables.

confidentiality and public
    peril 175–6
confirmation
    responses to 40
    in therapeutic presence **31**, 40
confrontations remaining
    caring 32
Congdon, C. 201
congruence in helpers 268
conscience in nursing care **70**, 73
consumers, patients as 17
control
    negotiation outcomes in
        communication 116
    patients' lack of, in encounters
        with doctors 116
Cook, M. 295
Copp, L. A. 182
Corey, G. 144, 147, 151, 155, **157**,
    163, 294
Cornell, J. 205
cost-effectiveness in NHS 57
counselling
    central position of clients in 142
    definitions of 140, **141**
    distinction from interpersonal
        and other skills 140, 143
    for effective practice 133–68
    guidance on 143
    nature of 134–40
    provision of 139, 140–4
    purpose of 140
    roles and boundaries in 142
    skills as subset of interpersonal
        skills 139
    skills, use of 137–40
    suppressing desire to make
        decisions for clients 140–2
    see also counselling, criticisms of;
        counselling practice;
        counselling theories
counselling, criticisms of 156–9
    attributes of counsellor in 156,
        157
    curriculum and course content
        in 158
    dependency on therapist in 158
    difficulty of measuring
        effectiveness in 156
    exploitation of clients in 158

impossibility of resolving wider
    social issues in 158
lack of theoretical foundation
    in 156
need for counselling in 157–8
quality of counselling in 158–9
sparsity of research in 156
theoretical underpinnings
    in 156–7
see also counselling; counselling
    practice; counselling theories
counselling practice, effective
    avoidance of inappropriate
        delegation in 160
    based on assessment of
        individual 161
    competences required for 160
    coordinated interventions
        in 160
    evaluating success of 163
    guidelines for 159–64
    managerial support for 160
    preliminary questions for 161
    pressure for quantitative
        evaluation of 164
    records for 163
    roles and boundaries in 163
    seven principles of
        (Burnard) 162, **162**
    see also counselling; counselling,
        criticism of; counselling
        theories
counselling theories 143–4, 144–51
    key differences between 144,
        150
    see also behavioural approach;
        cognitive approach; combine
        approach; person-centred
        approach; psychoanalytic
        approach
Coupland, J. 110
Coupland, N. 110
Courtney, R. 37
Cox, B. D. 66
Crean, P. 2
Crockford, E. 112
Croft, S. 18
Crute, V. 92
cultural barriers to
    communication 120–2

316

cultural context in organisational
model 99
cultural grouping (Hofstede) 120
cultural norms in personal
interactions 121
cultural values and health 68
'Cultures, The Two' *see* 'Two
Cultures'
Cupach, W. 85
Curtis-Jenkins, G. 159

Dabbs, J. M. 296
Daft, R. L. 183
Dale, N. 134
Dallmayr, F. R. 26
Dalton, P. 273, 274
Daly, J. 93
Darley, J. 196, 198
Davidhizar, R. 109
Davies, C. 57, 59
Davis, H. 85, 119
Dawes, R. 194, 197
day surgery, in NHS 58
decision tree analysis 180
Delaney, F. 228
demographic barriers to
communication 109–11
Department of Health (DoH) 9,
25, 37, 179
dependency on care provider 33
Derlega, V. 115
DeVito, J. 104
dialogicalism (Buber) 25, 27–9
Dickson, D. 10, 16, 86, 92, 96,
103, 134, 203, 208, 261, 263,
264
DiClementi 244
difficult clients *see* challenging
communication
Dillard, J. 93
Dillon, R. S. 38
Di Matteo, M. R. 101, 102, 105,
119, 302
Dimbleby, R. 102
Dinkmayer, D. 94
disability as barrier to
communication 102
displacement in psychoanalytic
counselling theory 145

dispositional barriers to
communication 117–18
DoH *see* Department of Health
Dollard, J. 200
Donahue, W. 209
Dornan, M. C. 170
Downie, R. S. 71, 180, 235
Dreyfus, H. L. 56
Dryden, D. 144, 164
Dryden, W. 140, 141, 142, 150, 151
Dubos, R. 230
Dunne, A. 265
Dunnington, G. 120

economics as driving force of new
managerialism 58
Education for Mutual
Understanding (EMU)
(Northern Ireland) 205
efficiency in NHS 57
Egan, G. 141, **154**, 266, 270, 271,
272, 280
egocentricity as barrier to
communication 117, 118
Einzig, H. 159
Eliot, George 84
Ellesworth, P. C. 296
Elliot, R. 265, 271
Ellis, A. 151, 181
Ellison, C. 202
Emmett, D. 71
emotional barriers to
communication 111–114
emotional defensiveness 112
empathy 35
and egocentricity 117
in nursing care **70**, 73
and positive therapeutic
outcomes 117
empowerment in nursing care **70**,
75–7
Endler, N. 98
engagement and detachment in
communication 113–14
environmental barriers to
communication, physical 103
environment in health promotion,
supportive 234
Epstein, J. 202
Epstein, R. 119

317

319

Health Service Commissioner 15, 101
  annual report of 86–7
health service
  not illness service 18
  reorientated, towards health promotion 234
health status, model of 230–3, **231**, 241
  coping mechanisms and 232
  physical 231, **231**
  physical environment in **231**, 232–3
  psychosocial 231–2, **231**
  social environment in **231**–3
  spiritual **231**, 232
Health and Wellbeing into the Millennium (DHSSNI) (1996) 236
Healthy Cities 236
Heidegger, M. 27, 50, 69, 71
Heider, F. 107
Heidt, P. 32
Heimann, P. 220
helping skills 136–7
Henderson-King, E. 195
Henderson, M. 300
Heppner, P. 265
Hermonssen, G. 278
Heron, J. 4, 136
Hewison, A. 116–17
Heyman, R. 170, 177, 180
Higgins, B. H. 38
Highland Centre for Human Caring (Inverness) 59
Hill, C. 114, 262, 265, 271
Hinshelwood, R. D. 223
Hinton, P. 95, 108
HIV/AIDS 261
Hofstede, G. 120
Hogstel, M. 107
Hollander, M. H. 300
Holley, S. 119
Holli, B. 102, 103, 118
Holmes, J. 220, 225
Homans, H. 230
honesty
  and health promotion 34
  and information 34
  in therapeutic presence **31**, 33–5

and trust 33
  see also communication, ethical; truth
Hopson, B. 279
Horowitz, L. M. 299
hospital
  environment as barrier to communication 103
  length of stay in 24
Hovland, C. 200
Howard, A. 139, 156, 158
Howell, P. 275, 276
Hugo, Victor 74
humanistic paradigm, difficulties in changing to 179
humour in therapeutic presence 32
Hunt, G. 171
Hunter, J. 199
Husserl, E. 27

Ignatieff, M. 17
'I-It' relationships (Buber) 27–28, 30, 40, 70–1
Illich, I. 56, 60
illness, national differences in concept of 121
income generation in NHS 58
information
  and community health care 15
  deficiency in collection of 16
  deficiency in provision of 16, 67
  gathering from patient 100–1
  giving to patient 101
  overload/underload in communication model 99
  patient preference for psychologically supportive 302
  quantity of 16
  requirements as areas of potential misunderstanding 301
  symbolised as compassionate nursing care 302–3
Ingham, H. **269**
Inman, M. 193
Inskipp, F. 134, 160, 162
intellectualisation as barrier to communication 113

321

322